INTEGRATED FOOD SAFETY AND VETERINARY PUBLIC HEALTH

Integrated Food Safety and Veterinary Public Health

Sava Buncic

School of Veterinary Science
University of Bristol

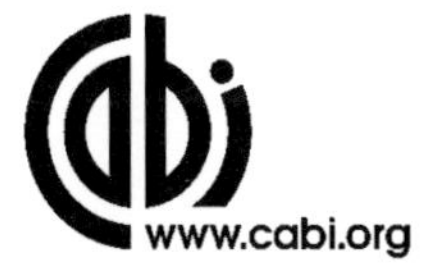

CABI is a trading name of CAB International

CABI Head Office
Nosworthy Way
Wallingford
Oxfordshire OX10 8DE
UK

Tel: +44 (0)1491 832111
Fax: +44 (0)1491 833508
E-mail: cabi@cabi.org
Website: www.cabi.org

CABI North American Office
875 Massachusetts Avenue
7th Floor
Cambridge, MA 02139
USA

Tel: +1 617 395 4056
Fax: +1 617 354 6875
E-mail: cabi-nao@cabi.org

A catalogue record for this book is available from the British Library, London, UK.

Library of Congress Cataloging-in-Publication Data

Buncic, Sava.
Integrated food safety and veterinary public health / Sava Buncic.
p. cm.
Includes bibliographical references and index.
ISBN-13: 978-0-85199-908-1 (alk. paper)
ISBN-10: 0-85199-908-5 (alk. paper)
1. Food of animal origin—Quality control. 2. Food industry and trade—Quality control. 3. Veterinary public health. I. Title.
RA601.S28 2005
664′.902--dc22

2005024107

ISBN-10: 0-85199-908-5
ISBN-13: 978-0-85199-908-1

Typeset by Columns Design Ltd, Reading, RG4 7DH, UK
Printed and bound in the UK by Cromwell Press, Trowbridge

Contents

Contributors

Guest Contributors on Selected Topics

Aabo, Søren, *Department of Microbiological Food Safety, Danish Institute for Food and Veterinary Research, Mørkhøj Bygade 19, DK-2860 Søborg, Denmark. email: saa@dfvf.dk*

Avery, Sheryl, *Microbiology Research Division, Direct Laboratories Ltd., Wergs Road, Wolverhampton WV6 8TQ, UK. email: mahiafireplace@hotmail.com*

Maijala, Riitta, *National Veterinary and Food Research Institute (EELA), Department of Risk Assessment, PO Box 45, 00581 Helsinki, Finland. email: riitta.maijala@helsinki.fi*

Nørrung, Birgit, *Danish Institute for Food and Veterinary Research, Mørkhøj Bygade 19, DK-2860 Søborg, Denmark. email: bin@dfvf.dk*

Nute, Geoffrey, *Division of Farm Animal Science, School of Veterinary Science, University of Bristol, Langford, Bristol BS40 5DU, UK. email: geoff.nute@bristol.ac.uk*

O'Brien, Sarah, *Health Sciences and Epidemiology, University of Manchester, Clinical Sciences Building, Hope Hospital, Stott Lane, Salford M6 8HD, UK. email: sarah.o'brien@manchester.ac.uk*

Small, Alison, *Division of Farm Animal Science, School of Veterinary Science, University of Bristol, Langford, Bristol BS40 5DU, UK. email: a.h.small@bristol.ac.uk*

Vågsholm, Ivar, *Swedish Zoonoses Center, Department of Disease Control, National Veterinary Institute, Uppsala S 751 89, Sweden. email: ivar.vagsholm@sva.se*

Voysey, Phil, *Microbiology Department, CCFRA, Chipping Campden, Gloucestershire GL55 6LD, UK. email: p.voysey@campden.co.uk*

Warriss, Paul, *Division of Farm Animal Science, School of Veterinary Science, University of Bristol, Langford, Bristol BS40 5DU, UK. email: p.d.warriss@bristol.ac.uk*

Wilkin (née Reid), Carol-Ann, *Division of Farm Animal Science, School of Veterinary Science, University of Bristol, Langford, Bristol BS40 5DU, UK. email: c.a.reid@bristol.ac.uk*

Wood, Jeffrey, *Division of Farm Animal Science, School of Veterinary Science, University of Bristol, Langford, Bristol BS40 5DU, UK. email: jeff.wood@bristol.ac.uk*

Wotton, Steve, *Division of Farm Animal Science, School of Veterinary Science, University of Bristol, Langford, Bristol BS40 5DU, UK. email: steve.wotton@bristol.ac.uk*

Preface

The importance of food for human health has been widely recognized; eating optimal quantities of nutritious and safe food is a major precondition for a happy and productive life.

The safety of foods of animal origin is particularly relevant because the large majority of food-borne diseases are derived from poultry-, egg-, meat-, dairy- and fish-based foods. Understandably, farm animals are one of the key factors affecting human health in several ways:

1. Animals can convert inedible plants to edible protein.
2. Foods of animal origin represent a total complement of essential proteins.
3. Healthy animals produce healthy food that produces healthy people.

Connections between health problems in animals and those in people were probably recognized early in human history, but the first written proofs of such considerations can be traced to Aristotle and Hippocrates. Later, progress in medical sciences and better understanding of the significance of food safety led to the beginnings of meat inspection in Europe: in France in the mid-12th century, in England in the early 14th century, and in Germany in the late 14th century. Subsequently, the traditional meat inspection system was fully developed in Germany in the mid-19th century; this was adopted by most other European countries, and spread wider. It has been used without major changes until today. Naturally, the major contributions of veterinarians to the control of animal diseases and food (meat) safety, and hence to human health, have a long history. In addition to its animal health and welfare goals, veterinary medicine also has human health aims that can be summarised as:

- Primary: zoonoses prevention, food protection, medical research;
- Other: environmental protection, administration, health education, contribution to protection of mental/emotional status of animal owners.

Veterinarians working in the areas of protection of public health from animal-related hazards and food safety (i.e. Veterinary Public Health: VPH) have to use knowledge and information from different scientific disciplines on a regular basis. A range of competencies ranging from medicine to food production and technology is required by those dealing successfully with food safety. Since no single profession is qualified in-depth in all these competencies, a multidisciplinary approach with cohesive teamwork is necessary in food safety. Nevertheless, among all professions, veterinarians are in the best position to take a lead in this multidisciplinary area, due to their medical education and close familiarity with animal and food production.

I have worked in the VPH (food safety) area for many years, in a combined veterinarian–academic–researcher capacity and in different countries, including Serbia (Belgrade University), New Zealand (MIRINZ-AgResearch) and the United Kingdom (University of Bristol). These experiences, as well as my engagement in the European College of Veterinary Public Health, have helped me to understand that the basic principles and concepts of food safety and VPH are universal and applicable under varying conditions; some specifics, whilst they may be important, are often of 'local' relevance and/or very changeable.

For these reasons, my main intention with this book is to provide core, concise reading material on the basic principles and concepts of Food Safety and Veterinary Public Health for undergraduate students of veterinary medicine. With the UK model, more practical specifics and detailed related legislation are expected to be provided by post-University courses, for those veterinarians who wish to work as Official Veterinary Surgeons. An Official Veterinarian (or Official Veterinary Surgeon) is the one qualified to work within the VPH sector. Therefore, the content of this book reflects the curriculum of the VPH course as currently taught at the Bristol School of Veterinary Science. The content is more heavily oriented towards meat-related issues, compared with other types of foods, but this is more a reflection of the reality than a personal choice.

Nevertheless, practising and Official Veterinary Surgeons may wish to use the book as a refresher source; some parts of the book may also be useful to individuals with other professional profiles dealing with food hygiene and safety.

I have been privileged and very pleased that several colleagues from the University of Bristol, as well as from other European countries, kindly accepted my invitation to contribute to the book on selected topics; their names are listed and also indicated in the relevant chapters. I am deeply thankful for these contributions.

Also, I am very grateful to Professor Jovan Raseta, who was my first teacher on food (meat) hygiene, and to Professor Niels Skovgaard, who introduced me to scientific work in food microbiology and safety.

I would also like to express my warmest gratitude to my wife Sheryl and to my son Veljko, without whom I would not be who I am, and to my parents and sister, for always being there for me.

Sava Buncic
June 2005
Bristol, UK

I On-farm Phase in the Context of the Food Chain

1 Food Chain and Health Hazards

1.1 Characteristics of the Food Chain and Associated Hazards

Sufficient knowledge has been accumulated to understand that, in modern times, food production and food safety have to be approached simultaneously. The commercial success of the former is unachievable unless the latter is assured; food safety cannot be achieved unless related control measures are incorporated within all phases of the production. The reasons for that include:

- public health hazards can enter the food chain at different and often multiple points;
- the total number of public health hazards potentially contaminating food is very large, and they differ considerably by their nature;
- therefore, for each hazard of a specific nature, the entering point(s) and entering route(s) must be identified and their relationship with the phase of the production process must be understood;
- what happens at a given point (phase) of the food chain inevitably affects adjacent points (either preceding, subsequent or both) so individual phases of the food production cannot be considered 'in isolation';
- if something goes wrong at a given point in the food chain, it can negate any successes achieved at other points, so all the activities along the whole food chain must be integrated and coordinated.

The strong inter-relationship between food production chain and food quality/safety is being increasingly recognized and accepted by major food retailers (e.g. supermarket chains). By doing so, they represent a commercial motor for the vertical integration of food producers. Examples of good integration include the poultry chain and the milk/dairy chain, in which a single company often owns all production phases: animal feed–animal farms–primary food production–food processing–retailing.

In such systems, approaches to associated public health hazards and their controls can be, and often are, similarly integrated. The main phases of the food production and associated hazards are illustrated in Fig. 1.1 using the example of the meat chain. When considering the complexity of the chain, diversity of the hazards and necessity of understanding their inter-relationship, it becomes clear that the approach to protection of the consumer's health must be science-based and multidisciplinary. In the following chapters, essential information required for assessing the public health risks and their controls along the food chain will be given, leading to the final chapter summarizing the framework for longitudinal and integrated food safety assurance.

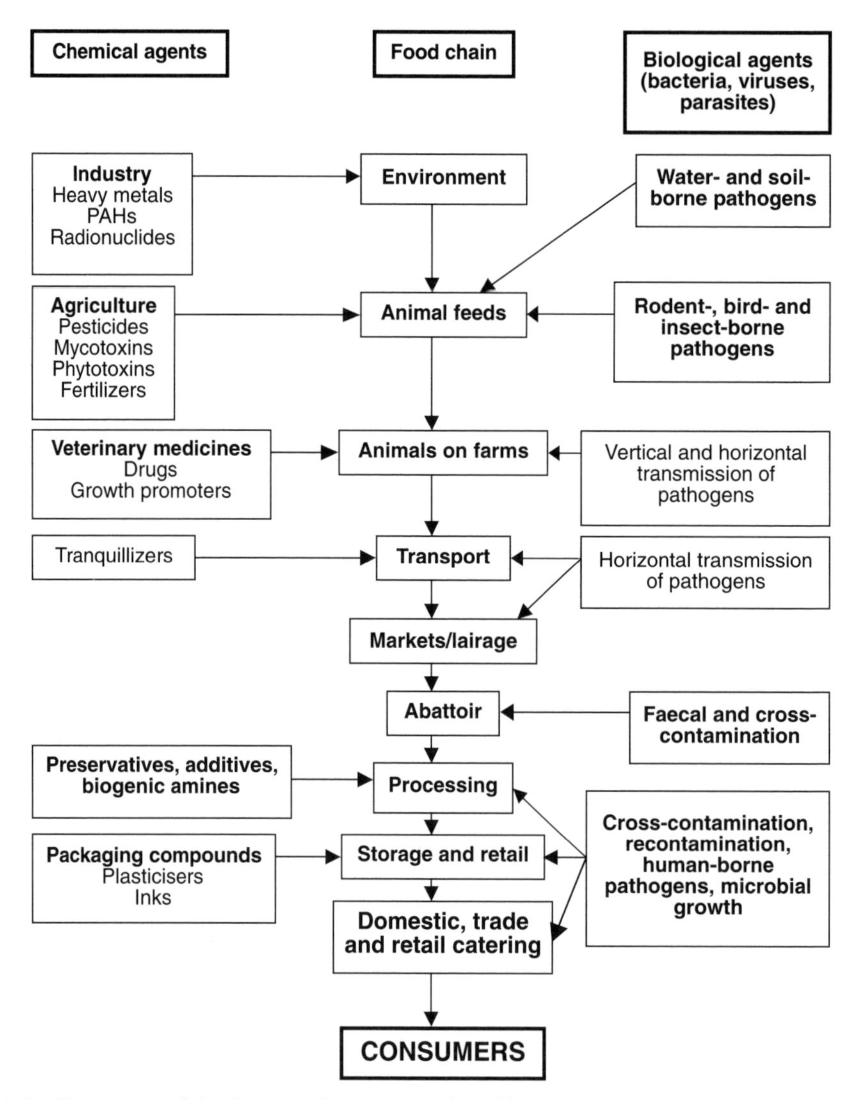

Fig. 1.1. The nature of the food chain and associated hazards.

1.2 Microbial Food-borne Pathogens

SHERYL AVERY

There are three categories of microbial food-borne diseases:

1. Invasive infection, in which the organism invades and penetrates intestinal mucosa.
2. Toxico-infection, in which the organism produces toxin while in the intestinal tract.
3. Intoxication, in which the organism produces specific toxins or toxic metabolite(s) in the food that is ingested.

Classification of disease by symptoms may be misleading from an aetiological point of view, because more than one organism can be responsible for similar clinical symptoms. For example, haemolytic uraemic syndrome (HUS) can be caused by *E. coli* O157, other stx-producing *E. coli*, *Shigella* and *Campylobacter*.

Agents for food-borne disease have generally been recognized because of the occurrence of large numbers of cases from a common source and with similar symptoms (a disease outbreak) or clusters of cases (two to a few individuals). During outbreaks, epidemiological investigators examine suspect foods, recover bacterial isolates and compare those with patient isolates using genetic typing techniques (commonly Pulsed Field Gel Electrophoresis). However, most food-borne illness occurs sporadically – where only one patient has symptoms. Investigation of disease is more difficult for sporadic cases, as isolating the causative organism from food is problematic. Sporadic cases constitute most of the worldwide food-borne disease burden.

The source of bacterial pathogens existing in food includes many harvest or post-harvest sources and may not be confined to the food itself (livestock, livestock products or plants). Although some food-borne bacterial pathogens are zoonotic agents (e.g. *Salmonella, Listeria*), their presence on/in food is not necessarily a direct result of their spread from livestock during harvest. Food handlers can be a source of food-borne pathogens, as they may harbour some pathogens asymptomatically, be infected or have hands contaminated from other sources (e.g. *Listeria* from drains). To establish a zoonotic link, matching isolates should be recovered from the animal in question, which is not often possible. Contamination of food by food handlers via faeces, vomit, skin lesions or mucus is a likely source of many food-borne bacteria, while viral pathogens may originate from human faeces or vomit. Fomites may also be vehicles for the spread of bacterial pathogens to foods.

Gram-negative Bacterial Pathogens

An important group of Gram-negative bacteria found in the GIT of humans and animals are classified in the bacterial family Enterobacteriaceae. Genera from this family, which can be food-borne pathogens, are *Salmonella*, *Escherichia*, *Shigella* and *Yersinia*.

Measures to control specific food-borne pathogens, discussed below, do not generally include on-farm hygiene measures, nor adjustment to food processing parameters.

Campylobacter

Campylobacter jejuni (the most common species) and *C. coli* cause the invasive infection campylobacteriosis. The pathogen is found in the GIT of livestock, poultry and other animals including pets (Blaser *et al.*, 1979; Stern and Line, 2000), so is commonly spread by faeces and faecally contaminated water. Asymptomatic faecal carriage occurs occasionally in humans. *Campylobacter* cause between 5 and 14% of all diarrhoeal illness worldwide (Anon., 2000a,b), and are the most common laboratory isolates from humans with gastroenteric symptoms in most developed countries (Table 1.1).

Campylobacter are spiral, curved or winged motile rods (Smibert, 1984). *Campylobacter* have a t_{opt} of between 37 and 45°C, but do not grow well, if at all, below 25°C. *Campylobacter* is micro-aerophilic, with optimal growth in 10% CO_2 and requiring a low O_2 concentrations of around 5%. They are salt-sensitive, being mostly inhibited by 2% NaCl. The pathogen grows best at pH 6.5 to 7.5. *Campylobacter* survive in foods at 4°C, but are sensitive to drying and heating (ICMSF, 1996).

The incubation period is typically 2 to 5 days (Stern and Line, 2000). Symptoms include fever, malaise, abdominal pain (can be severe, mimicking appendicitis), diarrhoea – which can be bloody (Blaser *et al.*, 1979) and headache. Sequelae include reactive arthritis, while Guillain-

Table 1.1. Incidence of laboratory isolations of selected pathogens from humans with disease symptoms, by country (isolations per 100,000 population).

Country, year of report	*Campylobacter*	*Salmonella*	*E. coli* O157	*L. monocytogenes*	Reference
Australia, 2003[a]	113	40.3	0.1	0.3	(Anon., 2003a)
Canada, 2000	40.1	18.4	8.8[b]	nr	(Anon., 2000b)
Denmark, 2003	65.8	32	0.5	0.4	(Anon., 2004a)
New Zealand, 1998–2000	320	49.6	1.3	0.5	(Anon., 2000a)
Switzerland, 2003	77.8	30.5	0.8	0.6	(Anon., 2003b)
UK, 2002	88.7	27.6	1.4	0.3	(Anon., 2002)
USA, 2003	12.6	14.5	1.1	0.33	(Anon., 2004b)

[a] Calculated as food-borne illnesses.
[b] Isolations of all shiga toxin-producing *E. coli* serovars.
nr = not reported.

Barré syndrome may develop 1 to 3 weeks after *C. jejuni* infection (Stern and Line, 2000). HUS also can occur. Campylobacteriosis is more common in children or young adults than in others. The disease is self-limiting and typically lasts up to 10 days, but individuals can shed the pathogen for up to 2 months post-resolution of symptoms (Anon., 1992a). Infants and young adults are most at risk.

Campylobacter jejuni invades the large and small intestine (Beery *et al.*, 1988), produces toxin and forms abscesses in the crypts of the villi. Infection of the appendix may occur.

As the infectious dose appears low, around 500 CFU (colony-forming units), growth of the pathogen in food is not necessary. Foods that have caused campylobacteriosis include unpasteurized milk, water and undercooked poultry. Foods which appear to have been cross-contaminated from known *Campylobacter* sources are often implicated.

Measures to control campylobacteriosis include:

1. Cook poultry and meats thoroughly.
2. Pasteurize milk and dairy products; don't consume unpasteurized products.
3. Prevent cross-contamination of heat-treated foods.
4. Prevent cross-contamination of utensils.
5. Use only potable water in food production; consume only potable water.
6. Control birds and rodents.

Salmonella

Salmonella causes two types of food-borne human disease. First, salmonellosis is most commonly caused by *S. enterica* subsp. *typhimurium* or *S. enterica* subsp. *enteritidis* (World Health Organization, 1995; D'Aoust, 2000). Secondly, *S. enterica* subsp. *typhi* and *S. enterica* subsp. *paratyphi* are the causes of typhoid fever or paratyphoid fever, respectively (Anon., 1992c). *Salmonella* can replicate both inside the vacuoles of host cells (Garcia-del Portillo and Finlay, 1994) and in the external environment. *Salmonella* are the second most common pathogens isolated from humans with gastroenteric disease in developed countries (Table 1.1).

Salmonella are non-sporing, motile rods, and are facultatively anaerobic (Le Minor, 1984). *Salmonella* have a t_{opt} of 37°C, but this is strain-dependent; growth occurs between 5 and 47°C. Grow best at pH 7, but can grow in relatively acidic conditions, pH 4.0 to 5.4. Nitrite and high salt concentrations are inhibitory at low pH. *Salmonella* survive very well in dried foods, particularly those with protective fats and proteins. *Salmonella* are not heat-tolerant, so will be destroyed by thorough cooking.

Salmonellosis

Salmonella typhimurium and *S. enteritidis* occur in the GIT of animals, including livestock. The pathogen is spread by faeces to the environment and to foods. Faecal–oral transmission is normal, but person-to-person transmission can occur, particularly in institutions.

The incubation period is typically 6 to 48 h (Yoshikawa, 1980). Symptoms include mild fever, nausea, vomiting, headache, aching limbs, abdominal pain and diarrhoea lasting from a few days to one week. The disease is self-limiting, but can be severe in young, elderly or otherwise IC (immunocompromised) people (Anon., 1992c; World Health Organization, 1995).

Salmonella invade epithelial cells in the ileum and proliferate in the *lamina propria*. Profuse, watery diarrhoea results. Some isolates produce a heat-labile enterotoxin, which initiates diarrhoea. Sequelae include post-enteritis reactive arthritis and Reiter's syndrome (D'Aoust, 2000), and systemic infection can result. Individuals can develop carrier status of up to 6 months in duration (Anon., 1992c).

The infectious dose varies, from only a few CFU to >10^5 CFU, so growth of the pathogen in foods has not been a factor in all cases of food-borne salmonellosis, but appears to have been in some. Foods known to have been vehicles of salmonellosis include poultry, eggs, meat, milk, chocolate, coconut and frog legs. However, any faecally contaminated food can be implicated. As *Salmonella* are heat sensitive, raw or undercooked foods are more likely to cause infection.

Measures to control salmonellosis include:

1. Cook foods thoroughly.
2. Pasteurize milk and dairy products; avoid consumption of unpasteurized products.
3. Prevent cross-contamination of heat-treated foods.
4. Avoid undercooked or raw eggs.
5. Store heat-treated foods at <4°C or >60°C to prevent growth.
6. Reduce carriage of livestock by vaccinating or dosing with antibiotics or probiotics.
7. Exclude infected or carrier-status individuals from handling food.
8. Control rodents and insects.
9. Dispose of sewage in a sanitary manner.

Typhoid fever and paratyphoid fever

Salmonella typhi and *S. enterica* subsp. *paratyphi* cause the systemic diseases typhoid fever and paratyphoid fever, respectively. These pathogens occur in human faeces, and are spread via human faeces to the environment and to foods. Person-to-person transmission is common.

The disease symptoms of typhoid and paratyphoid fevers are dissimilar to those of enteric salmonellosis. The incubation period is typically 10 to 20 days, but ranges from 3 to 56 days. Symptoms include fever, headache, abdominal tenderness, constipation, rose-coloured spots on the body, possibly followed by diarrhoea.

Salmonella penetrate the intestinal epithelium, possibly proliferating in macrophages and polymorphs, pass into mesenteric lymph nodes, liver or spleen then cause septicaemia. Peritonitis and subsequent death can occur. Ulceration of the ileum can occur if organisms multiply in the bile of the gall bladder and cause reinfection.

The infectious dose ranges from 10^3 to 10^6 CFU. Any food could be a vehicle of infection if contaminated with human faeces. Foods known to have been vehicles of typhoid fever include raw milk, shellfish and meat. However, typhoid fever is predominantly spread by water contaminated with human faeces.

Measures to control typhoid and paratyphoid fevers include:

1. Use only potable water in food production; consume only potable water.
2. Dispose of sewage in a sanitary manner.
3. Avoid consumption of raw shellfish.
4. Use good personal hygiene practices when handling foods.
5. Cook food thoroughly.
6. Prevent cross-contamination of heat-treated foods.
7. Exclude infected or carrier-status individuals from handling food.
8. Give antibiotic therapy to prevent long-term carrier status developing.

Escherichia coli O157

Escherichia coli O157 causes toxico-infections, producing enteric and/or systemic illnesses. Although this disease is relatively infrequent (Table 1.1) it can have severe consequences, including haemorrhagic colitis (HC), haemolytic uraemic syndrome (HUS) and thrombotic thrombocytopaenic purpura (TTP).

Shiga toxin (stx)-producing *E. coli* O157 are carried in the GIT of healthy livestock. Cattle are a suspected main reservoir (Chapman *et al.*, 1992), but the organism can be found in the GIT of sheep, deer, goats, poultry, horses, dogs, rats, flies, birds and humans. Asymptomatic faecal carriage occurs in both animals and people. Other stx-producing *E. coli* are also carried extensively in the GIT of healthy cattle, but are less common human pathogens and, to date, have only rarely been proved to be food-borne. The most common route of *E. coli* O157 infection is person-to-person, but other routes of infection include food-borne and animal-to-person.

E. coli O157 are non-sporing, facultatively anaerobic rods that are usually motile (Ørskov, 1984). The organism is a member of the family Enterobacteriaceae, so grows optimally at 37°C and pH 7.0 (Anon., 1992b). Although the organism does not grow at refrigeration temperature, it survives well in refrigerated food. Growth can occur as low as 7 to 8°C, in the pH range 4.4 to 9.0, and in 6.5% NaCl. *E. coli* O157 are similarly acid resistant as serovars of *E. coli*, most of which appear to be quite acid tolerant. *E. coli* O157 are not heat-tolerant, so will be destroyed by thorough cooking. *E. coli* O157 survive well in livestock wastes and soils (months, up to 1 year).

The incubation period is typically 3 to 8 days, and ranges from 1 to 11 days (Anon., 1992b). The infectious dose appears extremely low, around 10 to 100 CFU. Symptoms are very varied, including watery diarrhoea and HC with severe abdominal pain, sometimes accompanied by vomiting. HUS can occur, with symptoms of kidney failure, reduced white cell count and anaemia (Nataro and Kaper, 1998). TTP typically has similar symptoms to HUS, but the CNS is also involved, and bleeding into tissues and organs can develop, with blood clots in the brain. Young children are at greatest risk of HUS. HUS typically lasts days or weeks, and requires hospitalization, blood transfusions and dialysis. Coma and death occur frequently in target populations of the young (HUS) and the elderly (TPP) (Nataro and Kaper, 1998).

Ingested bacteria adhere to the large intestine where they probably proliferate and produce stx 1 and/or stx 2. Stx may be translocated to target organs (kidneys, CNS) by unknown means, and to cells containing active binding sites for stx. Stx binds to the cell surface, moves through the cell membrane to the endoplasmic reticulum and halts protein synthesis, causing cell death.

As the infectious dose can be extremely low, growth of the pathogen in foods is not necessary. Foods that have been proven vehicles of infection include meats, particularly if minced or comminuted and then undercooked, e.g. beefburger (Anon., 1992b). Ready-to-eat meats including salami, jerky and cooked meats have caused outbreaks, as have unpasteurized apple juice, unpasteurized milk, unpasteurized cheese, yoghurt, salad sprouts, well water and lake water (Park *et al.*, 1999).

Measures to control *E. coli* O157 include:

1. Use GHP and HACCP in meat production.
2. Cook meat thoroughly until >72°C in the centre, instantaneously.
3. Pasteurize juice and dairy products; don't consume unpasteurized products.
4. Prevent cross-contamination of heat-treated foods.
5. Exclude infected individuals from handling foods.
6. Use only potable water in food production; consume only potable water.
7. Prevent young children contacting livestock and farm environments.
8. Avoid eating in areas that could be contaminated with animal faeces. Wash hands thoroughly before eating.
9. Do not use organic waste or faecally-contaminated water on ready-to-eat crops.
10. Control rodents, insects and birds.

Shigella

Shigella sonnei, *S. dysenteriae*, *S. boydii* and *S. flexneri* cause the invasive infection shigellosis. *Shigella* are found only in the GIT of humans and higher primates, where they are mostly carried asymptomatically (Lampel *et al.*, 2000). Transmission occurs via the faecal–oral route and person-to-person.

Shigella are non-sporing, motile rods, and are facultatively anaerobic. The organism is a member of the family Enterobacteriaceae (Rowe and Gross, 1984), so grows in the range of 6 to 48°C, but t_{opt} is 37°C and pH 7. *Shigella* can grow in 5% NaCl.

The incubation period is typically 48 h, but ranges from 1 to 7 days (Anon., 1992d). *Shigella* causes a variety of symptoms, from mild to severe. Symptoms include mild diarrhoea, typically lasting for one to two weeks, and are self-limiting (Anon., 1992d). Dysentery is more severe, with high fever, chills and dehydration. Convulsions can occur in children under 4 years old. Sequelae include HC, neurological symptoms and HUS. Severe cases of dysentery can require hospitalization, and blood transfusion or kidney dialysis may be necessary in the case of HUS. Individuals can develop carrier status, lasting for months.

Shigella proliferate within epithelial cells in the ileum and colon, producing the milder symptoms. If surfaces of the *epitheliae* become inflamed, causing necrosis and ulceration, red blood cells and serum proteins can subsequently infiltrate the lumen, producing dysentery.

As the infectious does is typically ~100 CFU, but may be as few as 10 CFU in susceptible individuals, growth of the pathogen in food is not necessary. Shigellosis is not necessarily a zoonosis; any food requiring substantial handling can be a non-specific vector. Foods involved are raw foods including fruits and salads, as well as food handled before incorrect cooking or after cooking (chicken, shellfish, egg products, puddings). Poor hygiene amongst infected/carrier food handlers and faecal contamination of water supplies are common factors contributing to outbreaks.

Measures to control shigellosis include:

1. Use good personal hygiene practices when handling foods.
2. Exclude infected or carrier-status individuals from handling food.
3. Use only potable water in food production; consume only potable water.
4. Dispose of sewage in a sanitary manner.
5. Cook food thoroughly to inactivate *Shigella* on raw food.

Vibrio cholerae

Vibrio cholerae O1 classic biotypes, El Tor biotype and *V. cholerae* O139 are the cause of cholera, a toxico-infection (Anon., 1992e). *V. cholerae* primarily inhabit marine water, estuaries and salt marshes. The most common source of cholera is faecally contaminated water (Kaysner, 2000).

All *Vibrio* are facultatively anaerobic halophilics, straight or curved, motile rods. Seawater or 2 to 3% (range 0.5 to 10%) NaCl is required for survival and growth of most *Vibrio* (Kaysner, 2000). Growth occurs from 5 to 43°C, but growth t_{min} in waters is around 10 to 19°C. Growth occurs over a wide pH range, from pH 4.8 to 11.0, but they are alkalophilic, with pH_{opt} of 7.8 to 8.6. *Vibrio* are sensitive to heat: cooking to 65°C kills this pathogen.

The incubation period is typically 6 h to 5 days (Kaysner, 2000). Symptoms include profuse watery diarrhoea with 'rice water' stools, containing flakes of mucus, epithelial cells and large numbers of *V. cholerae*. Abdominal pain and vomiting occur later. Fluid loss can lead to severe dehydration, acidosis, shock and circulatory collapse. Death can occur, and be very rapid (within a few hours), if patients are not rehydrated.

Ingested *V. cholerae* probably colonise the small intestine by attaching to intestinal epithelial cells, where they proliferate and excrete a potent enterotoxin. Secreted enterotoxin enters intestinal epithelial cells and activates adenylate cyclase. Intracellular cAMP levels increase, while H_2O, Na^+, K^+, Cl^- and HCO_3^- are secreted into the lumen of the small intestine, producing diarrhoea.

The infectious dose is high, around 10^6 CFU. Typically, water-borne cholera is spread by poor sanitation, producing contaminated water supplies, which can also subsequently produce contaminated filter-feeding shellfish. Seafood, including raw, lightly cooked or recontaminated shellfish or fish, is the most common source of food-borne cholera.

Measures to control cholera include:

1. Consume only potable water.
2. Dispose of sewage correctly.
3. Use only potable water in seafood harvesting and preparation.
4. Do not harvest seafood from waters containing *V. cholerae*.
5. Avoid raw seafoods.
6. Chill seafood to <4°C at harvest and after.
7. Exclude infected individuals from handling food.

Vibrio parahaemolyticus

Vibrio parahaemolyticus causes enteritis, and like *V. cholerae*, is an inhabitant of marine environments (see above). Marine animals can carry this organism, and asymptomatic carriage can occur in humans. Characteristics of this pathogen are described above.

The incubation period for *V. parahaemolyticus* enteritis is typically 12 to 24 h, but ranges from 4 h to 4 days (Anon., 1992f). Symptoms include diarrhoea, cramps, nausea, sometimes vomiting, low fever, chills and headache. The disease is usually self-limiting. Sequelae may include reactive arthritis.

V. parahaemolyticus enteritis is probably an infection with an unknown toxin produced in the GI tract. Invasion probably occurs via blood. They produce a heat-stable haemolysin (Kanagawa factor), which may be involved in pathogenicity, amongst other possible factors. However, toxins can also be formed in food.

The infectious dose is not known, but may be around 10^4 CFU (or greater for healthy individuals). In Japan, *V. parahaemolyticus* is the leading cause of food-borne disease, where consumption of raw, contaminated seafood is the major cause. In the USA, most cases occur via cross-contaminated seafood.

Measures to control *V. parahaemolyticus* enteritis include:

1. Do not harvest seafood from contaminated waters.
2. Chill seafood to <4°C at harvest and after.
3. Prevent cross-contamination.
4. Avoid raw seafoods particularly those harvested from estuaries during summer.

Vibrio vulnificus

Vibrio vulnificus causes septicaemic invasive infection and, like other *Vibrio* (see above), occur in marine environments, including seawater and marine sediments.

The incubation period is typically 16 to 38 h, but ranges from 7 h to several days (Anon., 1992g). Symptoms include fever, chills, nausea and hypotension. People with higher than normal iron levels are more susceptible. Necrotic skin lesions appear in most patients, with oedema, tissue necrosis and death frequent. Amputation is often required.

The infectious dose is $<10^2$ CFU for susceptible individuals. Raw oysters have caused this food-borne infection, while other seafoods do not normally harbour *V. vulnificus*. They can cause septicaemia via skin lesions or wounds.

Measures to control *V. vulnificus* food-borne septicaemia include:

1. People with liver disease or other chronic disease should not eat raw shellfish, particularly oysters.
2. Avoid raw seafoods, particularly those harvested from estuaries during summer.

Yersinia enterocolitica

Yersinia enterocolitica serogroups O3, O5, O8 and O9 cause the invasive infection termed yersiniosis. *Y. enterocolitica* is very common in the throat, tonsils and faeces of pigs, but is also found in water, soil and dogs. Dogs may be a reservoir for non-food-borne yersiniosis.

Y. enterocolitica are facultatively anaerobic rods, non-motile at 37°C, but usually motile at 30°C (Bercovier and Mollaret, 1984). The pathogen can grow at refrigeration temperature (t_{min} −2°C) but t_{opt} is around 30°C. Grows in 5% NaCl, and survives alkaline pH well (Bercovier and Mollaret, 1984).

The incubation time is typically 24 to 36 h, but may be 3 to 11 days (Anon., 1992h). Symptoms include abdominal pain, fever and diarrhoea; nausea and vomiting are less frequent. Abdominal pain can be severe, and may be mistaken for appendicitis, and enteric symptoms can last for months. Sequelae include reactive arthritis, Reiter's syndrome and septicaemia. The young, elderly and IC individuals are most at risk.

Y. enterocolitica produce a local inflammatory response after internalization in intestinal epithelial cells. A heat-stable enterotoxin can be produced *in vitro*, but has not been found *in vivo*, and its role is unknown.

The infectious dose is not known (Nesbakken, 2000). Foods involved have included putatively pasteurized milk and flavoured milk, water, chow mein and tofu. Pork meats are often implicated as the source of infections (Nesbakken, 2000). However, although pork meats – including tongue and chitterlings (intestines) – frequently contain *Y. enterocolitica*, these have not yet been proven as vehicles of food-borne yersiniosis.

Measures to control yersiniosis include:

1. GHP in food production.
2. Pasteurize milk and dairy products; don't consume unpasteurized products.
3. Use only potable water in food manufacturing; consume only potable water.
4. Cook meats thoroughly.
5. Prevent cross-contamination of heat-treated foods.
6. GHP when handling domestic pets.

Gram-positive Bacterial Pathogens

Listeria monocytogenes

Listeria monocytogenes cause the invasive infection listeriosis, a disease of humans and livestock, although non-invasive disease can also occur in humans (see below). *L. monocytogenes* can be carried asymptomatically in the GIT of livestock, other animals and humans, and can be shed in the milk of cows with or without mastitis symptoms (Farber and Peterkin, 2000). The pathogen is ubiquitous in the environment, including food processing plants, refrigerators, drains, soil, water, sewage, dust and on plant tissues (Seeliger and Jones, 1986). *L. monocytogenes* has been found in improperly fermented silage, which is suspected as being a source of listeriosis in livestock.

L. monocytogenes are rods, motile at 25°C, but usually non-motile at 37°C (Seeliger and Jones, 1986). The organism is a facultative anaerobe, but prefers a microaerophilic atmosphere if O_2 is present. *L. monocytogenes* is capable of growth on food at −1.5°C, and can grow *in vitro* up to 45°C. The pathogen can proliferate at pH 4.1 to 9.6, and in 10% NaCl. *L. monocytogenes* is very resistant to drying, can form persistent biofilms in food manufacturing plants, and can survive 1 year in 16% NaCl.

Listeriosis

Two forms of human listeriosis are recognized, and both are commonly food-borne. Invasive listeriosis symptoms include septicaemia, meningitis, encephalitis and spontaneous abortion (Anon., 1992l). People at high risk of invasive listeriosis are IC individuals (pregnant women, AIDS patients, cancer patients, young, elderly) and those with diabetes, heart or hepatic disease (Farber and Peterkin, 2000). In pregnant women, spontaneous abortion usually occurs in the third trimester, resulting in death of the infant. Non-invasive listeriosis symptoms are mostly enteric and include diarrhoea, mild fever, headache and myalgia, and the disease has a short incubation period (1 to 3 days). Healthy individuals are at risk for non-invasive listeriosis. However, due to its environmental ubiquity, it follows that *L. monocytogenes* is regularly consumed via foods by healthy people without causing illness.

In invasive listeriosis, *L. monocytogenes* passes through intestinal epithelia, probably via intestinal epithelial cells or Peyer's Patches (Farber and Peterkin, 2000). Subsequent spread via the blood and lymphatic systems to the liver and spleen occurs, after which the pathogen is largely killed by macrophages, and cleared from the circulatory system. However, if the immune response in the liver is inadequate, surviving *L. monocytogenes* proliferate intracellularly within liver macrophages. *L. monocytogenes* then commences a process of cell-to-cell spread, inducing cell death, and spreading to the CNS, heart, eyes or foetus. In non-invasive listeriosis, the pathogen is probably efficiently cleared from the circulatory system by immune response macrophages.

The infectious dose is not known, but for invasive listeriosis appears low (>100 CFU) for IC individuals, so growth of the pathogen in food is not necessary. Generally, high doses ($>10^5$ CFU) of *L. monocytogenes* appear to be involved in non-invasive listeriosis, so prevention of *L. monocytogenes* growth in foods is a priority in avoiding this form. Foods that have been proven vehicles of infection include soft cheese, raw and pasteurized milk, ready-to-eat meat products (paté), poultry products (turkey frankfurters), seafood products, vegetables and fresh salads.

Measures to control listeriosis include:

1. Use GHP and HACCP in food production.
2. Immunocompromised individuals and other target populations should avoid high-risk foods.
3. Pasteurize milk and dairy products; don't consume unpasteurized products.
4. Prevent cross-contamination and recontamination of heat-treated foods.
5. Completely separate raw and cooked products during meat product manufacture.
6. Re-heat ready-to-eat foods adequately.
7. Do not use organic waste or faecally contaminated water on ready-to-eat crops.
8. Use the hurdle concept to limit growth of *L. monocytogenes* in foods.
9. Use correct starter cultures in cheese and meat fermentations.

Staphylococcus aureus

Staphylococcus aureus causes the food-borne intoxication staphyloenterotoxicosis. *S. aureus* produces a range of enterotoxins in food (A, B, C_1, C_2, C_3, D, E, F) (Baird-Parker, 2000). Most human food-borne disease is caused by type A enterotoxin (Anon., 1992m). *S. aureus* is harboured in the anterior nares of up to 50% of people, but is also a common environmental contaminant found in dust, air, water, vegetation and on environmental surfaces (Kloos and Schliefer, 1986). *S. aureus* primarily causes enteric illness, but also causes skin and throat lesions in man and animals.

S. aureus are non-motile, facultatively anaerobic cocci. Growth occurs at 6.7 to 48°C and at pH 4.0 to 9.8. *S. aureus* survives desiccation extremely well, tolerates up to 20% NaCl, and can grow in a_w of 0.83 (Kloos and Schliefer, 1986). Enterotoxin is not produced below 8°C, but enterotoxin A is produced in 10% NaCl. *S. aureus* enterotoxins are extremely heat stable and are typically not destroyed by boiling for 30 minutes, so their formation in food must be prevented.

The incubation period is typically 1 to 6 h (Anon., 1992m). Symptoms include nausea, vomiting, abdominal cramps, diarrhoea, sweating, headache and possibly a drop in body temperature. Fluid does not accumulate, but the CNS is stimulated, triggering the emetic centre in the brain, thus inducing vomiting.

Growth of the pathogen in food is necessary, as large numbers of *S. aureus* ($>10^5$ CFU/g per g, but commonly 10^7 CFU/g) are required to produce enough toxin (<1 μg) in food to cause illness. Poor hygiene amongst food handlers with skin infections, or those who carry the pathogen in their nostrils, is frequently a primary factor in outbreaks of food-borne staphyloenterotoxicosis. Foods that have been proven vehicles of infection include cold, cooked and handled cream- and custard-filled bakery products, custard, cream-based desserts, milk, meat, canned fish, seafood and fermented sausages.

Measures to control staphyloenterotoxicosis include:

1. Use good personal hygiene practices when handling foods.
2. People with skin infections should not handle foods.
3. Use GHP when handling foods.
4. Chill cooked food rapidly in small quantities.
5. Store cooked or heat-treated foods at <4°C or >60°C.
6. Avoid extensive handling of foods.
7. Avoid delays between cooking and eating.

Clostridium perfringens

Clostridium perfringens causes the toxico-infection perfringens food poisoning. Perfringens food poisoning is most commonly caused by organisms producing type A enterotoxin. Other types of enterotoxin (B to G) do not normally cause food-borne disease (Labbé, 2000). *C. perfringens* is ubiquitous in the environment, and is frequently detected on spices, raw meats, soil (levels up to 10^4 CFU/g), water, sewage and dust. Asymptomatic faecal carriage occurs in animals (Cato *et al.*, 1986).

C. perfringens are spore-forming rods which prefer a low redox potential (*Eh*) environment (usually anaerobic). Spores are resistant to environmental extremes. Growth occurs between 15 and 50°C, with t_{opt} between 40 and 45°C, and at pH 5.5 to 8.0. Growth is usually inhibited in 7 to 8% NaCl (Cato *et al.*, 1986). Enterotoxin is produced optimally at 35 to 40°C.

The incubation period is typically 8 to 22 h (Anon., 1992k). Symptoms include severe abdominal pain with profuse diarrhoea. Vomiting, nausea or fever are rare. The young and elderly are more at risk. Infection with type C can cause necrosis and haemorrhage in the small intestine. This type is common in Papua New Guinea, and is rare, but does occur, in other countries.

Ingested vegetative cells sporulate in the small intestine, releasing enterotoxin. Enterotoxin damages the brush border of epithelial cells, disrupting water and ion flux, and producing fluid movement and diarrhoea (Labbé, 2000). The illness may last for up to 2 days, and recovery is usually complete.

The infectious dose is believed to be high, $>10^6$ CFU/g, indicating that growth in foods is necessary. Some cases appear to have ingested pre-formed toxin (probably as well as vegetative cells), which may have induced shorter than normal incubation times. A common chain of events involves contaminated foods, cooked in bulk and inadequately cooled. The cooking procedure activates *C. perfringens* spores which germinate in the anaerobic conditions. The pathogen proliferates once the dish has cooled to an appropriate temperature, leading to ingestion of large numbers of vegetative cells. Foods involved are meat and poultry dishes, particularly those containing gravy, and those with long, slow cooking. Cooking foods in bulk and in advance is frequently a contributing factor, so perfringens food poisoning is mostly associated with bulk catering.

Measures to control perfringens food poisoning include:

1. Cook food thoroughly to kill vegetative cells.
2. Chill cooked food, especially meat dishes, rapidly in small quantities.
3. Store cooked food at <5°C or >60°C to prevent growth.
4. Limit the storage interval for cooked food to reduce growth of survivors.
5. Reheat food to at least 75°C to kill vegetative cells and to inactivate toxin if pre-formed in food.
6. Remove soil and dust from food to reduce spore contamination.

Bacillus cereus

Bacillus cereus causes two types of food-borne human disease. Emetic syndrome is an intoxication, while diarrhoeal syndrome is a toxico-infection. *B. cereus* is a common inhabitant of soil, water, dust, vegetation, spices, dried foods and human faeces.

B. cereus are facultatively anaerobic, spore-forming rods; most strains are motile. Growth occurs between 10 to 50°C, t_{opt} is 28 to 35°C. *B. cereus* grows at pH 4.9 to 9.3 (Claus and Berkeley, 1986). Spores are heat resistant.

B. cereus *emetic (vomiting) syndrome*

The incubation period is quick, typically 1 to 6 h (Anon., 1992i). Symptoms include nausea, vomiting and malaise. Diarrhoea may occur later. The symptoms can appear similar to *S. aureus* food poisoning. The emetic toxin is very heat- and acid-stable.

The infectious dose is believed to be high, around 10^8 CFU/g of food, so the pathogen must grow in the food. A frequent chain of events involves contaminated foods, cooked in bulk and inadequately cooled, enabling spores which have survived cooking to germinate and proliferate. Pre-formed toxin is ingested. Foods which have been involved include fried rice (boiled first, then stored and subsequently flash-fried), boiled rice, potato and pastas. Any foods prepared in bulk and improperly cooled could be a risk.

Measures to control *B. cereus* emetic syndrome include:

1. Prepare food in small batches.
2. Chill cooked food rapidly in small quantities.
3. Store cooked food at <5°C or >60°C.
4. Re-heat cooked foods thoroughly to kill vegetative cells.

B. cereus *diarrhoeal syndrome*

The incubation period is typically 8 to 16 h. Symptoms include nausea, abdominal pain and watery diarrhoea. Vomiting is rare. Spores or vegetative cells are ingested, and toxin is produced in the GIT.

The infectious dose is usually 10^5 to10^8 CFU/g of food, so faults allow *B. cereus* growth to occur. Proteinaceous foods, vegetables, sauces and puddings have been implicated.

Measures to control *B. cereus* diarrhoeal syndrome are the same as for emetic syndrome.

Clostridium botulinum

Clostridium botulinum causes two types of food-borne human disease. Botulism is an intoxication, whereas infant botulism (floppy baby syndrome) is a toxico-infection. *C. botulinum* is an environmental contaminant and is found typically in damp soils and muddy sediments, marine and fresh waters (Lund and Peck, 2000). Asymptomatic carriage occurs in the GIT of animals and humans (Cato *et al.*, 1986).

C. botulinum are spore-forming rods which proliferate in low E_h environments (usually anaerobic). The spores are resistant to environmental extremes, but spores may germinate even if oxygen is present (Lund and Peck, 2000). Conditions for growth and toxin production are very strain-dependent. Some strains grow at 3°C, others as high as 48°C (Cato *et al.*, 1986). *C. botulinum* grows in 5% NaCl, but not in 10% salt or below pH 4.6. Nitrite and competitive microorganisms on foods are inhibitory. The toxin is heat labile, so can be destroyed by heating.

Botulism

Ingestion of *C. botulinum* toxin types A, B, E and F is the usual cause of food-borne botulism, although four other toxin types are known and have occasionally been involved (Anon., 1992j; Lund and Peck, 2000). The incubation period is typically 12 to 36 h, but ranges up to 8 days, and probably depends on the level of toxin ingested. Botulinum toxin is very potent: it is estimated that only 0.1 to 1.0 μg can cause food-borne disease (Anon., 1992j). Symptoms include nausea and vomiting followed by dizziness, difficulty swallowing, slurred speech, blurred vision and headache. Fatigue, muscle weakness, paralysis and respiratory impairment can occur. Respiratory failure can cause death (the mortality rate is 30 to 60% in hospitalized individuals).

Botulinum toxin is absorbed into the body by unknown means, attaches to neuromuscular junctions, becomes internalized, and prevents release of acetylcholine. Prognosis is normally improved by rapid administration of antitoxin (Lund and Peck, 2000).

As toxin must be pre-formed in food, growth of the pathogen in food is necessary. This mostly occurs in anaerobic environments, so in Western countries, home-canned, and sometimes commercially canned, non-acid foods (fish, shellfish, meats, vegetables, fungi) are the most common source of botulism. Growth of the pathogen in canned foods is not necessarily evident, as off-odours or can-blowing do not always occur. Other proven sources of botulism include chopped garlic in oil, hazelnut purée, sausages and fish eggs. Fermented fish products and bean products, in Japan and China, respectively, are more frequent sources than other foods. Sea mammal products are common sources of infection in Inuit populations.

Measures to control botulism include:

1. Avoid home canning of vegetables, fish and meats.
2. Discard cans with faulty seals.
3. Heat any suspect food to 80°C for 15 minutes to destroy toxin.
4. Store home-canned foods at <3°C.
5. Use the hurdle concept for home canning of food.

Infant botulism

Infant botulism produces neuromuscular symptoms similar to botulism, resulting in constipation, weak cry and respiratory distress. Infant botulism is usually mild, but depends on the individual patient. Children under 1 year old do not have established gut microflora, so the pathogen may colonize more easily than in other individuals. Infant botulism has occurred in adults, when it has been associated with abnormal GIT function (Lund and Peck, 2000).

The organism is ingested and proliferates in the GIT, producing toxin. Honey is the most common source, and batches from outbreaks have contained up to 10^4 spores/kg (Lund and Peck, 2000). Powdered formula milk caused one case in the UK, in July 2001. Theoretically, any foods that are not heat treated could be a vehicle of infection.

Measures to control infant botulism include:

1. Do not feed honey to babies or infants.
2. Do not feed infants non-heat treated foods.

References

Anon. (1992a) *Campylobacter jejuni*. United States Food and Drug Administration and the Center for Food Safety and Applied Nutrition, http://www.cfsan.fda.gov/~mow/chap4.html (accessed 11 October 2004).

Anon. (1992b) *Escherichia coli* O157:H7. United States Food and Drug Administration and the Center for Food Safety and Applied Nutrition, http://www.cfsan.fda.gov/~mow/chap15.html (accessed 11 October 2004).

Anon. (1992c) *Salmonella* spp. United States Food and Drug Administration and the Center for Food Safety and Applied Nutrition, http://www.cfsan.fda.gov/~mow/chap1.html (accessed 11 October 2004).

Anon. (1992d) *Shigella* spp. United States Food and Drug Administration and the Center for Food Safety and Applied Nutrition, http://www.cfsan.fda.gov/~mow/chap19.html (accessed 11 October 2004).

Anon. (1992e) *Vibrio cholerae* Serogroup O1. United States Food and Drug Administration and the Center for Food Safety and Applied Nutrition, http://www.cfsan.fda.gov/~mow/chap7.html (accessed 11 October 2004).

Anon. (1992f) *Vibrio parahaemolyticus*. United States Food and Drug Administration and the Center for Food Safety and Applied Nutrition, http://www.cfsan.fda.gov/~mow/chap9.html (accessed 11 October 2004).

Anon. (1992g) *Vibrio vulnificus*. United States Food and Drug Administration and the Center for Food Safety and Applied Nutrition, http://www.cfsan.fda.gov/~mow/chap10.html (accessed 11 October 2004).

Anon. (1992h) *Yersinia enterocolitica*. United States Food and Drug Administration and the Center for Food Safety and Applied Nutrition, http://www.cfsan.fda.gov/~mow/chap5.html (accessed 11 October 2004).

Anon. (1992i) *Bacillus cereus* and other *Bacillus* spp. United States Food and Drug Administration and the Center for Food Safety and Applied Nutrition, http://www.cfsan.fda.gov/~mow/chap12.html (accessed 11 October 2004).

Anon. (1992j) *Clostridium botulinum*. United States Food and Drug Administration and the Center for Food Safety and Applied Nutrition, http://www.cfsan.fda.gov/~mow/chap2.html (accessed 11 October 2004).

Anon. (1992k) *Clostridium perfringens*. United States Food and Drug Administration and the Center for Food Safety and Applied Nutrition, http://www.cfsan.fda.gov/~mow/chap11.html (accessed 11 October 2004).

Anon. (1992l) *Listeria monocytogenes*. United States Food and Drug Administration and the Center for Food Safety and Applied Nutrition, http://www.cfsan.fda.gov/~mow/chap6.html (accessed 11 October 2004).

Anon. (1992m) *Staphylococcus aureus*. United States Food and Drug Administration and the Center for Food Safety and Applied Nutrition, http://www.cfsan.fda.gov/~mow/chap3.html (accessed 11 October 2004).

Anon. (2000) Foodborne Diseases. National Institute of Allergy and Infectious Diseases, http://www.wrongdiagnosis.com/artic/food-borne_diseases_niaid_fact_sheet_niaid.htm (accessed 11 October 2004).

Anon. (2000a) Microbial pathogen data sheets. New Zealand Food Safety Authority, http://www.nzfsa.govt.nz/science-technology/data-sheets/ (accessed 28 October 2004).

Anon. (2000b) Notifiable diseases on-line. Public Health Agency of Canada, http://dsol-smed.hc-sc.gc.ca/dsol-smed/ndis/index_e.html (accessed 2 November 2004).

Anon. (2002) Zoonoses report United Kingdom 2002. Department for Environment, Food and Rural Affairs, http://www.defra.gov.uk/animalh/diseases/zoonoses/zoonoses_reports/zoonoses2002.pdf (accessed 2 November 2004).

Anon. (2003a) Foodborne disease in Australia: incidence, notifications and outbreaks. Annual report of the OzFoodNet network, 2002. The OzFoodNet Working Group Vol 27 No 2, June 2003, http://www.health.gov.au/internet/wcms/Publishing.nsf/Content/cda-pubs-cdi-2003-cdi2702-htm-cdi2702g.htm (accessed 2 November 2004).

Anon. (2003b) Swiss zoonoses report 2003; *Salmonella*, *Campylobacter*, STEC, *Listeria*. FVO-magazine Information Service, http://www.biret.admin.ch/info-service/e/publikationen/magazin/1_index.html (accessed 28 October 2004).

Anon. (2004a) Annual report on zoonoses in Denmark 2003. Ministry of Food, Agriculture and Fisheries, http://www.dfvf.dk/files/filer/zoonosecentret/publikationer/annual%20report/annual_report_2003-endelig.pdf (accessed 28 October 2004).

Anon. (2004b) Incidence of cases of infection with nine pathogens under surveillance by the Foodborne Diseases Active Surveillance Network, by site, compared with national health objectives for 2010 – United States, 1996, 1998 and 2003. Centers for Disease Control and Prevention, http://www.cdc.gov/mmwr/preview/mmwrhtml.mm5316a2.htm#tab (accessed 28 October 2004).

Baird-Parker, A.C. (2000) *Staphylococcus aureus*. In: Lund, B.M., Baird-Parker, A.C. and Gould, G.W. (eds) *The Microbiological Safety and Quality of Food, Vol. II*. Aspen Publishers Inc, Gaithersburg, Maryland, pp. 1317–1335.

Beery, J.T., Hugdahl, M.B. and Doyle, M.P. (1988) Colonization of gastrointestinal tract of chicks by *Campylobacter jejuni*. *Applied and Environmental Microbiology* 54, 2365–2370.

Bercovier, H. and Mollaret, H.H. (1984) Genus XIV: *Yersinia*. In: Kreig, N.R. and Holt, J.G. (eds) *Bergey's Manual of Systematic Bacteriology, Vol. 1*. Williams and Wilkins, Baltimore, Maryland, pp. 498–506.

Blaser, M.J., Berkowitz, I.D., LaForce, F.M. *et al.* (1979) *Campylobacter* enteritis: clinical and epidemiologic features. *Annals of Internal Medicine* 91, 179–185.

Cato, E.P., George, W.L. and Finegold, S.M. (1986) Genus *Clostridium*. In: Sneath, P.H.A., Mair, N.S., Sharpe, M.E. and Holt, J.G. (eds) *Bergey's Manual of Systematic Bacteriology, Vol. 2*. Williams and Wilkins, Baltimore, Maryland, pp. 1141–1200.

Chapman, P.A., Siddons, C.A., Wright, D.J., Norman, P., Fox, J. and Crick, E. (1992) Cattle as a source of verotoxigenic *Escherichia coli* O157. *Veterinary Record* 131, 323–324.

Claus, D. and Berkeley, R.C.W. (1986) Genus *Bacillus*. In: Sneath, P.H.A., Mair, N.S., Sharpe, M.E. and Holt, J.G. (eds) *Bergey's Manual of Systematic Bacteriology, Vol. 2*. Williams and Wilkins, Baltimore, Maryland, pp. 1105–1139.

D'Aoust, J.-Y. (2000) *Salmonella*. In: Lund, B.M., Baird-Parker, A.C. and Gould, G.W. (eds) *The Microbiological Safety and Quality of Food, Vol. 2*. Aspen Publishers, Inc., Gaithersburg, Maryland, pp. 1233–1299.

Farber, J.M. and Peterkin, P.I. (2000) *Listeria monocytogenes*. In: Lund, B.M., Baird-Parker, A.C. and Gould, G.W. (eds) *The Microbiological Safety and Quality of Food, Vol. 2*. Aspen Publishers, Inc., Gaithersburg, Maryland, pp. 1178–1232.

Garcia-del Portillo, F. and Finlay, B.B. (1994) Invasion and intracellular proliferation of *Salmonella* within non-phagocytic cells. *Microbiologia SEM* 10, 229–238.

ICMSF (1996) *Campylobacter*. In: Roberts, T.A., Baird-Parker, A.C. and Tompkin, R.B. (eds) *Micro-organisms in Foods, Vol. 5*. Blackie Academic and Professional, London, pp. 45–65.

Kaysner, C.A. (2000) *Vibrio* species. In: Lund, B.M., Baird-Parker, A.C. and Gould, G.W. (eds) *The Microbiological Safety and Quality of Food, Vol. 2*. Aspen Publishers Inc., Gaithersburg, Maryland, pp. 1336–1362.

Kloos, W.E. and Schliefer, K.H. (1986) Genus IV: *Staphylococcus*. In: Sneath, P.H.A., Mair, N.S., Sharpe, M.E. and Holt, J.G. (eds) *Bergey's Manual of Systematic Bacteriology, Vol. 2*. Williams and Wilkins, Baltimore, Maryland, pp. 1013–1035.

Labbé, R.G. (2000) *Clostridium perfringens*. In: Lund, B.M., Baird-Parker, A.C. and Gould, G.W. (eds) *The Microbiological Safety and Quality of Food, Vol. 2*. Aspen Publishers Inc, Gaithersburg, Maryland, pp. 1110–1135.

Lampel, K.A., Madden, J.M. and Wachsmuth, I.K. (2000) *Shigella* species. In: Lund, B.M., Baird-Parker, A.C. and Gould, G.W. (eds) *The Microbiological Safety and Quality of Food, Vol. 2*. Aspen Publishers, Inc, Gaithersburg, Maryland, pp. 1300–1316.

Le Minor, L. (1984) Genus III: *Salmonella*. In: Kreig, N.R. and Holt, J.G. (eds) *Bergey's Manual of Systematic Bacteriology, Vol. 1*. Williams and Wilkins, Baltimore, Maryland, pp. 427–458.

Lund, B.M. and Peck, M.W. (2000) *Clostridium botulinum*. In: Lund, B.M., Baird-Parker, A.C. and Gould, G.W. (eds) *The Microbiological Safety and Quality of Food, Vol. 2*. Aspen Publishers, Inc., Gaithersburg, Maryland, pp. 1057–1109.

Nataro, J.P. and Kaper, J.B. (1998) Diarrheagenic *Escherichia coli*. *Clinical Microbiology Reviews* 11, 142–201.

Nesbakken, T. (2000) *Yersinia* species. In: Lund, B.M., Baird-Parker, A.C. and Gould, G.W. (eds) *The Microbiological Safety and Quality of Food, Vol. 2*. Aspen Publishers, Inc., Gaithersburg, Maryland, pp. 1363–1393.

Ørskov, F. (1984) Genus I. *Escherichia*. In: Kreig, N.R. and Holt, J.G. (eds) *Bergey's Manual of Systematic Bacteriology, Vol. 1*. Williams and Wilkins, Baltimore, Maryland, pp. 420–423.

Park, S., Worobo, R.W. and Durst, R.A. (1999) *Escherichia coli* O157:H7 as an emerging foodborne pathogen: a literature review. *Critical Reviews in Food Science and Nutrition* 39, 481–502.

Rowe, B. and Gross, R.J. (1984) Genus II: *Shigella*. In: Kreig, N.R. and Holt, J.G. (eds) *Bergey's Manual of Systematic Bacteriology, Vol. 1*. Williams and Wilkins, Baltimore, Maryland, pp. 423–427.

Seeliger, H.P.R. and Jones, D. (1986) Genus *Listeria*. In: Sneath, P.H.A., Mair, N.S., Sharpe, M.E. and Holt, J.G. (eds) *Bergey's Manual of Systematic Bacteriology, Vol. 2*. Williams and Wilkins, Baltimore, Maryland, pp. 1235–1245.

Smibert, R. (1984) Genus *Campylobacter*. In: Kreig, N.R. and Holt, J.G. (eds) *Bergey's Manual of Systematic Bacteriology, Vol. 1*. Williams and Wilkins, Baltimore, Maryland, pp. 111–118.

Stern, N.J. and Line, J.E. (2000) *Campylobacter*. In: Lund, B.M., Baird-Parker, A.C. and Gould, G.W. (eds) *The Microbiological Safety and Quality of Food, Vol. 2*. Aspen Publishers, Inc., Gaithersburg, Maryland, pp. 1040–1056.

World Health Organization (1995) WHO surveillance programme for control of foodborne infections and intoxications in Europe. Federal Institute for Health Protection of Consumers and Veterinary Medicine, Berlin.

Yoshikawa, T.T. (1980) Clinical spectrum and management of salmonellosis. *Western Journal of Medicine* 133, 412–417.

Viral Pathogens

Most food-borne viral diseases are caused by consumption of molluscan shellfish. During filter-feeding of seawater, molluscs concentrate viral particles, originating from human faeces, in their tissues. Many viruses are host-specific, so do not cause disease in both humans and animals. Methods for detection of viruses in foods are generally lacking, although routine PCR-based methods may be developed in the future. DNA or RNA sequence-based typing methods are used, but are not suitable for routine use. The only virus for which standard methods for its detection in foods have been developed is *Norovirus* in shellfish. Contamination of other foods, which have been implicated in outbreaks of food-borne viral disease, probably occurs via faeces or vomit from infected food handlers either directly or in aerosols, or via faecally contaminated water.

Noroviruses

Norovirus (family *Caliciviridae*) are a group of related, ssRNA viruses. *Norovirus* were previously described as Norwalk virus (the prototype), Norwalk-like viruses (NLV), Small Round Structured Viruses (SRSV) or calicivirus. *Norovirus* cause viral gastroenteritis, believed to be a very common cause of enteritis worldwide. Other members of *Caliciviridae* include *Sapovirus* – which can cause enteric symptoms in young children, *Vesivirus* and *Lagovirus*.

Norovirus are normally transmitted person-to-person by the faecal–oral route, but may also be water-borne. However, it has been detected in shellfish implicated in outbreaks, particularly oysters, clams and shrimps.

The incubation period is typically 1 to 3 days. Symptoms include nausea, projectile vomiting, diarrhoea (watery, voluminous) and abdominal pain. The disease is normally self-limiting. Elderly and IC individuals are most at risk.

Norovirus replicates in the mucosa of the small intestine and is shed in large numbers in faeces.

The infectious dose is not known. Any foods that require extensive handling could be vehicles of infection. Foods most commonly involved are shellfish, but fruits and salads have also been associated with infection.

Measures to control *Norovirus* include:

1. Don't consume raw shellfish.
2. Prevent faecal contamination of food, even pre-harvest.
3. Dispose of sewage in a sanitary manner.
4. Infected individuals should not handle food.
5. Prevent cross-contamination from shellfish to other foods.

Hepatitis A virus

Hepatitis A virus (HAV) is a ssRNA virus of the family *Picornaviridae*.

The incubation period is typically 2 to 9 weeks, so food may become contaminated with HAV before the onset of symptoms, but after faecal shedding has commenced. Early symptoms are anorexia, fever, malaise, nausea and abdominal discomfort. Vomiting and fever can occur. Sequelae include liver damage, seen in patients when jaundice develops. Hepatitis E virus (HEV) causes similar human disease, but belongs to the family *Hepeviridae*. While HEV has potential to be food-borne it is believed to have caused water-borne disease.

HAV is absorbed through the gastrointestinal mucosa and carried via the blood to the liver. HAV then binds to receptor sites on the hepatocyte surface and penetrates cells. Viral replication occurs, HAV is excreted in bile, and shed in faeces.

Food-borne transmission appears to have occurred in some HAV outbreaks, but the virus has not been detected in any foods. The long incubation period frequently means suspect foods are unavailable, and in-food detection methods have not been developed. HAV is transmitted person-to-person by the faecal–oral route. The infectious dose is unknown but likely to be low: perhaps ten to 100 virus particles. Implicated foods include water, shellfish, salads, fruits, cold meats, sandwiches, fruit juices, milk, milk products and iced drinks.

Measures to control HAV include:

1. Prevent faecal contamination of food even pre-harvest.
2. Infected individuals should not handle food.
3. Dispose of sewage in a sanitary manner.
4. Prevent overcrowded living conditions.
5. Use good personal hygiene measures.

Rotavirus

Rotavirus is a dsRNA virus, of the family *Reoviridae*. Rotavirus is transmitted person-to-person by the faecal–oral route, and causes viral gastroenteritis. Believed to have only rarely caused food-borne disease, but may be more commonly water-borne. Rotavirus has not been isolated from foods.

Rotavirus is the most common cause of viral gastroenteritis in children < 2 years old, and most or all children contract this virus after birth.

The incubation period is typically 1 to 3 days, and vomiting can last from 4 to 8 days after symptoms commence. Symptoms include vomiting, watery diarrhoea and low-grade fever. Rotavirus is normally self-limiting but, in severe cases, rehydration of patients is necessary.

Rotavirus replicates in the mucosa of the jejunum or ileum and is shed in faeces in large numbers.

The infectious dose is unknown but probably is ten to 100 virus particles. Water is most commonly implicated, but any foods that require extensive handling could be vehicles of infection. Implicated foods include salad, cold foods, shepherd's pie and school lunches. Poor personal hygiene is frequently a contributing factor.

Measures to control rotavirus include:

1. Infected individuals should not handle food.
2. Dispose of sewage in a sanitary manner.
3. Prevent faecal contamination of food.

1.3 Chemical Hazards in Foods

Chemicals can occur in the food chain due either to their existence in the environment through unintentional contamination of food, or to their intentional use somewhere along the food production chain (Table 1.2). Generally, industrial pollutants are unintentional contaminants of foods, so, even if regulated, may be difficult to control. Agricultural chemicals are deliberately applied to land or crops during production, so their use can be both regulated and controlled. Some toxic chemical compounds can occur naturally in foods and in the environment.

The rate of ingestion of chemical hazards by food animals can be either higher or lower than the rate of their excretion. In the former case, accumulation of chemicals occurs. In the latter case, animals have a 'decontaminating' effect from the public health perspective. Hazards that accumulate can be a greater public health risk than those which do not accumulate, because if animals are exposed even only to low levels of accumulating hazards but over extended time, their tissues can finally contain levels that pose a risk to consumers. With chemical hazards that accumulate, older animals are a higher risk than younger animals.

Industrial pollutants

Heavy metals

Heavy metals which can occur in foods include lead, arsenic, mercury, cadmium, copper, fluorine and selenium.

Lead

Lead can occur in animals grazing close to lead-smelting plants or after ingestion of paints or lead-containing substances. Paint (typically older types of paint) on animal housing and fences may contain lead and be licked/chewed by farm animals. Animals accumulate lead in the bones, and acute exposure results in high lead levels in the liver and kidney. After chronic poisoning, softening and cavitation of the CNS can be found.

Arsenic

Food animal exposure typically occurs via feeds or liquids contaminated with arsenical herbicides, rodenticides or insecticides. Arsenical compounds have been used as antiparasitics in the past, but are now largely obsolete. Accumulation of arsenic occurs in the liver and kidney, when fatty degeneration can be seen. Arsenic also accumulates in the bones of animals.

Table 1.2. Main groups and typical examples of chemical hazards in foods.

Industrial pollutants	Agricultural chemicals	Growth promoters	Veterinary medicines	'Natural' substances	Food additives	Packaging compounds
Heavy metals	Insecticides	Hormones and hormone-	Antimicrobials	Mycotoxins	Curing agents	Plastics
Lead	*Chlorinated hydrocarbons*	like substances	*Antibiotics*	Aflatoxins	Nitrites	VC-monomers
Arsenic	DDT	*Synthetic hormones*	Penicillins	Ochratoxins	Polyphosphates	Plasticizers
Mercury	Endrin	Diethylstilboestrol (DES)	Aminoglycosides		Sodium chloride	
Cadmium	Aldrin/Dieldrin	*Natural hormones*	Tetracyclines		Antioxidants	
Copper	BHC	Oestradiol	Cephalosporins	Algal toxins	Gallates	Pigments/inks
Fluorine	*Organophosphates*	Progesterone	Macrolides	Microcystin	BHA	
Selenium	Coumaphos	Testosterone	Quinolones	Exo-/Endo-	BHT	
	Malathion	*Fungal oestrogens*	*Nitro-compounds*	neurotoxins		
Halogenated	Diazinon	Zearalenone	Nitroimidazoles	Phyocyans	Preservatives	
hydrocarbons		*β-agonists*	Nitrofurans	PSP	Sulphite	
Polychlorinated biphenyls (PCBs)	Herbicides	Trenbolone	*Sulphonamides*	DSP	Benzoate	
Polychlorinated naphatelenes	2,4-D; 2,4,5-T; MCP	*Thyreostatics*	Sulphamethazine	ASP	Sorbic acid	
(PCNs)	Dioxins					
Dioxins					Smoke	
					compounds	
	Fungicides	Antimicrobial feed	Antiparasitics	Plant toxins	Polycyclic aromatic	
	Dichloran	additives	Salicilanides	Mushroom toxins	hydrocarbons	
	Folpet	Virginiamycin	Thiabendazole	Phytohaemagglutinin	Colours	
		Bacitracin	Benzimidazole	(red kidney beans)	Many	
	Rodenticides	Polymyxin B	Probenzimidazole	Grayanotoxin (honey		
	ANTU	Sulphonamides	Fenbendazole	from rhododendrons)	Emulsifiers	
	Warfarin		Oxfendazole		Many	
			Ivermectins			
	Fertilizers		Levamisole		Sweeteners	
			Tranquillizers		Saccharin	
			Azaperon		Acesulfame K	
			Phenothiazine		Aspartame	
			Promazines			
					Flavour enhancers	
					Many	

Mercury

Documented, but rare, cases of mercury poisoning (enlargement of internal organs, petechiation) have occurred in animals fed with seed grains treated with mercury-based anti-fungal dressings. Inorganic mercury is stored in the liver and kidneys, but organic is more widely distributed throughout the body.

Cadmium

Cadmium is an increasing problem in farm animal production. Unacceptably high cadmium levels can occur in animals, particularly cattle, after grazing pasture irrigated with aerobically digested sludge. High levels of cadmium are a major concern in fish and shellfish hygiene, since the metal is a major water contaminant. Cadmium accumulates in body tissues and can ultimately cause kidney failure in humans. However, significant time is required to reach this toxic level, and the presence of cadmium in animals is difficult to detect.

Halogenated hydrocarbons

This group of reactive compounds includes polychlorinated biphenyls (PCBs), polychlorinated naphatelenes (PCNs) and dioxins.

PCBs, PCNs

Common sources of PCBs and PCNs are electrical machinery, industrial plants, lubricants, paints and some insecticides. These pollutants are extremely stable, and do not break down readily in the environment or in food. PCBs and PCNs accumulate in the liver. Their toxicity primarily relates to teratogenic and carcinogenic effects.

Dioxins

Dioxins have industrial origins similar to PCBs and PCNs. The main source of dioxins is the burning of chlorine-based compounds with hydrocarbons (chlorinated wastes). Two industries which produce or use significant quantities of dioxins are paper mills, which use dioxin-containing compounds for bleaching, and plastics (PVC) manufacturing. Dioxins are extremely stable, and do not break down in the environment. The compounds accumulate in fat (beef, dairy, chicken, pork, fish, eggs, milk, humans). Their toxicity primarily relates to teratogenic and carcinogenic effects.

Agricultural Chemicals

Agricultural chemicals are intentionally used in agriculture i.e. food production, so in principle their use can generally be controlled by legislation or codes of good practice. Generally, most herbicides, fungicides, fertilizers and rodenticides are used well in advance of harvest and are not used directly on animals, so should not occur frequently in foods. However, insecticides can be used on crops nearer to harvest, and also on animals and animal-related environments to control insects/ectoparasites.

Insecticides

Insecticides encompass a large group of chemicals, some of which are extremely environmentally stable and toxic, and so can be found in foods. Insecticides are the most widely used agricultural chemicals, and therefore represent the greatest risk of food contamination. Main groups of insecticides include chlorinated hydrocarbons (DDT, Endrin, Aldrin/Dieldrin, BHC) and organophosphates (Coumaphos, Malathion, Diazinon), both of which can contaminate foods.

Chlorinated hydrocarbons

DDT is the best known and the most successful of the synthetic insecticides. DDT was used very successfully in the past for mosquito, animal ectoparasite and plant insect control in many countries. However, it has been banned since 1972. DDT is extremely durable, persistent and accumulates in tissues, so still occurs in the food chain in some previously heavily contaminated regions, even though it has not been in use for decades. Chlorinated hydrocarbons are CNS stimulants, and can cause congestion of internal organs and focal centrilobular necrosis of the liver.

Organophosphates

This is the largest class of insecticide in use today, both industrially and domestically. Organophosphates are extremely efficient, but are also extremely toxic to mammals. These compounds produce non-pathognomonic (acute) symptoms or chronic congestion of the lungs. Organophosphates successfully led to eradication of warblefly, with few adverse effects. These insecticides produce very little tissue residues and they are much less persistent in the environment than are organochlorines, so they are a lower risk to food safety than are the chlorinated hydrocarbons. However, organophosphates are an occupational hazard, particularly for people using them in agriculture.

Herbicides

Herbicides, including 2,4-D, 2,4,5-T, MCP or dioxins, are not normally used on food crops or livestock. However, when herbicide-treated products are used for animal bedding, residue problems can result. Auxin herbicides (hormone weedkillers) contain dioxins, which are extremely potent and stable chemicals (discussed above). Most other types of herbicides are not normally very toxic, although some of their derivative break down products can be highly toxic to humans. Many countries have factories producing herbicides for agriculture, the production of which should be controlled since the chemical processes can be rapidly altered to production of chemical weapons.

Fungicides

Fungicides, including dichloran and folpet, are used to control growth of moulds and yeasts, but do not normally occur as residues in foods. Fungicides can contain heavy metals. The compounds themselves are normally coloured, to enable identification of treated seed grains. However, treated grains may be mistakenly fed to animals or used in the preparation of cereal foods, and several cases of poisoning have been documented.

Fertilizers

Fertilizers can impact significantly on the environment, and can be problematic if their use on-farm results in contaminated run-off waters. Fertilizers can induce growth of toxic algae in river, lake or coastal waters resulting in contamination of shellfish, and in the death of indigenous biota in fresh and marine waters. If suitable pre-grazing or pre-harvest precautions are taken, fertilizer residues present no major problem in foods.

Rodenticides

Rodenticides, including Antu and Warfarin, are common in agricultural environments. When used under controlled and prescribed conditions, they should not be found in foods.

Growth Promoters

Animal growth promoters are used for commercial reasons, but do not have any health benefits for the animals or for consumers. The two major classes of growth promoters are hormone-like compounds and antimicrobials, which cause differing food safety-related problems. Growth promoters are not permitted in the EU, but are allowed in other countries, including the USA.

Hormone-like growth promoters

Hormones and hormone-like substances include synthetic hormones (Diethylsibesterol: DES), natural hormones (Oestradiol, Progesterone, Testosterone), fungal oestrogens (Zearalenone), β-agonists (Trenbolone) and thyreostatics. Hormonal growth promoters are not permitted for use in food animal production in the EU, but they are permitted in the USA, where they are in relatively widespread use. However, the risks associated with hormone growth promoters are difficult to evaluate. It can be difficult to differentiate natural hormones (used as growth promoters) from hormones that occur in animals, and in people consuming animal-derived foods, so tracing them in the food chain is difficult. Synthetic hormones may not be detectable in animals, particularly if they have been used in young animals which are slaughtered when older.

DES is used as an implant in food animals. However, two incidents in the public domain raised awareness of the potential dangers of this compound. First, after DES was used to prevent miscarriages in women, a proportion of girls born subsequently developed cervical adenocarcinomas. Secondly, DES in pork meat was linked to premature puberty in girls. The use of hormones for growth-promoting of food animals banned within the EU has caused an ongoing 'trade war' with the USA.

Antimicrobial growth promoters

Antimicrobial growth promoters are not permitted for use in the EU, but some antimicrobials are permitted in the USA. Low, but continuous, doses are typically given to animals via feed additives, producing more rapid growth of livestock. The mechanism of antimicrobials promoting animal growth is not known, but suppression of undesirable microorganisms within the gastrointestinal tract, or innate anabolic effects of some antimicrobials themselves, have been proposed. These compounds probably affect the composition of indigenous flora and behaviour of microorganisms in animals' gastrointestinal tracts. Virginiamycin, bacitracin, polymyxin B and sulphonamides are among those commonly used.

Veterinary Medicines

Antimicrobials

Antimicrobial residues in foods are generally regarded as unacceptable. Therefore, treatment of animals with antimicrobials requires a balance between desirable health effects in the animal and undesirable effects if residues occur in food. Undesirable effects of antimicrobial residues in food include the possibility of development of microbial resistance, which can be transmissible between differing strains of the organisms. Humans can develop allergic reactions after ingestion of antimicrobial residues (e.g. penicillin) via foods, particularly milk. Ingestion of antimicrobial residues could alter human gut microflora. Finally, high levels of residues could produce toxic reactions in people consuming contaminated foods.

Antimicrobial medicines including antibiotics (Penicillins, Aminoglycosides, Tetracyclines, Cephalosporins, Macrolides, Quinolones), nitrocompounds (Nitroimidazoles, Nitrofurans) and sulphonamides (Sulphamethazine) are used to treat diseases in animals. Antimicrobials can also be used in other circumstances. Previously, antimicrobials have been allowed as growth promoters in food animals in the EU (see above). In addition, antimicrobials can justifiably be prescribed for preventative measures to reduce infections in the case of outbreaks of animal disease. Limits on the levels of antimicrobials in foods are based on different considerations (see later), but include the sensitivity of methods for their detection.

Antiparasitics

Examples of antiparasitics include Salicilanides, Thiabendazole, Benzimidazole, Probenzimidazole, Fenbendazole, Oxfendazole, Ivermectins and Levamisole. Some metabolites or derivatives of parent antiparasitics are stable in animals, so these compounds should be prescribed and used with care. Residues can occur in meat, and teratogenic effects have been observed in sheep.

Tranquillizers

These compounds can be used to reduce animals' stress levels, which could be beneficial during transport and to handlers at slaughter. Compounds sometimes used include Azaperon, Phenothiazine and Promazines. It is not known whether tranquillizers produce residues in foods, or whether the consumption of foods derived from tranquillized animals has undesirable effects.

Toxic Substances Occurring Naturally in Foods

A wide range of naturally occurring substances can contaminate foods, including toxic biogenic amines, mycotoxins, algal toxins and plant toxins.

Biogenic amines

Toxic biogenic amines, important in food-borne intoxication (e.g. histamine, tyramine), can be produced by decarboxylation of free amino acids in any food. Intoxication occurs if excessive quantities of amines are ingested (perhaps > 500 ppm). Intoxication also results if the natural detoxifying enzymes monoamine oxidase (MAO) or diamine oxidase (DAO) are ineffective.

Histamine intoxication causes an allergic-type reaction with lowered blood pressure, and is associated primarily with fish (see Chapter 9.3); the prevalence of histamine intoxication in human populations is normally quantifiable.

Tyramine intoxication causes a sharp increase in blood pressure, specifically in the brain. Tyramine poisoning occurs primarily via ripened cheeses, fermented sausages (see Chapter 7.4), red wine and chocolate. Some people who suffer from migraine can be sensitive to tyramine in foods, but the prevalence of tyramine intoxication in human populations is unclear.

Mycotoxins

Toxigenic fungi (moulds) produce mycotoxins naturally during their growth. Toxigenic fungi are problematic if they grow in animal feeds, and livestock are fed mouldy, toxin-containing feed. Subsequently, food (milk/meat) derived from these animals may contain mycotoxins. Toxigenic fungi may also grow on some foods after harvest, so the presence of mycotoxins in human food can develop later in the food chain. Being strictly aerobes, fungi grow only on the surface of the food; in such a case the food safety question is whether the mycotoxins have diffused into the deeper layers of the product.

Two classes of mycotoxins are of concern. Aflatoxins produced by *Aspergillus flavus* and *A. parasiticus* (AFB1, AFB2, AFG1, AFG2) are carcinogenic for both animals and humans. Lesions may be observed in the liver of animals and humans. Ochratoxins are produced by *Penicillium* spp. and some *Aspergillus* strains. These toxins affect the kidney, and are most commonly associated with pigs. Derivatives of ochratoxins (Ochratoxin M) can also be detected in cows' milk.

Aflatoxins commonly occur in some foods, even without obvious mould growth. For example, peanuts contain aflatoxins derived from fungi growing in association with the plant root, so aflatoxin contamination of the crop occurs even pre-harvest.

Algal toxins

A number of algae growing in certain coastal regions can produce toxins, that can subsequently be accumulated in shellfish filter-feeders (see Chapter 9.3) and cause paralytic shellfish poisoning (PSP) and related intoxications in humans.

Plant toxins

Some edible plants can produce toxins, e.g. mushroom toxins that are heat-stable, phytohaemagglutinin (red kidney beans) that is destroyed by cooking, and grayanotoxin (honey from rhododendrons).

Food Additives

Chemical compounds used as food additives are present in foods due to intentional and presumably controlled use, and their presence in foods is considered as 'normal' if in concentrations predetermined as posing no significant risk for consumers. They include curing agents (e.g. nitrites, polyphosphates, sodium chloride), smoke compounds, antioxidants (e.g. gallates, BHA, BHT), and preservatives (e.g. sulphite, benzoate, sorbic acid). Food additives are not usually discussed in the context of chemical contaminants of foods, which are present in foods 'abnormally' and unintentionally (e.g. pesticides, industrial pollutants, etc.) and which are considered as a serious threat to consumers. Nevertheless, because food additives are chemical compounds artificially added to foods, and also because some of them can represent a health hazard if ingested in too high concentrations and/or at too high frequencies, they are addressed in this chapter.

Additives used primarily to affect sensory qualities of foods

A very large number of various additives are used in some highly processed foods to make their sensory qualities more acceptable and/or desirable to the consumers. They include food colours (dyes), emulsifiers, sweeteners (e.g. saccharin, acesulfame K, aspartame) and flavour enhancers (e.g. Na glutamate). The main intention of adding these additives to food is of a commercial nature, whilst generally they do not provide food safety benefits. Potential public health concerns associated with this group of food additives are not well defined yet, but have been expressed in some scientific publications, and include potential association of their regular ingestion with behavioural problems (e.g. hyperactivity) in young children.

Nitrites and nitrates

There are two main uses for nitrites in meat, at concentrations ranging from <100 to 200 mg/kg (see Chapter 7.2). First, NO_2 reacts with meat pigment (myoglobin) producing a bright red, attractive and thermo-stable compound. Secondly, nitrites are a remarkably effective inhibitor of the outgrowth of clostridial spores in cured meats, particularly sausages.

Nitrites are toxic in concentrations higher than those typically used in cured meat production, so their levels should be monitored. These compounds can react with certain amines from meat and produce nitrosamines, known carcinogens. The risks from consuming nitrites in meat products produced under controlled conditions may be small, and outweighed by the benefit of *C. botulinum* control achieved. In addition, tobacco smoke and plant foods (e.g. spinach) contain much higher levels of nitrites than do meat products. However, strict control of nitrites is necessary but not always easy to achieve during production of meat products. In addition, there is a risk that meat products could be inadvertently overdosed with these compounds.

Polyphosphates

Polyphosphates, used at <0.5% (w/w) concentration, are added to meats for commercial reasons (see Chapter 7.2). Polyphosphates increase the ability of meat proteins to bind water. This property enables incorporation of additional water, perhaps up to 30%, in some products (frankfurters, bologna). Polyphosphates do not have any public health benefits. The main health concern is the potential disturbance of the balance of phosphorus and calcium in the body, and subsequent insufficient utilization of phosphorus, due to increased intake of phosphates. This could be particularly problematic in children, who have high calcium demands and metabolism due to rapid bone growth.

Smoke

Smoke flavours are commonly used in dairy, seafood and meat products, and produce desirable organoleptic qualities, e.g. flavour, colour (see Chapter 7.2). Some smoke compounds (e.g. organic acids, phenols) have antimicrobial properties, and so may contribute to food safety. However, some smoke compounds are potent carcinogens. Carcinogenic polycyclic aromatic hydrocarbons (e.g. 3,4 benzpyrene) are produced during smoking at temperatures >300°C; the higher temperatures the higher the concentrations. These temperatures can be reached and the toxic compound generated over open fire, which includes the use of home barbeques – if organic compound fossil fuels are burnt. The toxic compounds in smoke can be removed and the desirable compounds filtered into a liquid smoke product. Liquid smoke is commonly used, since it is regarded as a safer and more controllable way of obtaining the desirable organoleptic qualities of smoke without the risks of carcinogen production.

Plastic Packaging Compounds

Many plastic packaging materials are produced from basic raw carcinogenic vinyl chloride (VC) monomers, which in the process are converted into safe, non-toxic polymeric vinyl chloride (PVC). PVC manufactured by some less advanced methods and processes can contain traces of VC monomers. In modern food production, much consumer-level food is wrapped or packed in plastics (see Chapter 7.2), so migration of plastic compounds from such materials into the foods could occur. On the other hand, if food is placed in non-microwave-safe plastic material during heating in a microwave oven, some plastic compounds can react with food fats producing toxic derivatives. In addition, some pigments or inks used for labelling of plastic packages may carry a risk of their migration into foods. Therefore, plastics used in contact with food must be manufactured under stringent quality assurance procedures, and should be declared as safe for use with foods and whether they are microwave-safe.

Calculation of Residue Limits

The level of any residue allowed in foods is called the acceptable daily intake (ADI). The methods for determination of ADI is:

$$\text{ADI (mg/kg/day)} = \frac{\text{NOEL}}{\text{SF}} \quad (1)$$

SF = safety factor.

The no observable effect level (NOEL) is the dose (mg/kg) at which no adverse effects are observed during animal bioassay toxicological studies using the most sensitive testing methods available in the most sensitive animal species, e.g. teratogenicity, carcinogenicity, mutagenicity or immunopathological effects. NOEL is divided by a chosen safety factor of 100–1000, to take account of the fact that humans may have a lower threshold for the residue than the test animal species.

The maximum acceptable total residue level (TRL, see below) is calculated from the ADI and is based on the assumption that an average person of 60 kg body weight will consume a certain amount (g) of a given food per day.

$$\text{TRL (mg/kg)} = \frac{\text{NOEL}}{\text{SF}} \times 60 \times \text{CF} \quad (2)$$

CF = consumption factor; 60 = body weight; SF = safety factor.

The TRL is the combined residue level of the parent compound, plus any harmful derivatives of that compound formed during storage, cooking, or after ingestion of the parent compound. TRL refers to the safe concentration of total residues.

The maximum residue level (MRL) is frequently used by regulatory agencies to state the maximum permissible level of one particular marker residue. The marker residue is the drug-related substance (parent compound or metabolite) that is feasible to quantify by laboratory methods, which enables the level of total residues of toxicological concern in the target tissue to be monitored. MRL is always lower than the TRL, since it refers only to one compound in the food, whereas TRL refers to the total of related compounds in a food.

Further Reading

Anon. (1986) *The Control of Pesticides Regulations 1986 (as amended)*. (COPR), The Pesticides (Maximum Levels in Crops, Food and Feedingstuffs) (England and Wales).

Anon. (1991) EC Council Directive 91/414/EEC. European Commission, Brussels.

Anon. (1998) Annual Report on Pesticide Residues by the Working Party. MAFF Publications, London.

Anon. (1999) The Control of Substances Hazardous to Health Act 1999 (COSHH), London.

Dabrowski, W.M. and Sikorski, Z.E. (2005) *Toxins in Foods*. CRC Press, London.

UK Veterinary Medicines Directorate (VMD), http://www.vmd.gov.uk/

1.4 Genetically Modified Foods

Veterinary surgeons are increasingly becoming involved in the issue of genetically modified (GM) foods. A major responsibility for veterinarians relates to advising on safety of feedstuffs used to produce healthy livestock on-farm. More and more, organic meat/milk producers require assurance of GM-free feeds on their farms. In addition, a proportion of the public will require GM-free food for companion animals, and the family veterinarian will also have to respond to the need for information on this topic.

Genetic modification technically started thousands of years ago, with animal selection during livestock breeding and cross-pollination of edible plants. However, there is a significant difference between such forms of genetic modification – which have been historically accepted – and the modern commercial production of GM plants and animals using molecular bioengineering. The historical approach was very limited, and also was applied only within the same species, or between very closely related species. In contrast, modern genetic modification can produce transgenic plants and animals, where organisms carry genes derived from different species, or even different genera and families.

The first GM food widely available to consumers was a potato, which was marketed during the 1960s in the USA, and used for the production of chips. Later, it was found that that product developed solanine toxin, and the potato was withdrawn from the market. This was the first public failure of a genetically modified food. In 1979, cows carrying recombinant somatotrophin (rPST – a growth hormone) were produced. It was planned that calves bred from these cows would carry rPST, and the increased levels of growth hormone would lead to better overall productivity. During the 1980s transgenic plants, with inserted genes from microorganisms, were produced. The 1990s saw the production of genetically modified cheese rennet-producing organisms, store-ripening tomatoes, and porcine rPST, all of which were foods produced for the US market.

GM Foods: *Pro* and *Contra*

Consumers are divided into two opposing groups: GM supporters and GM opponents. Although GM technology originated in Europe, the most comprehensive consumer opposition occurs in the EU countries, particularly the UK. However, the basic principle of consumer choice requires that people have the right to know what foods they are eating. On a wider scale, individual countries have the right to know if foods they are importing have been genetically modified, and to ensure that legal standards are adhered to. Therefore, the issue of GM foods affects relationships between multinational companies, scientists, farmers and regulators. Arguments centred on the rights or wrongs of this controversial subject can sometimes be politically based, instead of being based in science.

One criticism of genetic modification is that it has the potential to limit biological diversity. This is true if only very few, genetically modified, species are used for food production, and means that the larger number of non-GM species not being used will not be conserved; i.e. the genetic material they harbour will disappear. This can potentially have a negative effect on food security, as traditional species will not be available to turn back to if any problem occurs. Also, potential problems with GM technology are centred on spread of antibiotic resistance via GM organisms produced by methods involving use of antibiotics (see below), and development of resistance in pests and weeds against insecticides and herbicides produced by GM organisms. In addition, production of non-GM food on a single farm is not sustainable if all surrounding growers are using GM technology. Finally, although developing nations may be able to grow and harvest GM foods, they will lack the skills and resources to develop them. Ultimately, therefore, developing nations could become increasingly dependent on developed nations for agricultural development.

On the positive side, food production may be increased if GM foods become commonplace, while production costs should decrease. The sensory qualities of GM foods could be better than non-GM foods. Also, it is claimed that some health benefits may occur due to consumption of specific GM foods. In many countries, genetic modification is widely and increasingly used and espoused in medical biotechnology, and this clearly contrasts with the situation in food production, where the needs and benefits of genetic modification are not yet well accepted. This conflicting situation may have arisen because relatively small proportions of the population (i.e. diseased) would be exposed to medical genetic modification techniques, whereas the whole population requires health-giving foods to eat.

Genetic Modification of Crops

The main aims of genetic modification of crops are to produce foods with higher performance characteristics or to facilitate plant breeding – both are commercial considerations. In plants, herbicide resistance, insect resistance and production of sterile males to allow cross-fertilization in order to produce higher value nutrient contents (e.g. vitamins) are common forms of GM. Novel genetic material is usually introduced into host plants using bacterial plasmids, or by electroporation, using bombardment by accelerated DNA-coated particles propelled by high-energy electrical or magnetic fields.

Genetic Modification of Animals

Animals are most likely to be modified to enhance growth-related gene activity, either by introducing new genes or by increasing expression of existing genes (e.g. growth hormone, growth hormone-releasing factor or insulin-like growth factor). Genetic modification has also been used to introduce novel genes into animals' intestinal epithelium. The enzyme phytase, which increases phosphorus uptake, and bacterial enzymes for synthesis of cysteine – an essential amino acids – have been introduced into animals. To produce transgenic animals, foreign DNA is micro-injected into the egg pronucleus of mammals, or into the egg cytoplasm of fish. The DNA can be modified pre- or post-injection, and the techniques can be used to introduce autonomous artificial chromosomes into a host cell. Introduction of DNA by micro-injection into gametes produces permanent and heritable alterations in the host. For somatic cell modifications (gene therapy) electroporation or vectors, including retroviruses or plasmids, are used.

Safety Considerations of GM Foods

Whether GM foods are safe is a controversial question; the answer is presently unclear, although new information is being accumulated rapidly.

Substantial equivalence

The principle of substantial equivalence is used to compare a GM food to its non-GM counterpart. If substantial equality is established, the GM food is considered safe. However, how to assess substantial equivalence remains a fundamental problem with this approach.

For crops, for example, comparisons may be made between phenotype or compositional characteristics, or toxin production. One problem of assessing equality in plants is due to the large sample sizes required. Small changes may remain hidden except in the face of extensive sampling. For the same reason, crop sampling must be conducted in varying locations and seasons. It could be presumed, in general, that more profoundly modified crops probably present greater risks from unintended modification effects than do less modified crops.

For animals, establishing equality between GM- and non-GM organisms is also a guiding principle in establishing GM safety. If the inserted DNA is well characterized, it can be extracted from the host animal post-modification, and compared with the original insert. The gene products of inserted DNA can be studied (up-regulation or down-regulation of the inserted gene), as can other differences between GM and non-GM animals. One aspect of genetic modification in animals that needs attention is the technique of modification for disease resistance. Although such animals should not develop disease, they may represent a risk to human health by carrying the disease or disease agent asymptomatically. In such a case, overall, they may produce greater risks of human infection via the meat chain. Also, compositional analysis could be applied in equality studies, although novel methods may be required, as should the consequences of under- or over-expression of genes. There are few peer-reviewed data on the equivalence of GM and non-GM foods. Only one human feeding trial has been published, in which fish (tilapia) modified with growth hormone were fed to humans and, simultaneously, monkeys were injected intravenously with the produced growth hormone. No adverse effects were observed in this human feeding trail. In a second trial, fish (carp) modified with growth hormone were fed to mice. No adverse effects were found. Nonetheless, these trials were relatively limited in focus, and do not provide any wider conclusion about the safety of GM foods.

Animal welfare is another issue to be addressed when considering the safety of GM; there should be equivalence in all aspects of animal welfare between GM- and non-GM animals.

Allergens

Allergic reactions can be life-threatening, and GM technology could increase the risk that individuals are exposed to allergens without their knowledge. A FAO/WHO decision tree is used to assess the allergenicity of GM foods. First, sequence comparison of the expressed protein with very well-characterized, sequenced allergens is conducted (e.g. strawberry or groundnut proteins, known to be frequently allergenic). Second, if the gene source is a known allergen, its reaction with sera from allergic patients is examined. This is followed by further testing with sera from patients allergic to organisms broadly related to the gene source. Third, the effects of *in vitro* digestion with the stomach protease pepsin are studied. Finally, *in vivo* animal testing is required to complete the examination of allergenicity in a GM food. Some animal products contain substantial amounts of allergens (e.g. cows' milk, the shrimp protein tropomyosin); there are concerns whether these would be increased by gene modification of the animal itself. In contrast, experimental GM crops with reduced concentrations of intrinsic allergens have been created.

Gene transfer

The issue of gene transfer as a result of genetic modification of foods requires attention. Antibiotic resistance genes were often used in the production of some GM micro-organisms. Chosen antibiotic resistance genes, combined with the gene of interest, are inserted into a bacterial plasmid (highly mobile genetic elements, which can transmit easily from one bacterium to another). The GM plasmid is inserted into bacterial cells which are cultured on media containing the antibiotics. The GM plasmid itself can then be purified and used for plant modification. There is a risk that antibiotic resistance genes and the gene of interest could be transferred to other bacteria after consumption of the GM crop. Within the EU, the only gene initially approved for this procedure was for kanamycin resistance. Recently, however, the practice has been banned altogether within the EU, where the problem of antibiotic resistance gene transfer is perceived to be a very serious issue.

During genetic modification of animals, antibiotic resistance genes are not frequently used, although there is the potential for some problems to occur even without their use. First, wild plasmids can naturally harbour antibiotic resistance genes, and if such plasmids are used to prepare GM animals, the resistance genes could transfer unintentionally. GM animals could shed resistance genes in epithelial cells from the gastrointestinal tract mucosa and, subsequently, the genes may be transferred to bacteria in the GI tract. Also, inserted retroviral sequences in animals (GM poultry) could combine with wild-type viruses, potentially creating new retroviruses. Retroviruses are a common vector for genetic modification of animals, and attempts are being made to produce artificial retroviruses not prone to recombination.

Pre-market and post-market assessments

Safety assessment of any food should be conducted before it is released onto the market. However, in the case of GM foods, the question arises of what safety assessment to conduct if the food is already on the market.

Recent EU legislation requires that cultivated GM foods undergo monitoring and surveillance for substantial periods for unanticipated, undesirable long-term effects. In effect, this requires a programme for long-term surveillance and monitoring, including the time following the product's arrival on the market. Surveillance of plants or crops during normal trade and business is perhaps the hardest thing to achieve, as substantial mixing of ingredients, companies, places of origin etc. can occur. Due to their lack of traceability, GM crops could easily be 'lost', rendering surveillance or monitoring programmes defunct.

Animal traceability is already undertaken at a much higher level than with plants, so tracking GM animals for monitoring and surveillance should be less complex. However, legal definitions of GM animals as 'veterinary medicines' can confound the problem. Some producers have made the case that animals containing transgenic growth hormone should not be subjected to food legislation but, as a source of the growth hormone itself, should be subject to less stringent veterinary medicine legislation. Veterinarians must be aware, from a public health point of view, of such attempts to confound the intent of the law.

Regulatory aspects

The cultivation, trade and food and feed industry is subject to national regulations, with the safety assessments as part of the admission procedure. National regulations for cultivating GM crops can differ between countries, although GM crops are widely marketed. In the EU, legislation is generally more stringent compared with the USA, and a trade war has developed partially as a result of these differences. International harmonization initiatives are under way. Guidance documents by the Organisation for Economic Cooperation and Development (OECD) have been completed for soybean and oilseed rape; guidance documents for potato, sugarbeet, wheat, maize, rice, sunflower and cotton are under way. OECD guidance documents aimed at harmonization have been produced, including GM feed production for farm animals and GM feed production for pets. The *Codex Alimentarius* Intergovernmental Task Force on Foods Derived from Biotechnology is organizing expert consultations, and related risk analysis documents are being drafted; these will probably be adopted in a few years.

However, the production and use of GM animals has limited regulatory coverage. To date, two applications for GM animals to be marketed to consumers are known. In Australia, Bresatec pigs were found to contain transgenic growth hormone, designed to be 'switched on' when the livestock were fed zinc. The company abandoned the project when the relevant food safety authority declared itself not responsible for GM animals, and the supermarkets stated their reluctance. AquAdvantage salmon (USA) is transgenic for a growth hormone gene under the control of a promoter from the ocean eelpout's antifreeze protein gene. The application for this new animal drug, intended to be marketed as a human food, is pending and should involve numerous risk analyses including environmental risks (wastes, pens) and food safety risks.

In summary, existing data on the use of GM foods indicate:

1. Knowledge about the use and consequences of GM foods is limited.
2. Lack of evidence must not be interpreted to mean a GM food is safe.
3. Clear guidance on the suitability of assessing GM foods under existing food or drug legislation is required.
4. Methods for assessment of the safety of GM foods must be improved.
5. Proper labelling is essential, to provide consumers with choice, and to enable producers to emphasize improved product quality. Currently, labelling is not mandatory, and may be opposed by regulatory agencies on the basis of cost, stigmatization of products and logistical difficulties.

Further Reading

Anon. (2001) EU Directive 2001/18/EC on deliberate release into the environment of genetically modified organisms. *Official Journal of the European Commission* L106, 1–39.

Anon. (2004) Guidance document of the scientific panel on genetically modified organisms for the risk assessment of genetically modified plants and derived food and feed. *EFSA Journal* 90, 1–94.

Kleter, G.A. and Kuiper, H.A. (2002) Considerations for the assessment of the safety of genetically modified animals used for human food or animal feed. *Livestock Production Science* 74, 275–285.

OECD (1993) *Safety evaluation of foods derived by modern biotechnology: concepts and principles.* Organisation for Economic Cooperation and Development, Paris.

Schilter, B. and Constable, A. (2002) Regulatory control of genetically modified (GM) foods: likely developments. *Toxicology Letters* 127, 241–349.

WHO (1987) Principles for the safety assessment of food additives and contaminants in food. WHO Environmental Health Criteria No. 70, IPCS-Program, World Health Organization, Geneva.

1.5 Risk Assessment – Introduction

Phil Voysey

Today's consumers are looking for foods that are: healthier; more nutritious; longer lasting; and more convenient to prepare. To respond to this, the food industry has to be innovative in the development and production of its food and drink products. New developments in food production and manufacture can lead to differences in the pathogens encountered and in the general level of immunity in the population. This in turn puts increased emphasis on the need for food producers to know and understand more about the pathogens likely to occur in the products they are making, their origins, and the effects of processing and packaging techniques on those products.

To help food manufacturers tackle this consistently, Microbiological Risk Assessment (MRA) is now being applied as a systematic tool to allow effective decisions to be made in order to reduce the impact of pathogens on health.

Recent History of Microbiological Risk Assessment (MRA)

A number of MRAs have now been published. See, for example, the website of the World Health Organization: http://www.who.int/foodsafety/micro/links/en/

However, MRA is still a relatively recently developed science. The UK Government's Advisory Committee on Dangerous Pathogens (ACDP) set out the general principles of risk assessment as applied to microbiology in relation to public health issues in June 1996. This came in a document entitled *Microbiological Risk Assessment: an Interim Report*. Soon after the publication of this ACDP document, the Codex Alimentarius Commission (CAC) published a draft document *Principles and Guidelines for the Application of Microbiological Risk Assessment* in August 1996. The finished version of this document was published in 1999 (CAC, 1999). The document is of great importance because as a result of the GATT (General Agreement on Trade and Tariffs) and SPS (Sanitary and Phytosanitary Measures) agreements, guidelines and other documents produced by the CAC become reference standards for international trade.

A number of initiatives throughout the world are being taken to develop the field of MRA from a regulatory or governmental point of view. From the food manufacturer's point of view, Campden and Chorleywood Food Research Association (CCFRA) has published a guideline document on how to carry out an MRA (CCFRA, 2000). The second edition of this document is currently being written and will contain worked examples to act as guides for industry.

What is MRA?

MRA is one of three components of Risk Analysis, the others being Risk Management and Risk Communication. A diagrammatic representation of how these three components interact is given in Fig. 1.2. Put simply, Risk Assessment is the measurement of risk and the identification of factors that influence it. Risk Management is the development and implementation of strategies to control that risk, and Risk Communication is the exchange of information relevant to the risk among interested parties.

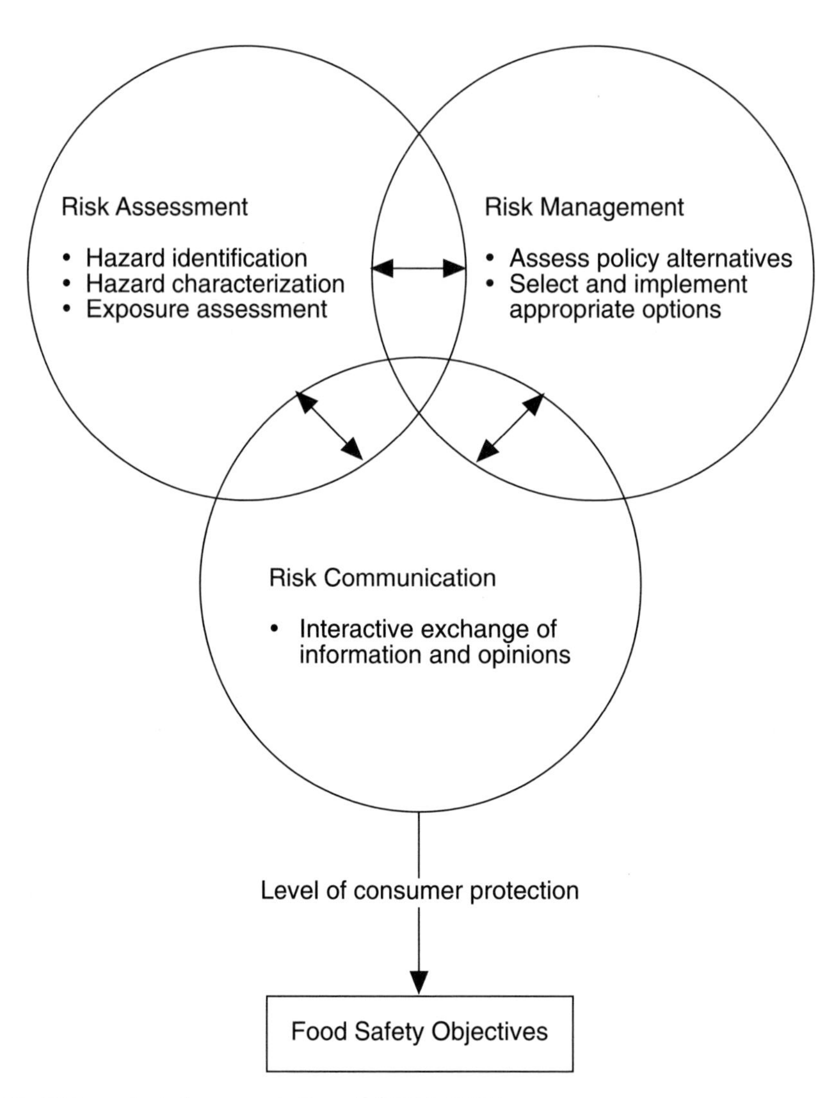

Fig. 1.2. Risk analysis framework (from CCFRA, 2000).

There are a number of important considerations to bear in mind when carrying out a risk assessment. These 'principles' are stated in CAC (1999) and are listed in Box 1.1.

Wherever and whenever possible, Quantitative Risk Assessments should be made. In other words, assessments where numbers and specific data are used. However, the quality of data available will have a bearing on whether this or a Qualitative Risk Assessment can be carried out. (Qualitative information is not based on specific numbers, but rankings: for example 'low', 'high', 'negligible' are qualitative terms). Qualitative Risk Assessment techniques have been used extensively in considering the chemical safety of foods. However, these techniques cannot easily be used in carrying out microbiological evaluations (Voysey, 1999).

Box 1.1. General Principles of Microbiological Risk Assessment (from CAC, 1999)

1. Microbiological Risk Assessment must be soundly based upon science.

2. There should be a functional separation between Risk Assessment and Risk Management.

3. Microbiological Risk Assessment should be conducted according to a structured approach that includes Hazard Identification, Hazard Characterization, Exposure Assessment and Risk Characterization.

4. A Microbiological Risk Assessment should clearly state the purpose of the exercise, including the form of Risk Estimate that will be the output.

5. A Microbiological Risk Assessment should be transparent. This requires: full and systematic documentation, statement of assumptions, value judgements and rationale, and a formal record.

6. Any constraints that impact on the Risk Assessment, such as cost, resources or time, should be identified and their possible consequences described.

7. The Risk Estimate should contain a description of uncertainty and where the uncertainty arose during the Risk Assessment process.

8. Data should be such that uncertainty in the Risk Estimate can be determined; data and data collection systems should, as far as possible, be of sufficient quality and precision that uncertainty in the Risk Estimate is minimized.

9. A Microbiological Risk Assessment should explicitly consider the dynamics of microbiological growth, survival and death in foods and the complexity of the interaction (including sequelae) between human and agent following consumption, as well as the potential for further spread.

10. Wherever possible, Risk Estimates should be reassessed over time by comparison with independent human illness data.

11. A Microbiological Risk Assessment may need re-evaluation, as relevant new information becomes available.

Components of an MRA

A quantitative MRA produces a mathematical statement that links the probability of exposure to an agent to the probability that the exposure will affect the test individual. This is coupled with a consideration of the severity of illness to yield an overall Risk Characterization. The components of an MRA are given in diagrammatic form in Fig. 1.3.

The first step is to decide on a *Statement of Purpose*. The specific purpose of the risk assessment needs to be clearly stated. The output and possible alternatives also need to be defined; for example, is the output to be the probability of infection in terms of cases per 100,000?

The second step is one of *Hazard Identification*. This identifies the micro-organism or microbial toxin of concern and evaluates whether the

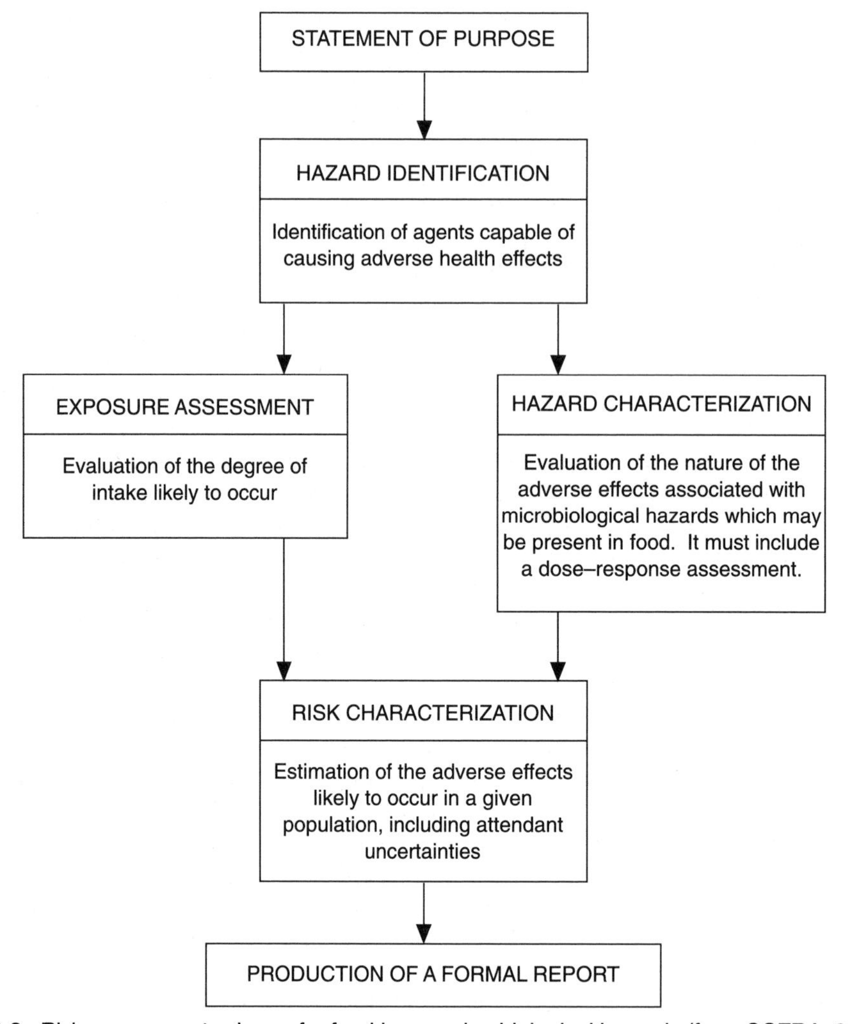

Fig. 1.3. Risk assessment scheme for food-borne microbiological hazards (from CCFRA, 2000).

agent is a hazard when present in food. If the focus of the Risk Assessment is on a pathogen, then available epidemiological and related data need to be used to determine if food-borne transmission is important to the disease and which foods are implicated. If a hazard identification is orientated towards the foods, then the focus will be to use available epidemiological and microbiological data to determine which pathogens could be associated with the product. To carry out hazard identification successfully, high-quality and relevant public health data and information on the occurrence and levels of pathogenic microorganisms in the foods of concern need to be readily available.

The next step in the Risk Assessment is *Exposure Assessment*. The ultimate goal of exposure assessment is to evaluate the level of microorganisms or microbial toxins in the food at the time of consumption. This may include an assessment of actual or anticipated human exposure. An accurate exposure assessment needs three types of information: (i) the presence of the pathogen in the raw ingredients; (ii) the effect that food processing, packaging, distribution, handling and preparation steps have on the pathogen; and (iii) consumption patterns, e.g. portion size. Because the occurrence of a specific pathogen tends to be heterogeneously distributed in food, both the frequency and extent of contamination are needed. Historical data on levels in raw commodities and finished products are useful in providing an estimate of the distribution of a pathogen. The methods used to determine levels and the statistical sampling for accumulation of data considering low levels of a specific organism are very important here. Each step in the manufacture and distribution of a food may have an impact on the levels of the microorganism of concern, hence they need to be considered. Well-validated/mathematical predictions can be useful here, e.g. in assessing the relative safety of thermal processes (Whiting and Buchanan, 1994).

The fourth step is *Hazard Characterization*, which is the qualitative and/or quantitative evaluation of the nature of the adverse effects on the consumer associated with biological, chemical and physical agents that may be present in foods. The important component of a hazard characterization step is a dose–response assessment. The purpose of hazard characterization is to provide an estimate of the nature, severity and duration of the adverse effects associated with harmful agents in food. Important factors to consider relate to the microorganisms, the dynamics of infection and to the sensitivity of the consumer.

It is well established that the virulence of closely related species of pathogenic bacteria may vary widely in terms of their hazard as a food poisoning bacterium, e.g. *Listeria monocytogenes* is known to be harmful to man; *Listeria ivanovii*, on the other hand, is not recognized as a human pathogen. A second important aspect to the dose–response assessment is the number of bacteria ingested. When the log of the number of bacteria ingested is plotted against the percentage of the population that becomes infected, a sigmoidal relationship is seen. From this a threshold level, below which ingestion of the organism does not produce infection, can be determined.

It is easy to see why it is difficult to obtain this type of information. Even if it does stem from human volunteer studies, which by its very nature it has to, the statistics relate only to healthy adults. Every population will contain more susceptible individuals than this, be they elderly, young or immunocompromised.

The integration of the exposure and dose–response assessment gives the fifth step of the process, the *Risk Characterization*. This gives an overall probability of occurrence and severity of health effects in a given population. To be meaningful, the risk characterization should include a description of statistical and biological uncertainties.

The final, sixth, step of the Risk Assessment is to produce a *Report*. This should contain a full and systematic record of the Risk Assessment. To ensure its transparency, the MRA report should indicate any constraints and assumptions relating to the Risk Assessment.

MRA and HACCP

The Hazard Analysis and Critical Control Points (HACCP) technique is the foremost system for the control of microbiological hazards in food. The first phase of both MRA and HACCP is the identification of hazards; consequently there is confusion between the two techniques. However, HACCP is really a Risk Management system, thus the role of Quantitative MRA is to provide the information HACCP system developers need to make more informed decisions. In addition to enhancing the hazard analysis phase of HACCP, Risk Assessment can be used to help identify critical control points (CCPs), establish the critical limits and determine the extent of hazard associated with product during periods of CCP deviation (ICMSF, 1998).

Examples of Quantitative Microbial Risk Assessments

The early MRAs that were carried out focused on establishing drinking water standards on a scientific basis (Macler and Regli, 1993). The hazardous organisms were bacteria, viruses and protozoa, and the target was to evaluate them against risks in using chlorine to control them. As the approach was developed, a quantitative Hazard Assessment for *L. monocytogenes* in milk processing was carried out to evaluate the efficacy of milk production and pasteurization practices (Peeler and Banning, 1994). Using this Hazard Assessment, the investigations concluded that there was less than a 2% probability that one *L. monocytogenes* would occur in 5.9×10^{10} gallons of pasteurized milk. More recent MRAs have improved in their degree of sophistication and reflect areas where there have been substantial food safety concerns, and in some cases disagreements, among international trading partners. Three areas that have received a great deal of attention are:

1. *Salmonella enteritidis* in eggs and egg products; see for example: http://www.fsis.usda.gov/ophs/risk/index.htm
2. *Listeria monocytogenes* in ready-to-eat foods; see for example: http://www.fao.org/es/esn/food/risk_mra_riskassessment_listeria_en.stm
3. Enterohaemorrhagic *E. coli* in ground beef; see for example: http://www.fsis.usda.gov/ophs/ecolrisk/pubmeet/index.htm

Conclusions

Although MRA is a powerful tool for levelling the playing field of food safety, it is apparent that no food can be considered to be risk free and each step in the processing of food from farm to fork has a role in assuring its safety. An important hurdle is to communicate this to the public in easily understood terms; MRA can assist with this. Currently there are large gaps in the amount of useful and useable data available; consequently the number of meaningful MRAs that can be carried out is limited. This area needs attention in terms of resources and these data gaps need to be filled; however, as a starter it is important that workers in the area of MRA all use the same definitions for terms used in MRA. Only in this way can communication of hazards and risks be meaningful to everyone.

References

CCFRA (2000) An Introduction to the Practice of Microbiological Risk Assessment for Food Industry Applications. CCFRA Guideline No. 28 (P. Voysey (ed.)). CCFRA, Gloucestershire, UK.

Codex Alimentarius Commission (1999) Principles and Guidelines for the Conduct of Microbiological Risk Assessment. Codex Alimentarius Commission GL-30, Rome.

ICMSF (1998) Potential application of risk assessment techniques to microbiological issues related to international trade in food and food products. *Journal of Food Protection* 61(8), 1075–1086.

Macler, B.A. and Regli, S. (1993) Use of microbial risk assessment in setting US drinking water standards. *International Journal of Food Microbiology* 18, 245–256.

Peeler, J.T. and Banning, V.K. (1994) Natural assessment of *Listeria monocytogenes* in the processing of line milk. *Journal of Food Protection* 57, 689–697.

Voysey, P.A. (1999) Aspects of Food Microbiological Risk Assessment. *New Food* 8, 10–12, 14, 15.

Whiting, R.C. and Buchanan, R.L. (1994) IFT. Scientific study summary: microbial modelling. *Food Technology* 44(6), 113–120.

2 On-farm Factors and Health Hazards

2.1 Principles of Epidemiology as Applied to VPH

Ivar Vågsholm

Epidemiology is a way of thinking and analysing problems with a view to increasing the knowledge of risks, risk factors, pathways of infections and contamination along the food chains, animal populations and environment, and is aimed at enabling community actions. VPH aims to apply veterinary knowledge to improve public health; thus, epidemiology is a building block in this endeavour.

To give a few examples of epidemiology applied to further public health it might be useful to start with John Snow's study of cholera in London in the Victorian era. John Snow worked as a doctor (anaesthetist) in Victorian London from 1840 to 1850. His pioneering studies were on the cholera epidemic in 1849, on which he published his studies in 1854. Today, we know cholera is a water-borne disease caused by the bacterium *Vibrio cholerae*. The organism harbours genes for producing cholera toxin, which is transmitted by sewage into water (rivers or lakes) subsequently used for consumption. In brief, the faecal–oral pathway of transmission can result in explosive epidemics, once the bacterium is introduced into the water system. It appears that certain crayfish can harbour the bacteria on their bodies, thus creating reservoirs for the cholera bacteria. In Snow's era, the prevailing wisdom specified miasma (foul air) or other vehicles to be the causes of cholera. Snow observed that during cholera outbreaks there were large differences in the number of cases (today one would say incidence or attack rate, i.e. the frequency of new cases during an outbreak) during cholera outbreaks in two similar areas of London. Two water companies supplied these separate areas. The water companies were supplying water for households through public pumps (outlets). During his investigations, Snow discovered that the water companies had their water intakes in the river Thames upstream and downstream of the sewage pipe into the river. The company upstream had the lower cholera incidence. Snow deduced that cholera was connected to the water being contaminated with sewage. This was several years before bacteria were recognized as a source of disease. To test his hypothesis, he removed (illegally) the handle of the water outlet associated with suspected cholera risk during the next outbreak. It appeared that the cholera incidence was reduced in the previous high-risk area. To sum it up; Snow did not know what caused the disease, but by applying principles of epidemiology comparing exposed with non-exposed populations he verified the hypothesis that cholera was connected with sewage contamination of drinking water. By intervention aimed at removing the exposure he could prove his hypothesis, albeit there was no prevailing knowledge of the true cause of the disease. This illustrates that epidemiology enables us to assemble enough knowledge to intervene in containing public or animal health risks long before we know all the relevant facts. The principles of comparison either of exposed *versus* not exposed with regard to disease incidence (cohort studies) or of the exposure rates in cases *versus* controls, produce ideas about the exposure risks. Interventions aimed at reducing exposures may confirm, or rather gather, further supporting evidence for the disease risks. Consequently, epidemiology is the cutting edge of medicine and public health activities, enabling prevention before the exact causes are identified, as was illustrated by John Snow's work.

With mad cow disease or bovine spongiform encephalopathy (BSE) the same story could be told in a modern setting (see MAFF, 2000). During 1984 in the UK, a new syndrome emerged in cattle, with symptoms such as behavioural changes (losing rank in cow herd), sound sensitivity, ataxia and weight loss, with no response to treatments whatsoever. During the next 2 years more cattle with similar symptoms appeared in dairy herds in the UK. Wells *et al.* (1987) described the histopathological symptoms of BSE as being similar to those of scrapie. At that time, BSE was defined as a combination of clinical syndrome and histopathological findings. Then, to assess the risk factors, the usual suspects were rounded up and investigated including:

- contacts with sheep and goats; the risk factor was scrapie, which was known to be transmitted between animals;
- exposure to insecticides, i.e. organophosphates and pyrethrins;
- exposure to meat and bone meal;
- imported animals;
- vaccines;
- genetic mutations;
- unknown factors.

The challenge was now to assess the available evidence using sound epidemiological reasoning to sift through all possible hypotheses for the risk from BSE.

Disease Control Strategies With Regard to Veterinary Public Health

Disease control strategies could be seen as the aim of disease control efforts. By conventional wisdom they are grouped into three broad strategies:

- control strategy is when the aim is to live with the disease agent(s) but to keep the prevalence or concentration below an acceptable level;
- eradication strategy is when the aim is to eliminate the disease agent(s) within a geographical area or population, a primary production system and/or a part of the food chain;
- prevention strategy is when the aim is to prevent the introduction of disease agent(s) into a population and a food chain.

Veterinary public health is often defined as veterinary activities aimed at protecting and/or improving public health in a broad sense by employing one or a combination of these strategies.

Food safety is a veterinary public health activity employing all three strategies. With the advent of meat inspection during the last century, several zoonoses such as tuberculosis, and parasites such as trichinosis, could be controlled. However, it was soon recognized that food safety could not be assured by end product testing alone. This insight led to the development of the HACCP (hazard analysis critical control points), to supplement Good Agricultural Practice (GAP), Good Hygiene Practice (GHP) and Good Manufacturing Practice (GMP).

The HACCP system was conceived by the Pillsbury Company, together with the National Aeronautics and Space Administration (NASA), and the US Army Laboratories at Natick developed this system to ensure the safety of astronauts' food during the 1960s (WHO, 2003). In the 40 years since then, the HACCP system has become the generally accepted method for food safety assurance. The recent growing worldwide concern about food safety by public health authorities, consumers and other concerned parties – and the continuous reports of food-borne outbreaks – have given further impetus to the application of the HACCP system. The HACCP system achieves process control by identifying hazards and critical control points in the process and establishing critical limits at these control points for the identified hazards (i.e. microbiological criteria), establishing systems for monitoring the critical control points and indicating suitable corrective actions if the critical limits are exceeded, and establishing suitable verification and documentation procedures.

The purpose of a critical control point (CCP) might be to control the growth of bacteria by keeping the food cold stored or frozen, e.g. *Salmonella* spp. or VTEC O157, and to have procedures to ensure that the cold-chain integrity is kept. Another purpose might be to eradicate pathogens from the food, e.g. pasteurization of milk.

The food chain could be seen as a consequence of the HACCP approach. Many HACCP plans had as their first critical control point the raw material – how to ensure that the raw material was safe. Thus, food processors and food safety authorities started to require that farmers and feed producers also had food safety assurance programmes. At the end of the day it appeared that there were critical control points both in primary production and in feed production, as well as in processing.

Instead of thinking of feed production, animal husbandry and production, abattoirs, cutting, dairying and other processing as separate and independent activities aimed at processing raw materials that might end up on the plate, the modern approach is that everybody along the food chain is producing food. Previously, for example, milk on the farm was considered as a raw material that was transported and changed into a foodstuff only after pasteurization. Now, it is regarded as a food that must be protected all the way from the pastures to the consumers. Consequently, the quality and safety requirements and the supervision along the food chain should be seamless and integrated. The slogans 'farm to fork', or 'from the fields to the plates' were used to illustrate this new thinking. Inevitably, this has changed the way veterinary surgeons work. Previously, our main goal was to cure sick animals. This is still our main task today but now, in addition, we must ensure that healthy animals produce healthy foods and that our cures for sick animals will not harm the safety of any food produced.

The BSE and dioxin crises within the EU originated due to problems in feed production: in particular the rendering practices in regard to the BSE epidemic, and the raw materials used for feedstuff production in regard to the dioxin crisis. Both crises contributed to this radical overhaul of how we work in food safety. The European Commission (2000) outlined this new approach in its White Paper (http://europa.eu.int/comm/dgs/health_consumer/library/pub/pub06_en.pdf). In the new EU general food law regulation (Council and Parliament Regulation 178/2002/EU) it is stated that all food business operators are responsible for producing safe food. Food business operators are defined as all those involved, from feed producers, farmers and food processors to caterers and supermarkets. Another challenge is to regard animal health and public health as two sides of the same coin.

In the food chain one might apply the same tool but be pursuing different strategies. For example, vaccination will be used to control some diseases (like *Salmonella* in layers), to control and eradicate other diseases like pseudorabies (Aujeszky's disease) and to prevent introduction of Newcastle disease into a poultry flock.

The remit of veterinary public health activities is wide – which makes this field the most satisfying in which to work in veterinary medicine. There are always new challenges awaiting. One interesting development is the issue of conservation medicine (Daszak *et al.*, 2004), where one links the prevention of zoonoses with the conservation of wildlife and ecosystems, with sustainability of agriculture and economic and social development all based on as sound an epidemiological knowledge as possible. The conservation medicine approach to emerging diseases integrates veterinary, medical, ecological and other sciences in interdisciplinary teams. These teams investigate the causes of emergence, analyse the underlying drivers and attempt to define common rules governing emergence for human, wildlife and plant emerging infectious diseases. The ultimate goal is risk analysis that allows us to predict future emergence of known and unknown pathogens. Then, the disease control strategies can be employed as appropriate.

Many zoonoses normally thought of as food-borne can be transmitted by direct contact with animals or through the environment, or from person to person. One example is *E. coli* O157 or enterohaemorrhagic *E. coli* (EHEC) – also referred to as shigatoxinlike (STEC) or verotoxin-producing *E. coli* (VTEC), as reviewed by Mead and Griffin (1998), and also verotoxigenic *E. coli* (VTEC) in foodstuffs, in the opinion of the Scientific Committee of Veterinary Public Health (2003). Hence, any disease control strategies employed must take a holistic view of the disease problem. To prevent person-to-person transmission the public health authorities may require that children in kindergartens with diarrhoea stay at home until the clinical symptoms cease. When visiting farms or herds visitors are obliged to wash their hands to avoid transmission of EHEC after direct animal contacts.

For some years it has been recommended in Sweden that children under 5 years of age should not visit farms during the summer, when the risk of catching EHEC is highest. EHEC poses a challenge since it can be eradicated at the processing stages of the food chain using heat treatment, while in the primary production stage the challenge is to control the bacteria and to prevent the clinical disease in humans.

I hope this and the following chapters will induce readers to pursue a career in veterinary public health. Although no promises about gold and glory can be given, your professional life will not be boring.

References

Daszak, P., Tabor, G.M., Kilpatrick, A.M., Epstein, J., Plowright, R. (2004) Conservation medicine and a new agenda for emerging diseases. Annals of the New York Academy of Sciences 1026, 1–11.

European Commission (2000) http://europa.eu.int/comm/dgs/health_consumer/library/pub06_en.pdf

MAFF (2000) *The BSE Inquiry*. http://www.bseinquiry.gov.uk

Mead, P.S., Griffin, P.M. (1998) *Escherichia coli O157:H7*. *Lancet* 352, 1207–1212.

Scientific Committee of Veterinary Public Health (2003) http://europa.en.int/comm/food/fs/se/sev/out58_en.pdf

Wells, G.A., Scott, A.C., Johnson, C.T., Gunning, R.F., Hancock, R.D., Jeffrey, M., Dawson, M. and Bradley, R. (1987) A novel progressive spongiform encephalopathy in cattle. *Veterinary Record* 121, 419–420.

WHO (2003) http://who.int/fsf/Micro/haup.htm

2.2 Zoonotic Diseases in Farm Animals

Basic Parameters for Describing Disease

Disease is an abnormal status that can be detected in clinical form by our senses (vision, palpation, smell, etc.) or in sub-clinical form only by specific tests. Zoonoses are diseases infecting animals that also can be naturally transmitted to humans.

With respect to their frequency of occurrence, zoonotic diseases can occur in the following forms:

- epidemic: a sharp increase in occurrence above the status that is, under given conditions, considered as 'normal';
- pandemic: a worldwide epidemic;
- endemic: regularly present in a given population;
- outbreak: a sudden epidemic affecting ≥ 2 or a high number of related individuals; and
- sporadic: a disease occurring as single cases in unrelated individuals.

To describe general disease patterns, some basic parameters can be used:

- incidence: number of new cases of a disease, expressed as a proportion of the 'at-risk population' within a given period;
- at-risk population: part of a population particularly susceptible to a given disease; and
- prevalence: diseased individuals as the proportion of the total population at a given time.

Information needed about a given disease often includes whether it is present or absent. Absence of disease can be proved only by testing all susceptible animals; this normally poses numerous practical difficulties. Rather, this is commonly handled through testing of a sample of the animals in the location. The sample size chosen will depend on the particular circumstances, such as size of the animal population and nature/prevalence of the disease, but the most important factor is which confidence level is expected from the results (most commonly 95%). Sampling and testing programmes can be:

- monitoring: ongoing testing to detect changes in disease prevalence; and
- surveillance: continuous testing, often of the same population section, to detect early cases for disease control purposes.

Notifiable Diseases

Notifiable disease are those designated in official lists issued by national (e.g. UK Government, Table 2.1) and/or international regulatory authorities (e.g. OIE; Table 2.2) and which, immediately after their

Table 2.1. Notifiable diseases in the UK (from DEFRA, 2005).

Notifiable Disease	Species affected	Last occurence
African Horse Sickness	Horses	Never
African Swine Fever	Pigs	Never
Anthrax	Cattle and other mammals	2002
Aujeszky's Disease	Pigs and other mammals	1989
Avian Influenza (Fowl plague)	Poultry	1992
Bluetongue	Sheep and Goats	Never
Bovine Spongiform Encephalopathy (to BSE home page)	Cattle	Present
Brucellosis (*Brucella abortus*)	Cattle	2004
Brucellosis (*Brucella melitensis*)	Sheep and Goats	1956
Classical Swine Fever	Pigs	2000
Contagious agalactia	Sheep and Goats	Never
Contagious Bovine Pleuropneumonia	Cattle	1898
Contagious Epididymitis (*Brucella ovis*)	Sheep and Goats	Never
Contagious Equine Metritis	Horses	2003
Dourine	Horses	Never
Enzootic Bovine Leukosis	Cattle	1996
Epizootic Haemorrhagic Virus Disease	Deer	Never
Epizootic Lymphangitis	Horses	1906
Equine Infectious Anaemia	Horses	1976
Equine Viral Arteritis	Horses	2004
Equine Viral Encephalomyelitis	Horses	Never
Foot and Mouth Disease	Cattle, sheep, pigs and other cloven-hooved animals	2001
Glanders and Farcy	Horses	1928
Goat Pox	Goats	Never
Lumpy Skin Disease	Cattle	Never
Newcastle Disease	Poultry	1997
Paramyxovirus of pigeons	Pigeons	Present
Peste des Petits Ruminants	Sheep and Goats	Never
Rabies	Dogs and other mammals	1970
Rift Valley Fever	Cattle, Sheep and Goats	Never
Rinderpest (Cattle plague)	Cattle	1877
Scrapie (on DEFRA's BSE website)	Sheep and goats	Present
Sheep pox	Sheep	1866
Swine Vesicular Disease	Pigs	1982
Teschen Disease (Porcine enterovirus encephalomyelitis)	Pigs	Never
Tuberculosis (Bovine TB)	Cattle and deer	Present
Vesicular Stomatitis	Cattle, pigs and horses	Never
Warble fly	Cattle (also deer and horses)	1990
West Nile Virus	Horses	Never

detection or suspicion, must be reported to the authorities. Therefore, a given disease can be notifiable internationally, nationally or both. There are several reasons for inclusion of a disease in the 'notifiable' category:

- it can cause significant economic damage (the most common reason), e.g. foot and mouth disease;
- it can cause severe illness or death in humans, e.g. rabies, tuberculosis;

Table 2.2. Diseases notifiable to the OIE (from OIE, 2004).

- Multiple species diseases
  - Anthrax
  - Aujeszky's Disease
  - Bluetongue
  - Echinococcosis/hydatidosis
  - Foot and mouth disease
  - Heartwater
  - Leptospirosis
  - Lumpy skin disease
  - New World screw-worm (*Cochliomyia hominivorax*)
  - Old World screw-worm (*Chrysomya bezziana*)
  - Paratuberculosis
  - Q fever
  - Rabies
  - Rift Valley fever
  - Trichinellosis
  - Vesicular stomatitis
- Sheep and goat diseases
  - Caprine and ovine brucellosis (excluding *B. ovis*)
  - Caprine arthritis/encephalitis
  - Contagious agalactia
  - Contagious caprine pleuropneumonia
  - Enzootic abortion of ewes (ovine chlamydiosis)
  - Maedi-visna
  - Nairobi sheep disease
  - Ovine epididymitis (*Brucella ovis*)
  - Ovine pulmonary adenomatosis
  - Peste des petits ruminants
  - Salmonellosis (*S. abortusovis*)
  - Scrapie
  - Sheep pox and goat pox
- Swine diseases
  - African swine fever
  - Atrophic rhinitis of swine
  - Classical swine fever
  - Enterovirus encephalomyelitis
  - Porcine brucellosis
  - Porcine cysticercosis
  - Porcine reproductive and respiratory syndrome
  - Swine vesicular disease
  - Transmissible gastroenteritis
- Lagomorph diseases
  - Myxomatosis
  - Rabbit haemorrhagic disease
  - Tularaemia
- Cattle diseases
  - Bovine anaplasmosis
  - Bovine babesiosis
  - Bovine brucellosis
  - Bovine cysticercosis
  - Bovine genital campylobacteriosis
  - Bovine spongiform encephalopathy
  - Bovine tuberculosis
  - Contagious bovine pleuropneumonia
  - Dermatophilosis
  - Enzootic bovine leukosis
  - Haemorrhagic septicaemia
  - Infectious bovine rhinotracheitis/infectious pustular vulvovaginitis
  - Malignant catarrhal fever
  - Rinderpest
  - Theileriosis
  - Trichomonosis
  - Trypanosomosis (tsetse-transmitted)
- Equine diseases
  - African horse sickness
  - Contagious equine metritis
  - Dourine
  - Epizootic lymphangitis
  - Equine encephalomyelitis (Eastern and Western)
  - Equine infectious anaemia
  - Equine influenza
  - Equine piroplasmosis
  - Equine rhinopneumonitis
  - Equine viral arteritis
  - Glanders
  - Horse mange
  - Horse pox
  - Japanese encephalitis
  - Surra (*Trypanosoma evansi*)
  - Venezuelan equine encephalomyelitis
- Avian diseases
  - Avian chlamydiosis
  - Avian infectious bronchitis
  - Avian infectious laryngotracheitis
  - Avian mycoplasmosis (*Mycoplasma gallisepticum*)
  - Avian tuberculosis
  - Duck virus enteritis
  - Duck virus hepatitis
  - Fowl cholera
  - Fowl pox
  - Fowl typhoid
  - Highly pathogenic avian influenza
  - Infectious bursal disease (Gumboro disease)
  - Marek's disease
  - Newcastle disease
  - Pullorum disease

Continued

Table 2.2. *Continued*

Fish diseases
- Bacterial kidney disease (*Renibacterium salmoninarum*)
- Channel catfish virus disease
- Enteric septicaemia of catfish (*Edwardsiella ictaluri*)
- Epizootic haematopoietic necrosis
- Epizootic ulcerative syndrome
- Gyrodactylosis (*Gyrodactylus salaris*)
- Infectious haematopoietic necrosis
- Infectious pancreatic necrosis
- Infectious salmon anaemia
- Oncorhynchus masou virus disease
- Piscirickettsiosis (*Piscirickettsia salmonis*)
- Red sea bream iridoviral disease
- Spring viraemia of carp
- Viral encephalopathy and retinopathy
- Viral haemorrhagic septicaemia
- White sturgeon iridoviral disease

Crustacean diseases
- Crayfish plague (*Aphanomyces astaci*)
- Infectious hypodermal and haematopoietic necrosis
- Spawner-isolated mortality virus disease
- Spherical baculovirosis (*Penaeus monodon-type baculovirus*)
- Taura syndrome
- Tetrahedral baculovirosis (*Baculovirus penaei*)
- White spot disease
- Yellowhead disease

Bee diseases
- Acarapisosis of honey bees
- American foulbrood of honey bees
- European foulbrood of honey bees
- *Tropilaelaps* infestation of honey bees
- Varroosis of honey bees

Mollusc diseases
- Infection with *Bonamia exitiosus*
- Infection with *Bonamia ostreae*
- Infection with *Candidatus xenohaliotis californiensis*
- Infection with *Haplosporidium costale*
- Infection with *Haplosporidium nelsoni*
- Infection with *Marteilia refringens*
- Infection with *Marteilia sydneyi*
- Infection with *Mikrocytos mackini*
- Infection with *Mikrocytos roughleyi*
- Infection with *Perkinsus marinus*
- Infection with *Perkinsus olseni/atlanticus*

Other diseases
- Leishmaniosis

- it cannot be differentiated from another disease, e.g. swine vesicular disease;
- it is a newly introduced disease with expected significant, or yet to be assessed, impact – e.g. caseous lymphadenitis in the UK; and
- it is important for tradition – or public opinion-related reasons.

Understandably, in practice, notification of a given disease is useful only if it is diagnosable by an appropriate test, and is controllable.

Actions Following Disease Notification

Management of a number of notifiable diseases in the UK (and EU) is covered by related EU policies, and can include:

- isolation of affected or suspect animals;
- declaration of an infected premises and possibly an area;
- control of the movement of animal, people and vehicles;

- killing (slaughter) of all affected and in-contact animals (with compensation) within a certain geographical radius, for disease eradication purposes e.g. foot and mouth disease;
- slaughter of an infected animal with compensation, e.g. tuberculosis, BSE;
- treatment, e.g. anthrax in pigs;
- vaccination, e.g. rabies, Newcastle disease; and
- related cleaning and sanitation regimes.

Understandably, necessary pre-conditions for successful management of notifiable diseases include individual and/or herd identification of animals and records of movement for relevant farm animal species. However, it should be noted that different countries may manage diseases differently. If a country declares (and proves) freedom from a given notifiable disease, then it can decide to import animals only from those countries that apply compulsory notification of that disease.

Principal zoonotic notifiable diseases in farm animals

Tuberculosis

This is a contagious, usually chronic disease, characterized by nodular lesions – tubercles with necrosis, caseation and calcification in lungs, lymph nodes or other organs. The infectious route is either mainly inhalation (e.g. cattle) or ingestion (e.g. pigs). Disease is caused by three different types of mycobacterium. *Mycobacterium tuberculosis* causes infections mostly in man, rarely in dogs, parrots and non-human primates. *M. bovis* causes tuberculosis mostly in cattle, but can also infect humans, goats and pigs; sheep and horses have high resistance. *M. avium* is found mostly in birds, and also in pigs, but it is still debatable whether can it infects humans. The main sources of infection of cattle appear to include wildlife, e.g. badgers in the UK – although this is still a controversial and debatable explanation – and opossums in New Zealand and Australia. In the EU, some countries are declared free from bovine tuberculosis, whilst in others prevalence of infected herds varies between <1% and 8%. In the UK at the beginning of 2001, around 900 animals were found to be reactors out of approximately 372,000 tested.

Diagnosis of bovine tuberculosis in live animals can be based on:

- culturing of respiratory tract secretions, but this gives positive results only in <20% of naturally infected animals;
- detection of antibodies, but antibody responses vary in magnitude and often cannot be detected until a few months after infection;
- cellular immune responses; infection stimulates strong responses, with delayed-type hypersensitivity reactions detectable 3–4 weeks after infection;
- tuberculin skin test; based on intradermal injection of a crude protein extract from supernatants of *M. bovis* and *M. avium* injected at two separate sites on the neck and measurement of the skin thickness after 72

hours. Sensitivity (% of infected animals correctly identified) of the tuberculin test is around 90%, and specificity (% of uninfected animals correctly identified) is around 99.9%;

- interferon-γ test (IFN-γ test); whole blood is cultured with PPD from *M. bovis* and *M. avium* and IFN-γ production is measured by ELISA after 24 hours. A field trial in Northern Ireland showed an IFN-γ test sensitivity of 84.3% whilst parallel tuberculin sensitivity was 83.1%.

Positive findings of tuberculous lesions (caseous lymphadenitis) at post-mortem meat inspection of tuberculin-positive slaughtered cattle can vary (40–70%). This variability can be affected by the interpretation criteria used for the tuberculin skin test, as well as by how detailed the meat inspection was. Tuberculous lesions in reactors are found mainly in lymph nodes draining the head and lungs (around 40 and 70%, respectively), but are found much less frequently in lung tissue or mesenteric lymph nodes (<10%). With respect to microbiological isolation of the pathogen, most lesions that are visible yield positive results. However, several weeks is required to obtain culture results. Carcass meat from cattle with only localized lesions found and removed is used for human consumption as in such cases there are no tuberculous lesions in muscles. However, the entire carcass is condemned in the case of spread or generalized tuberculous lesions. To date, there is not yet clear evidence of human *M. bovis* infection via meat or meat products.

Bovine tuberculosis had much higher implications for human health in the first half of 20th century, when neither herd testing nor milk pasteurization measures were implemented. For example, in the 1930s in the UK, 40% of cows were infected and 0.5% produced contaminated milk, leading to roughly 2000 human deaths per annum. However, since milk pasteurization and herd testing were introduced (1940s–1950s), the prevalence of positive herds decreased to 1.6–2.5% and human cases decreased to 32–34/year. Hence milk pasteurization prevents, to a large extent, the risks from food-borne tuberculosis, but it should be kept in mind that dairy products from unpasteurized milk dairy products are available on the market. Therefore, nowadays, occupational exposure to *M. bovis*, e.g. farmers, may represent a higher public health risk.

Mycobacterium paratuberculosis (*M. avium* subspecies paratuberculosis, *M. johnei*) causes Johne's disease (paratuberculosis) in cattle. Disease is characterized by enteritis and/or enlargement of mesenteric lymph nodes, often with haemorrhages. Diagnosis of paratuberculosis by blood tests (AGIDT, ELISA, CFT) is possible. Human infection with this pathogen (Crohn's disease) may be acquired primarily via contaminated milk, although the question of whether association between Johne's disease and corresponding Crohn's disease actually exists is still being debated.

Bovine Spongiform Encephalopathy (BSE)

This disease, caused by a proteinaceous agent called a 'prion', primarily affects cattle, in which it was first recognized in the mid-1980s in the UK.

However, a single case of BSE in a goat was confirmed in France in 2004; the implications of caprine BSE for overall BSE epidemiology have yet to be determined. Bovine BSE infections have been registered in a number of countries since the 1990s (Table 2.3). It is generally accepted that the initial source of infection was feeding of cattle with meat and bone meal which probably contained carcasses of sheep infected with scrapie in the 1980s. This was preceded by a change (lower temperature) in the rendering process. However, it seems that the vast majority of cases were caused by feeding cattle-derived material to cattle.

Clinical symptoms include apprehensiveness, occasional aggression, kicking when milked, high-stepping gait (particularly hind legs), skin tremors and loss of condition. Early studies on BSE looked for, and did not find, evidence that BSE was associated with pharmaceuticals, pesticides, genetic determinants, artificial insemination or direct contact with sheep/cattle.

Trends in the BSE epidemic in the UK are characterized by a sharp increase in new cases until the peak in 1992, when 1% of adult breeding cows per year were infected. Since then, the incidence has been decreasing by approximately 40% per year. The infection was associated primarily with dairy herds; 61% of all dairy herds were affected, comprising 81% of BSE cases. The intra-herd prevalence was relatively low (on average ≤2.7%).

Table 2.3. Incidence of BSE in cattle at the end of 2003 (adapted from OIE data).

Countries	First recorded case	Total cases
EU		
Ireland	1990	1,360
Portugal	1993	862
France	1991	897
Switzerland (non-EU)	1990	417
Germany	1994	298
Spain	1990	897
Belgium	1997	118
Italy	1994	119
Netherlands	1997	71
Denmark	1992	13
Luxembourg, Austria, Greece, Finland		1
Slovakia	2001	13
Czech Republic	2001	8
Slovenia	2001	3
Poland	2002	9
United Kingdom	1985?	182,482
Other countries		
Israel	2002	1
Japan	2001	9
Canada	1993	2
USA	2003	1

With respect to the spread of BSE, no evidence has been found either for horizontal transmission or for vertical transmission via the sire. However, vertical maternal transmission could be possible, as scrapie infection proved possible by feeding sheep with placenta from scrapie-positive sheep. Also, the calf offspring of clinical cases had a higher risk of BSE (9.6%), compared to those from non-BSE cases.

Currently available, or under development, diagnostic procedures for BSE (indeed, as well as for scrapie) include:

1. Post-mortem tests:
   - histopathology of brain samples, a gold standard against which all other tests are validated (EU Diagnostic Manual);
   - antibody-based tests for PrPSc protein: Western blot with brain; Immunocytochemistry (ICC) with brain, tonsil, third eyelid, ELISA with spinal cord, etc.; and
   - others.
2. Ante-mortem tests (in live animals):
   - clinical signs; however, these produce around 20% false positive diagnoses;
   - immuno-capillary Electrophoresis (ICE);
   - urine test (for metabolic markers); and
   - others.

Control measures for BSE used in the UK have focused on multiple aspects and were implemented both on-farm and on-abattoir:

1. Computerized cattle tracing system (CTS):
   - operated by the Government and holding the full history about birth, movement and death of all cattle in the UK since 28 September 1998 (and 1996–1998 retrospectively);
   - each animal entering the food chain has a passport; and
   - numerical ear tagging from 17 January 2000.
2. Feed controls that include:
   - prohibition of all mammalian protein (except milk, gelatin, amino acids, dried blood products, dicalcium phosphate) to ruminants;
   - prohibition of mammalian meat and bone meal (MMBM) to any farm stock;
   - ban of MMBM at feed-handling premises;
   - some exceptions include milk and milk products, fishmeal for animals other than ruminants, and (under specified conditions) non-ruminant gelatin for coating of additives, hydrolysed protein and dicalcium phosphate.
3. Slaughter of cattle over 30 months scheme (OTMS):
   - slaughter with compensation of bovines >30months;
   - only at licensed abattoirs; and
   - meat banned for human consumption is incinerated, or rendered and destroyed.

4. Beef Assurance Scheme (BAS):
- animals up to 42 months old can be slaughtered for human consumption under certain conditions;
- these animals are from only herds that have never had a BSE case;
- they are from only specialist beef herds;
- grass-fed only; no feeding of MMBM during the past 7 years, no feeding of concentrates during the past 4 years (unless from a mill not used for MMBM production); and
- animals tested and negative for BSE.

5. Accelerated slaughter scheme: slaughter of animals born between 1989 and 1993) that during first 6 months of life shared contaminated feed with BSE cases.
6. Offspring cull scheme: slaughter of animals born after 1996 (tight feed control), but at risk from infection from their dams.
7. Removal of Specified Risk Materials (SRMs) from the food chain: meat hygiene measures (at abattoir) to remove and destroy specified organs and tissues, potentially containing prions if the animal is infected, from all bovines intended for human consumption. For details, see Chapters 5 and 6.
8. Ban of pithing and, potentially in the future, mechanical stunning of ruminants (see same chapters).

Public health concerns associated with BSE have arisen since recognition of a new variant of the previously known transmissible spongiform encephalopathy in humans (Creutzefeld-Jacob disease: vCJD). Because it resembles BSE characteristics, it has been assumed that it is a result of meat-borne BSE infection. The incidence of vCJD is shown in Table 2.4. However, current knowledge of the possibilities and ways of contracting vCJD from BSE infected foods is insufficient. The main reason is that vCJD cases could not be clustered until relatively recently. Namely, one cluster of five cases of vCJD occurred in a village in the UK, which retrospectively could be linked to a local butcher, whose practices at the time could enable meat contamination by bovine brain tissue. Understandably, further intensive research on BSE–vCJD link is both ongoing and necessary.

Table 2.4. vCJD deaths in the UK (adapted from UK DEFRA data).

Year	Deaths
1995	3
1996	10
1997	10
1998	18
1999	15
2000	28
2001	20
2002	17
2003 (up to 6 May)	8

Anthrax

It is caused by *Bacillus anthracis*, an anaerobic bacterium that sporulates when exposed to air (oxygen), although the spores can survive in the environment for many years. Disease, principally in cattle, is characterized by sudden death with 'tarry' blood from body orifices. In pigs, anthrax can take sub-acute form. Anthrax is endemic in semi-tropical countries and sporadic in temperate areas; it is typically a food-borne disease. Diagnosis in animals is mainly based on microscopic identification of polychrome methylene blue-stained, square-ended bacilli in smear samples from blood; suspect dead animals are commonly sampled after cutting off an ear. Controls may include restrictions imposed on infected location, prohibition of certain feeds, moving animals off the premises and vaccination. In humans, anthrax is relatively rare and the majority of cases (e.g. 85% in the UK) are not food-borne but associated with occupational exposure, e.g. handling hides/skins. Human anthrax infections can take different forms: cutaneous anthrax (localized ulceration, black scab, fever, followed by septicaemia), inhalation anthrax (fulminating pneumonia) and intestinal anthrax (acute gastroenteritis).

Brucellosis

Other names include: in humans, Malta fever, undulant fever; in animals, Bang's disease, contagious abortion, epizootic abortion. The causative agent and main occurrence are as follows: *Brucella abortus* (cattle; worldwide), *B. canis* (dog; North America), *B. melitensis* (sheep, goat; Mediterranean, Middle East), *B. ovis* (sheep; New Zealand, Australia, Americas), *B. suis* (pig; Latin America, Europe) and *B. neotomae* (desert rat).

Brucellosis of cattle is caused by *Brucella abortus,* which also produces disease in humans. Brucellosis of cattle produces no characteristic post-mortem signs. Diagnosis is by laboratory testing of blood or milk samples and by laboratory culture of the pathogen from the placenta, vaginal discharge or the milk of infected cows. Since brucellosis of cattle is still present in many countries, including some in the EU, prevention in brucellosis-free UK relies on herd surveillance: monthly testing of bulk milk samples from dairy herds and blood testing of beef breeding herds every two years. All infected cattle and contacts which have been exposed to infection must be slaughtered.

Brucella melitensis infects sheep and goats and can cause a disease in humans known as 'Malta fever', usually after ingestion of affected milk. When infection is first introduced into a flock or herd, a very high number of abortions can occur, but signs also include fever, mastitis, arthritis, orchitis or nervous signs in both sheep and goats. There are no lesions which distinguish *B. melitensis*-affected animals from animals with other diseases which also cause abortion. *B. melitensis* is prevalent in Mediterranean and Middle Eastern countries, as well as in some areas of Asia, Africa and Central and South America. In the UK, annual surveys for

B. melitensis are carried out; blood samples are tested using ELISA and serum agglutination.

Brucella suis infects pigs but has no such public health relevance, as have *B. abortus* or *B. melitensis*.

Slaughter of animals infected with brucellosis is permissible only under conditions of special preventive measures (gloves, masks, etc.) to protect abattoir staff from potential infection.

Glanders

Two forms of this serious disease, mainly of equids (horses, mules and donkeys), are caused by the bacterium *Burkholderia mallei*. In 'glanders' the principal lesions are in the nostrils, submaxillary glands and lungs; in 'farcy' the main lesions are on the surface of limbs or body. This disease was eradicated from the UK in 1928, but is still present in parts of Europe, Asia, Asia Minor and North Africa. Glanders is an important zoonosis; humans can be infected from affected horses by inoculation through a wound. Without treatment, the mortality rate can reach 95%. Diagnosis can be made by taking samples from clinical cases and by the 'mallein' test, when a dose (0.1 ml) of antigen is injected into the tissue below the eye. Swelling at the injection site, often with a high temperature, often indicates a potential carrier state, and can be an aid to field diagnosis. Controls include immediate slaughter of infected horses and strict isolation of suspected cases and contact animals.

West Nile Virus (WNV)

WNV is a flavivirus, one member of a group of Arthropod-borne viruses (Arboviruses), and causes infection of birds, horses and humans. Poultry can be infected but do not usually develop the clinical disease. Although a range of other animal species, such as goats and sheep, can be infected, they develop only low levels of the virus. To date, there have been no reports of cattle having been affected by the virus. Disease is transmitted by the bite of infected mosquitoes, and takes the form of encephalitis or meningitis.

The disease has been recorded in Africa, the Middle East, West and Central Asia and the USA. In Europe, recent outbreaks occurred in Romania (1996), Italy (1998), Russia (1999) and France (2000). Infected humans can have a flu-like illness with fever; a small proportion of cases (less than 1%) develop meningo-encephalitis, which produces nervous signs and may be fatal. However, many infected people show no symptoms. In the USA in 2002, 4161 people were reported to be infected with the disease, with 277 fatalities. In the UK, antibodies against WNV were found in birds, suggesting exposure, but the virus itself has not been identified in horses or in humans.

The main route of transmission of WNV is through mosquitoes, and the risk of food-borne infection of humans via meat/milk from infected animals is considered to be extremely low. The virus is destroyed by normal cooking methods (at <100°C) and pasteurization, and there have been no reports of the virus infecting people following consumption of meat and milk from infected animals. However, it should be noted that a related viral disease, tick-borne encephalitis, has been proved to cause food-borne infection via unpasteurized goats' milk.

The main control measures are focused on control of the mosquito population, since control of migratory birds is very difficult. In addition, handling dead birds with bare hands should be avoided.

Rift Valley fever (RVF) virus

This virus belongs to the family *Bunyaviridae*, genus *Phlebovirus*, and causes disease in wild and domestic ruminants, dromedaries, some rodents, as well as in humans; it is a major zoonosis.

After incubation of 1–67 days, disease in animals is characterized by fever, abortion and diarrhoea; mortality can reach 70% (calves). In humans, infection is flu-like and recovery occurs within 1 week.

Infection is transmitted via many families of mosquitoes, which serve as competent vectors, *Aedes* mosquitoes are the main host reservoir. Sources of infection for animals are wild animals and mosquitoes; and for humans mosquitoes, blood, nasal secretion and vaginal secretion, but aerogenic and alimentary (meat, milk) routes of infection are also possible.

To date, RVF has been reported only in some African countries, particularly those with a humid climate and large mosquito populations. The only epidemics north of the Sahara were recorded in Egypt (1977, 1993) and in Mauritania (1987). However, few cases of laboratory infection have occurred in other countries; RVF is not yet present in Europe.

Control measures include hygiene and vector control, but so far have not shown a significant efficacy.

Avian influenza (AI) virus

Influenza has three types including type A, for which birds are the natural host. Type A is further divided into subtypes, based on haemagglutinin (HA, 15) and neuroaminidase (NA, 9). Avian influenza (AI) includes a sub-clinical type (LPAI; low mortality) and a high-pathogenicty type (HPAI; high mortality) which differ with respect to clinical symptoms and genetic characteristics. Although it is known that LPAI can become HPAI, it is unknown whether this is associated with pathogenicity for humans.

Transmission of AI is possible via direct contact, contact with faeces of infected animals (transport, cages), as well as via the airborne route, but it is not certain whether vertical transmission occurs.

When considering the zoonotic potential of AI, it should be stressed that no hard evidence for sustained transmission to humans has been found to date. However, it should also be noted that immunity against this disease (i.e. H5N1) does not exist in human population. Adaptation of H5N1 to human hosts, through close contact between infected animals and humans, would have represented the main potential risk for human population – ultimately enabling efficient human-to-human transmission.

Prevention of AI entering Europe is based on border controls, biosecurity (i.e. prevention of contact with flying wild birds, avoiding livestock markets) and surveillance systems for early detection. In the case of an HPAI epidemic, the contingency plans include slaughter of infected or suspect animals and destruction of the meat. In some cases, preventive slaughter of flocks neighbouring the infected flocks would be possible, as well as emergency vaccination.

Controls related to humans would include public information systems, protection of staff in the infected zone (physical protection, vaccination, antiviral treatments) and monitoring of contact from infected individuals. Poultry products, generally, should not pose a risk even if they contain the virus, because of both its non-alimentary transmission and the fact that only cooked poultry products are normally eaten.

Other zoonotic diseases associated with farm animals: microbial

Erysipeloid

Erysipeloid (erysipelas, diamonds) is disease, most often seen in pigs, caused by the bacterium *Erysipelothrix insidiosa* (*rhusiopathiae*) that is present in soil. Clinical features in animals include high fever, diamond-shaped lesions on the skin (acute form) or enlarged, painful joints and heart disease (chronic form). Transmission to humans occurs via contaminated cuts and abrasions during handling affected animals/meat, usually on the hand or forearm; human disease takes the form of localized erythema with pain or arthritis in finger joints; septicaemia can occur, but very rarely. Prevention measures include keeping pigs on concrete and vaccination of sows (twice yearly, 3–6 weeks before farrowing).

Listeriosis

Listeriosis (mononucleosis, circling disease) is a disease primarily of ruminants, but also occurs in humans. It is caused by the bacterium *Listeria monocytogenes* (sometimes *L. ivanovii* in sheep), which is widely distributed, excreted in the faeces of healthy food animals and humans, and ubiquitous in the soil/environment and in silage. In animals, listeriosis is commonly in the meningoencephalitis form (circling, paralysis) or the visceral form (abortion, with retained placenta) with fatality rates of 3–30%. Disease can be transmitted to humans directly from animals (rarely), or as food-borne from contaminated foods (see Chapter 1.2). It is characterized by sudden fever, headache, meningitis, pneumonia, septicaemia, abortion and stillbirth; primarily in pregnant and IC individuals.

Orf

Orf is an infection caused by a Parapox virus that can survive in environment for up to 20 years. Infection of sheep can occur via cuts and abrasions. Orf is often seen on the mouth, teat and udder; the virus has been isolated from the poll of rams. Can be transmitted to humans via direct contact, i.e. infection of fingers due to sheep milking.

Leptospirosis

Leptospirosis in humans is caused by *Leptospira hardjo* (Dairy Worker Fever) via infected cows' urine, with the organism entering through mucous membranes, cuts and abrasions. Another type of leptospirosis is caused by *L. icterohaemorrhagiae* (Weil's Disease) via infected rat urine and contaminated water. The human disease is characterized by flu-like symptoms and causes prolonged debilitation.

Q Fever

Q Fever in sheep and goats is caused by *Coxiella burnetti*, a rickettsial organism; it is very infectious for humans. Transmission routes include infected urine, faeces and afterbirths, as well as contaminated dust and unpasteurized milk. It is characterized by a general malaise.

Other zoonotic diseases associated with farm animals: parasitic

The main groups of zoonotic parasites relevant to meat hygiene and inspection include:

- nematodes (roundworms), e.g. *Trichinella*;
- cestodes (flatworms, tapeworms), e.g. *Taenia saginata*, *T. solium*, *Echinococcus granulosus*;
- trematodes (flukes), e.g. *Fasciola*, *Fascioloides*, *Dicrocoelium*;
- protozoa, e.g. *Toxoplasma gondii*, *Sarcocystis*, *Giardia/Cryptosporidia*;
- arthropoda (insects, lice, mites, bugs, linguatula).

Trichinellosis

Relevant species of this parasite include *T. spiralis* (main species affecting mammals), *T. pseudospiralis* (affecting birds and mammals), *T. nativa* (present in cold regions of Canada, Russia, Arctic regions) and *T. nelsoni* (present in Africa, but also in Europe). In food animals, the occurrence of trichinellosis is low (sporadic) in some countries in Europe and in the USA, exceptionally low in other countries such as Norway and Sweden, and the disease is declared eradicated in some countries such as Denmark, UK, Portugal and Canada. The main reservoirs of trichinellosis are numerous wild, meat-eating animals, as well as vermin (rats, mice); disease is transmitted only by ingestion of muscles containing viable encysted *Trichinella* larvae. Among animals from which meat is eaten by humans, the disease affects domestic pigs, wild boar, horses, bear and walrus.

The life cycle of the parasites comprises: (i) intestinal stage with adult parasites laying live larvae in gut wall; (ii) migration stage with non-infective larvae migrating via blood/lymph circulation or actively from gut to muscles; and (iii) muscular stage with larvae becoming encysted intracellularly in muscles and subsequently infective. The largest numbers of cysts (invisible to the naked eye) are present in respiratory muscles (diaphragm, intercostal), larynx and tongue. Animal hosts usually show no symptoms, whilst in humans the disease in its muscular stage is serious (severe muscle pain, swollen face/eyelids) and, in case of heavy infestation, can be life-threatening.

Modes of transmission in humans include consumption of undercooked meat or, most often, uncooked types of meat products (dried hams, salamis) domestically prepared from non-examined meat, in which the larvae can survive. Modes of transmission in pigs include eating carcasses of infected animals (wildlife, vermin), consumption of raw/undercooked meat containing skeletal/striated muscles, e.g. meat plant offal or uncooked food remains from kitchen (swill), as well as via cannibalism. Modes of trichinellosis infection in herbivores (e.g. horses) are unclear, but may include ingestion of feeds containing remains of infected rodent carcasses. The main controls for trichinellosis in animals can vary between countries, depending on the epidemiological situation and whether the meat will be exported to other countries requesting specified controls to be applied, but can include:

- rearing pigs in a *Trichinella*-free system, based on biosecurity measures to prevent infection (stock held indoors only, vermin controls, feed controls);
- immunological pre-slaughter (on-farm) testing for the infection (e.g. ELISA);
- examination of muscle samples (diaphragm) of slaughtered pigs and horses to detect larvae (by microscopy following artificial digestion of meat, see Chapter 6); and
- inactivating the larvae in meat by freezing or cooking to 77°C in the centre.

Taeniasis and cysticercosis

Humans infected with taeniasis can be the host for two species of *Taenia* tapeworms: *T. saginata* and *T. solium*. The lifecycles of the two are very similar. Humans carrying tapeworm(s) in their intestines excrete parasite eggs via faeces. *T. saginata* eggs ingested by cattle via faecally contaminated pasture/feed (defaecating humans, sewage, flooding) develop into the larval form (*T. saginata cysticercus*, previously called *Cysticercus bovis*), i.e. cysts (5–9 mm diameter) in the muscles and heart, causing cysticercosis. In cattle, the largest number of cysts is found in mastication muscles, heart and tongue. Similarly, pigs ingest *T. solium* eggs that subsequently develop into *T. solium cysticercus* (previously called *Cysticercus caelullose*) in the muscles. If humans ingest raw/undercooked meat containing either species of cysticerci, the larvae will become free in the intestines and develop to adult tapeworms. Only in the case of *T. solium*, humans can also become infected by an additional route, via ingestion of tapeworm eggs (faecal–oral route); in such a case humans can develop *T. solium* cysticercosis as well. *T. saginata* and bovine cysticercosis are common in Africa, have a low but constant prevalence in New Zealand, in the UK were unknown before the mid-20th century but appear more prevalent since then (many human cases may remain unreported), whilst they are declared as eradicated in some countries (e.g. Germany, Greece). *T. solium* and porcine cysticercosis have high prevalences in Africa, Mexico and South America; in Europe they are sporadic, and are declared as eradicated in Finland, Greece and Canada. The main control measures for taeniasis and cysticercosis include:

- personal hygiene and related education;
- prohibition of sewage effluent as fertilizer;
- prevention of livestock access to human faeces;
- identification and immediate treatment of infested humans;
- diagnostic testing of animals (e.g. Ag-ELISA methods);
- effective visual meat inspection (cutting and inspection of mastication muscles and heart in slaughtered cattle; carcass muscle surfaces in pigs); and
- effective cooking/freezing of meat to inactivate larvae.

Hydatid disease

The intestinally located tapeworm *Echinoccocus granulosus* infects dogs and other *Canidae,* which are definitive hosts. Infected definitive hosts (e.g. dogs) faecally excrete eggs that can contaminate animal feeds or human foods and be ingested. Subsequently, in intermediate hosts (e.g. farm animals, humans), hydatid cysts containing large number of larvae can develop in internal organs (e.g. liver, lungs) and brain, but are rarely in muscles. The cysts can vary in size from a marble to a small football, and in shape which depends on the shape of the organ where they are located. The symptoms and severity of disease depend on the location of cysts, i.e. whether vital organs are affected (e.g. brain). If dogs ingest these cysts, they develop the tapeworm; the disease is zoonotic but not meat-borne for humans. The occurrence of hydatid disease is worldwide; in the UK prevalence in sheep varies from 1% to 50%, whilst in farmers may be up to 30%. The main controls include:

- regular antiparasitic treatment of dogs;
- prevention of contamination (direct or indirect) of animal feeds/pasture and human foods with dog faeces;
- visual examination of organs at meat inspection and subsequent feedback to the farm of origin;

- appropriate disposal (including previous cooking) of rejected infected organs from slaughtered animals to prevent ingestion of viable cysts by dogs and wildlife (Canidae); and
- washing hands after handling dogs.

Fascioliasis

Fascioliasis (large fluke) is mainly a disease of domestic (cattle, sheep) and wild herbivores caused by the parasite liver fluke *Fasciola hepatica*. Adult parasites live in the bile ducts and lay eggs which are excreted via faeces. After hatching, the miracidium further develops within an intermediate host (a snail, *Lymnaeae truncułata*) and cercariae leave the snail to encyst on plants in stagnant waters. Animals can become infected through consumption and humans by inadvertently nibbling contaminated plants. In the duodenum, larvae are freed and develop into fluke in liver. The occurrence of fascioliasis is worldwide. It is quite common in the UK: more than 1 million sheep livers are condemned annually due to liver fluke, and around 30% of cattle are found infected.

Dicrocoeliosis

Dicrocoeliosis (small fluke; *Dicrocoelium dendriticum/lanceolatum*) is a similar disease of herbivores with a similar parasitic life cycle but involving two intermediate hosts: a snail and an ant. Infective cysts are formed in ants, and herbivores become infected by ingesting ants with pasture plants. Humans are accidental hosts (small fluke in bile ducts) after ingesting ants on fresh vegetables or occasionally whilst nibbling grass. Both fascioliasis and dicrocoeliosis are zoonotic diseases, but not meat-borne; the severity of these diseases in humans depends on the extent of the liver infestation. The main controls include:

- land management, including control of populations of intermediate hosts (e.g. snails) on pastures/feeds;
- examination of incised livers (bile ducts) at meat inspection of slaughtered herbivores, and feedback to the farms of origin; and
- education of people.

Toxoplasmosis

The definitive host for this protozoan parasite (*Toxoplasma gondii*), cats and wild felines, become infected via ingestion of raw meat or prey (birds/rodents) that contain larval forms (cysts) of the parasite. The infection is transmitted primarily via cat faeces to other mammals, birds and humans, but transmission cycles can involve different routes:

- rodent–vertical transmission–rodent–cat;
- cat–faeces–human;

- cat–faeces–sheep, cattle, horses–contact (placenta)–human;
- cat–faeces–sheep, cattle, horses–meat–human; and
- cat–faeces–pig–cannibalism (tail biting)–pig–meat–human.

In animals, toxoplasmosis does not usually cause symptoms. Cats can sometimes develop encephalitis, hepatitis or diarrhoea, in the case of heavy infestation. In sheep, the main characteristic is abortion later in pregnancy. In humans, the infection can be asymptomatic, but disease can also be vertically transmitted: congenital infection with encephalitis and hydrocephalus. Human toxoplasmosis in the form of cysts in the brain develops mainly in IC individuals (e.g. AIDS patients), whilst in pregnant women it may result in abortion. The occurrence of toxoplasmosis is worldwide, particularly in Africa. It is enzootic in the UK, with prevalence of up to 25% in food animals; some Asian countries declared it as eradicated (e.g. Singapore). The main controls include:

- prevention of contamination of animal feeds (fodder) with cat faeces;
- meat inspection to detect toxoplasmosis lesions such as granulomata in lungs, heart and brain (but they occur rarely) and microscopic meat examination (but this is not routinely conducted);
- freezing and (preferably) cooking of meat to inactivate cysts; and
- advising pregnant women to avoid contact with lambing ewes and cat faeces.

Sarcosporidiosis

These protozoan, coccidian parasites (sarcosporidia) are in the phylum *Apicomplex* and affect all animals, birds, reptiles and man. The two most relevant, zoonotic species are *Sarcocystis hominis* and *S. suihominis*, affecting cattle and pigs, respectively, as intermediate hosts. For both, definitive hosts are dogs, cats and humans. Transmission routes include:

- dog/cat faeces (sporocysts)–food or water–cattle, pigs–muscle (sarcocysts)–humans or dogs, cats; and
- humans–faeces (sporocysts)–food or water–cattle, pigs–muscle (sarcocysts)–humans or dogs, cats.

Infection in animals is normally asymptomatic, but clinical cases can occur in older animals, stall-fed cattle and swill-fed pigs. In humans, infection sometimes causes transient diarrhoea and abdominal pain. Occurrence of sarcosporidiosis is worldwide, but most reports are from North America, UK and Australia, with up to 75% of animals found to be infected. The main controls include:

- prevention of faecal contamination of food and water;
- meat examination (eosinophilic myositis), but it is rarely diagnosed macroscopically, and microscopic examination is not carried out routinely; and
- freezing or (preferably) cooking of meat to inactivate cysts.

Giardia/Cryptosporidia infections

These infections are caused by the protozoan parasites *Giardia intestinalis* and *Cryptosporidium parvum*, occuring in most domestic animals (e.g. young cattle) and humans. The occurrence is worldwide; indeed, these are so widespread that the parasites' oocysts are considered as 'environmental contamination'. Transmission is faecal–oral with a number of possible routes:

- young ruminants–faeces (oocysts)–animal handling–humans;
- young ruminants–faeces (oocysts)–water–humans;
- young ruminants–faeces (oocysts)–rodents–young ruminants;
- young ruminants–faeces (oocysts)–water–domestic animals; and
- humans–faeces–humans or domestic animals.

Humans most often become infected via contaminated water or raw vegetables (salads), but also via chicken salad, milk drinks and apple cider. Any food that could become faecally contaminated may be a source of infection. Usual symptoms include diarrhoea and possibly loss of weight, but the respiratory system or gall bladder of IC individuals can be infected. The main control measures include:

- treat livestock waste on-farm with raised temperatures and high ammonia levels;
- limit farm run-off into waterways;
- dispose of sewage in a sanitary manner;
- immunocompromised individuals to boil water before consumption; and
- use good personal hygiene measures and exclude infected/carriers from handling food.

Further Reading

Andrewes, C.H. and Walton, J.R. (1977) *Viral and Bacterial Zoonoses*. Baillière Tindall, London.

Anon. (2001a) *Zoonoses and Communicable Diseases Common to Man and Animals, Vols 1–3*. Pan American Health Organization, Pan American Sanitary Bureau, Regional Office of the World Health Organization, Washington, DC.

Anon. (2001b) *Trends and sources of zoonotic agents in animals, feedingstuffs, food and man in the European Union and Norway in 2001*. European Commission, Health and Consumer Protection Directorate-General, Brussels.

Anon. (2003) Tuberculosis in bovine animals: risks for human health and control strategies. *The EFSA Journal* 13, 1–52.

Anon. (2004) Design of a field trial protocol for the evaluation of new rapid BSE post mortem tests. *The EFSA Journal* 46, 1–11.

Bell, J.C., Palmer, S.R. and Payne, J.M. (1988) *The Zoonoses; Infections Transmitted from Animals to Man*. Edward Arnold, London.

DEFRA (2004) *Zoonoses Report – United Kingdom 2003*. DEFRA Publications, London.

DEFRA (2005) Notifiable diseases in the UK. http://www.defra.gov.uk/animals/diseases/notifiable.index.htm (accessed March 2005).

OIE (2004) http://oie.int/eng/maladies/en_classification.htmListeOIE (accessed December 2004).

Salman, M.D. (2003) *Animal Disease Surveillance and Survey Systems*. Iowa State Press, Ames, Iowa.

Thrusfield, M. (1995) *Veterinary Epidemiology*. Blackwell Science, Oxford, UK.

Toma, B., Dufor, B., Sanaa, M., Benet, J.-J., Ellis, P., Moutou, F. and Louza, A. (1999) *Applied Veterinary Epidemiology and the Control of Disease in Populations*. Maisons-Alfort, France.

2.3 On-farm Factors Affecting Food-borne Pathogens

Introduction

The main food-borne pathogens causing the majority of food-borne diseases in humans in modern times, e.g. *Salmonella*, *Campylobacter*, *E. coli* O157, originate from healthy farm animals that excrete them faecally. These pathogens enter the food chain by a variety of routes (e.g. guts–environment–contaminated animal coats–carcass–meat) and their control during the post-farm phase is neither easy nor always efficient. Therefore, it is important to understand their spread, and to consider any related controls, of these pathogens on farms. This could minimize further transference of food safety hazards to subsequent phases of the food chain. The significance of the on-farm presence of food-borne pathogens can be illustrated by data on the occurrence of *E. coli* O157 in healthy cattle: herd prevalence is highly variable and can be anything between 40% and 75%, whilst prevalence in individual animals may be between <1% and >20%. The main route of transmission for food-borne pathogens in farm animals is faecal–oral.

Role of animal diet/feeds

Contaminated feed can be a very important source of food-borne pathogens, e.g. *Salmonella* spp., particularly in poultry and pigs. Usually, the most persistent contaminants are 'local' *Salmonella* spp., whilst 'exotic' *Salmonella* spp. are often transient and associated with imported feed compounds or components (e.g. protein-based). Feeds can also be contaminated with pathogens excreted by vermin (rodents, birds). Therefore, feeds are sometimes fermented, e.g. liquid feeds for pigs in order to reduce the risk of *Salmonella* infection. Feeds can also be acidified by the addition of acidulants, or heat treated to reduce or eliminate pathogens. In fermented silage production, rapid fermentation by dominant lactic acid bacteria and suppression of food-borne pathogens is required. It is a two-step process, starting with aerobic fermentation, which consumes available oxygen and produces heat, followed by anaerobic fermentation and accumulation of lactic acid that lowers pH. If air is not properly (or rapidly) excluded, poor-quality silage can result, in which some pathogens such as *Listeria monocytogenes* can proliferate and be spread to animals.

Also, numerous studies have been published in which effects of the diet type on shedding of pathogens were examined, e.g. the ongoing debate about whether shedding of *E. coli* O157 is greater in grain-fed or hay-fed cattle. However, because faecal shedding of this or other pathogens is affected by numerous factors other than diet, but acting simultaneously, the actual relevance of diet itself is presently unclear. On the other hand, it had been advocated in the past that the total amount of faeces – and hence the prevalence or levels of food-borne pathogens excreted by animals – could be reduced by total withdrawal of feed for 1–2 days before slaughter. However, some studies have shown that feed withdrawal can actually increase shedding of pathogens, e.g. *E. coli* O157 in cattle.

With respect to animal diet-based control measures to reduce faecal shedding of pathogens on farms, two approaches have attracted significant attention:

- use of *probiotics*, which involves feeding animals viable pre-selected microorganisms (usually, lactic acid bacteria) to suppress targeted pathogen(s) within the animal gut either through changing the gut environmental factors or via production of antimicrobial compounds (e.g. bacteriocins); and
- use of *competitive exclusion*, which involves feeding animals with complex mixtures of bacteria that 'saturate' locations on the gut mucosa needed for attachment of pathogens, hence preventing/reducing colonization of the animal gut by the pathogens. For example, *Salmonella* spp. can be competitively excluded in intensively reared chicks by feeding them with diluted minced gut content of mature hens (anaerobically fermented gut contents).

Unfortunately, both approaches suppress faecal shedding of pathogens in monogastric animals (poultry and pigs) better than in ruminants. In ruminants, it is more difficult to change gut microflora via these oral treatments, due to physiological/microbiological processes occurring in the rumen. Nevertheless, attempts have been made to overcome such difficulties by application of the treatments via rumen-resistant boluses.

Role of stress

The gut microflora of animals start to establish from birth and, once stable and well-balanced, provide good protection against gut colonization by pathogens, e.g. *Salmonella* spp. However, stress (alone or in combination with antibiotic therapy) can disturb the balance of the microflora and render animals more susceptible to colonization. Therefore, it could be assumed that stress can cause an increase in shedding of pathogens. Stressors include parturition (e.g. calving/farrowing), weaning, sudden changes in diet that alter gut pH and select for particular bacteria, transportation (stress increases with journey length, unloading and reloading) and mixing of animals (on-farm and also at markets, lairage).

Effect of animal age

In some on-farm studies of *E. coli* O157, gut colonization was more frequent in young cattle. Experimentally infected calves can shed around

1 log higher levels, and also for around 3 months longer, than can adult cattle. Also, it is considered that the biggest reservoir of *Salmonella* spp. is growers and finishers, but younger animals are more likely to be affected.

Spread between animals

It is generally believed that indoor farming (i.e. group housing) increases horizontal transmission of pathogens, as compared to outdoor farming, due to closer contacts between animals (including social contact such as licking/grooming) and/or between animals and the contaminated environment. For example, oral secretions and regurgitation of organisms in cattle contribute to the spread of *E. coli* O157 between neighbouring animals and even between neighbouring pens. Vertical transmission can also occur, but is probably less important due to some protection from maternal antibodies for up to 7 weeks. In addition, introduction of novel shedding-positive animals to established groups increases on-farm spread of pathogens.

Role of vectors

Spread can occur between distant pens or indeed between farms via vermin, wild animals, farm staff and farm equipment. Humans, through their daily activities on-farm, are one of the biggest causes of on-farm spread of pathogens. Rodents (mice and rats) are also very important; a *Salmonella*-shedding mouse can excrete up to 5–7 logs of the pathogen's cells in its faeces in one day, which can be sufficient to infect an animal. Some studies found 1–3% of gulls from intertidal sediments harboured *E. coli* O157. A study carried out in the USA showed that *E. coli* O157 can be isolated from deer sharing grazing land with cattle.

Survival in the environment

Pathogens can survive for long periods in farm environment-related substrates such as soil, faeces and building materials for extended periods (days to weeks). Pathogens can be attached to dust particles and liquid droplets, and then carried by winds or aerosols (hosing, rain) for considerable distances. Generally, pathogens die off to a large extent when exposed to a combination of higher temperatures and drying, but at lower temperatures and in water (or damp substrates) they survive very well. All water drinkers used by more than one animal can serve as a route for between-animal spread. Water troughs are clearly proven as a source of *E. coli* O157 infections and re-infections on farms; the pathogen survives in the water for several months and can even multiply in the sediment. This means that the pathogen can survive between two grazing seasons (e.g. over winter).

Recycling of pathogens via organic fertilizers

Animal wastes, such as farmyard manure, slurry and certain abattoir wastes (lairage wastes and gut contents; see Chapter 2.4) often contain food-borne pathogens faecally shed by farm animals. Animal wastes in solid (manure) and liquid (slurry) form can be stored on the farm, transported for use elsewhere, or deposited directly onto land. Storage can reduce levels of pathogens; e.g. appropriate storage of farmyard manure can lead to their 'auto-heating' (composting) to pasteurization temperatures (e.g. >60°C), that can destroy vegetative forms of pathogens. Spreading untreated wastes on pasture or agricultural land for crop production can mediate further infections or re-infections of animals with pathogens through either grazing, or feeding contaminated feeds produced on contaminated land. Survival periods of pathogens in soil are variable and affected by numerous factors, but some studies indicate survival periods of >2 years for *Salmonella* spp. and around 10 months for *L. monocytogenes*. Pathogens' survival is better if the organic wastes are applied on land by the injection method (often used for odour control purposes) than by surface spreading; in the latter case, pathogens are more intensively exposed to antimicrobial factors, including drying and sunlight.

Summary of existing on-farm control measures

Presently, the main on-farm control measures for pathogens are based on hygiene and biosecurity incorporated in Good Farming Practices/Good Hygiene Practices (GFP/GHP) – and HACCP-based principles:

- operate an all-in, all-out policy;
- disinfect pens between batches of animals;
- avoid mixing animals (new or by age group);
- use a reliable pathogen-free source of livestock;
- disinfect vehicles used for transportation;
- train staff to disinfect boots and equipment, and keep work clothes on site;
- operate an effective programme for control of vermin;
- clean and disinfect water troughs regularly;
- avoid grazing animals on land newly applied with slurry or manure; ideally store waste for 3 months prior to application onto land;
- restrict access of visitors to units;
- manage feed properly; reliable source, proper production of silage;
- monitor pathogen presence in animals, e.g. 'ZAP' *Salmonella* programme in the UK; and
- vaccinate animals against pathogens, e.g. *Salmonella* in poultry.

Future on-farm control measures, that are not being routinely used but are under intensive research and development, include in particular: (i) vaccinations against a range of pathogens including such as *Campylobacter* and *E. coli* O157; and (ii) bacteriophage therapy based on viruses which attack and targeted pathogenic bacteria.

Further Reading

Anon. (2000) *Opinion of the Scientific Committee on Veterinary Measures Relating to Human Health on Food-borne zoonoses*. European Commission Health and Consumer Protection Directorate-General, Brussels.

Hinton, M.H. (2000) Infections and intoxications associated with animal feed and forage which may represent a hazard to human health. *Veterinary Journal* 159, 124–138.

Johnston, A.M. (2000) HACCP and farm production. In: Brown, M. (ed.) HACCP in the Meat Industry. Woodhead Publishing Ltd, Cambridge, UK.

Maunsell, B. and Bolton, D.J. (2004) *Guidelines for Food Safety Management on Farms*. Teagasc – The National Food Centre, Dublin.

Stanfield, G. and Dale, P. (2002) *Assessment of Risk to food Safety Associated with the Spreading of Animal Manure and Abattoir Wastes on Agricultural Land*. Final Report to the Food Standards Agency, Report No. UC6029, London.

2.4 Animal By-products, Wastes and the Environment

Animal by-products and wastes produced by abattoirs have not been well regulated in the past; many of them were frequently applied on agricultural land without any treatment. This practice carries the risk of re-cycling of public health hazards from shedding animals – through the environment – back to grazing animals or those fed by crops harvested from the environment. Additionally, these hazards can contaminate crops grown on the land and intended for human consumption, e.g. root vegetables, salads, etc.

Surveys of abattoir wastes conducted in the UK between 1999 and 2001 indicated that most abattoirs used to discharge effluents and wastes onto agricultural land, either directly or via sub-contraction to secondary companies. Abattoir wastes varied greatly with respect to: (i) types (e.g. lairage manure-based wastes, gut contents, blood, etc.); (ii) volume stored at the premises (e.g. 1–200 tonnes); (iii) conditions of storage (e.g. in tanks, hips, etc.); and (iv) the length of time they were stored on the premises before being disposed of (e.g. between 1 day and 2 years). These variations were much larger among red meat abattoirs, whilst wastes from poultry abattoirs were more uniform. In the surveys, particularly food-borne protozoan pathogens and, to a lesser extent, bacterial pathogens, were found in abattoir wastes, which confirms the public health relevance of abattoir waste handling.

Subsequently, EU regulation EC 1774/2002 has provided health rules concerning animal by-products not intended for human consumption. This new legislation divides animal by-products into three categories, described below.

Category 1 by-products

These by-products represent the highest risk category. The main hazard in Category 1 by-products are TSE-BSE agents, so the controls are designed to target particularly specified risk materials (SRM), i.e. to limit their spread. This category includes:

1. By-products from animals:
- infected by TSE;
- killed for TSE eradication;
- other than farmed or wild (pet, zoo, circus);
- including experimental animals;
- including wild animals suspected of harbouring communicable diseases; and
- with prohibited chemical residues.

2. Animal material collected in waste water treatment from Category 1 processing plants.

3. Catering waste from international transport. This is considered as high-risk material from a public health perspective, since effective, cross-border controls are non-existent.
4. Mixtures of Category 1 with Category 2 or Category 3 materials.

Disposal of Category 1 by-products

1. Directly incinerated in a registered plant.
2. Processed in a plant using any of methods 1 to 5 (Table 2.5)and then incinerated.
3. If the by-products do not contain SRM, those processed in a plant by method 1 must later be buried in a landfill.
4. Catering waste from international transport is disposed of by burial in a landfill.

Category 2 by-products

These by-products represent a medium risk to public health. The category of manure and digestive tract contents must be treated as if they contain organisms pathogenic to humans. If Category 2 by-products are contaminated with category 1 by-products, then their risk level increases and they must be treated as Category 1 by-products. This category includes:

1. Manure and digestive tract contents.
2. Animal material collected in waste water treatment from Category 2 processing plants, or from abattoirs other than those covered under Category 1.

Table 2.5. Treatment methods for animal by-products.

Method	Material first reduced to particle size (mm)	Treatments (°C/min)
1[a]	≤50	>133/≥20/≥3 bars
2	≤150	>100/≥125 or >110/≥120 or >120/≥50
3	≤30	>100/≥95 or >110/≥55 or >120/≥13
4	≤30	>100/≥16 or >110/≥13 or >130/≥3
5	≤20	>80/≥120 or >100/≥60
Other	If approved and validated	

[a]Method 1 is regarded as suitable for destruction of TSE agents. The particle size is a critical part of the processing, since varying particles will conduct heat to differing degrees.

3. Animal products containing residues of veterinary drugs or other contaminants.
4. Animal products other than Category 1, if imported but non-compliant.
5. From animals, other than under Category 1, that died not by slaughter for human consumption.
6. Mixtures of Category 2 and Category 3 materials.
7. Animal by-products other than Category 1 or Category 3.

Disposal of Category 2 by-products

In theory, all Category 2 by-products can be disposed of in the same manner as the higher-risk Category 1 by-products. However, these by-products can be commercially valuable, so may be treated by the following methods.

1. Directly incinerated in a plant.
2. Processed in a plant by any of methods 1 to 5 (Table 2.5).
3. Processed in a plant by method 1 and marked, followed by incineration or, in the case of rendered fats, further processed into organic fertilizers/improvers.
4. Processed in a plant by method 1 and marked, followed by:
- if proteinaceous, used as organic fertilizers/improvers if scientifically justified;
- used as raw material in biogas or compost production; or
- burial in a landfill.

5. Fish material ensiled or composted.
6. Manure, digestive tract contents (separated from the tract), milk and colostrums, if they originate from animals free from communicable diseases, can be disposed of:
- as raw material in biogas or composting plant; or
- by application to land as specified. The legislation specifically states that these wastes may be applied on agricultural land, but not on land used for grazing.

7. Wild animals with no communicable disease can be processed for trophy production in a plant.

Category 3 By-products

Category 3 by-products are the lowest public health risk, and originate from animals with no communicable diseases, which are fit for human consumption, or unfit parts if no communicable diseases. This category includes:

1. Hides and skins, hooves and horns, pig bristles and feathers; from the abattoir and from fit animals.
2. Blood from fit, non-ruminant animals; blood, hides and skins, hooves, feathers, wool, horns, hair and fur from animals with no communicable disease from abattoirs.

3. Raw milk and former foodstuffs of animal origin with no health risks; catering waste other than that covered under Category 1.
4. Fish and sea animals, except mammals from the open sea, for fishmeal.
5. Shells, hatchery by-products and cracked egg by-products from animals with no communicable disease.

Disposal of Category 3 by-products

1. Directly incinerated in a plant.
2. Processed in a plant by any of methods 1 to 5 (Table 2.5) and marked, followed by incineration in a plant.
3. Processed in a Category 3 plant.
4. Transformed into petfood or in a technical plant.
5. Transformed in a biogas or composting plant.
6. Catering waste can be transformed in a biogas plant or composted.
7. Fish origin material ensiled or composted.

Practical Implications of the By-products Regulations for the Animal and Meat Industry

1. Blood cannot be disposed of to land, but must be treated by approved methods.
2. Manure may be applied untreated to any land (in practice), including agricultural land and grazing land.
3. Digestive tract contents may be applied untreated to non-pasture land. However, some EU countries use a derogation from this rule, and allow digestive tract contents to be applied onto grazing land.
4. Sludge must be caught in 6 mm drain traps and the solids treated either as Category 1 (SRM) or Category 2 (no SRM). However, the waste water which passes through the 6 mm drain trap can be applied to agricultural land. If solids are not trapped and removed then the water and sludge combination is treated as Category 1 or 2. In effect, all sludge and water from cattle abattoirs must be treated as Category 1.
5. Feathers, skins, hooves, horns or pig hair cannot be disposed of to land, but must be treated by approved methods.
6. Organic fertilizers/soil improvers may be used on land including pasture, but holding periods, before the animals can be grazed, apply. Holding periods are 2 months for pigs and 3 weeks for other farm animals.

Nevertheless, it is important to stress that animal by-products disposal and the environment protection issues require further attention from the veterinary public health perspective. This relates particularly to major difficulties with identification and traceability of animal by-products/wastes, possibilities of between-waste cross-contamination, insufficiently defined environmental survival of hazards, standardization of methods for evaluation and validation of treatment methods, and the question of how the use of organic fertilizers/soil improvers relates to TSE global controls.

General Impact of the Food/Meat Industry on the Environment

The impact of abattoirs and food industry as a whole on the environment is much wider than just the issue of animal by-products and wastes. Other aspects of the impact include high usage of energy and water resources, release of undesirable/harmful gases and oxygen usage during wastes breakdown, as indicated in Tables 2.6, 2.7 and 2.8. Therefore, it is important to consider how to reduce the overall impact of the meat industry on the environment. The first step would be to ensure effective data capture and analysis. All plant inputs (e.g. water, energy) should be measured, at multiple points of each operation, to gain quantitative data on plant consumption. The outputs (e.g. potential pollutants) of each plant should be determined in a similar manner. These data would enable

Table 2.6. Impact, per animal, of abattoir operations on the environment.

Animal species	CO_2 (kg)	NH_3 (g)	Effluent (l)	Solids[a] (kg)	BOD[b] (kg)
Cattle (450 kg)	30	?	600	60	1.2
Pig (100 kg)	11	2.6	220	5	0.5
Broiler (1.9 kg)	?	?	12	0.1	0.2

[a] Excluding inedible by-products which are rendered.
[b] Biological oxygen demand.

Table 2.7. Impact, per tonne of carcasses produced, of abattoir operations on the environment.

Animal species	Water use (l)	Energy (kWh)	Nitrogen (kg)	Solids (kg)	BOD[a] (kg)
Cattle	2,200	180	0.8	300	5
Pig	2,500	300	0.9	50	5
Broiler	9,000	350	1.5	3.8	15
Mixed	12,000	475	1.5	?	15

[a] Biological oxygen demand.

Table 2.8. Impact, per tonne of product, of meat processing on the environment.

Product	Water use (l)	Energy (kWh)	Nitrogen (kg)	BOD[a] (kg)
Salami	5000	2100	0.4	6.5
Hams, sausages	5000	1500	?	11
Ready dishes	7500	1200	1	10
Lard, tallow	2000	600	?	?

[a] Biological oxygen demand.

effective analysis of technologies and techniques used, and subsequently the introduction of cleaner technologies that use fewer resources. To do this, industry staff must be motivated and responsible. To this end, the results of plants' input–output obtained need to be communicated effectively by both the companies and regulators. Only after necessary data are available, and all the participants in the abattoir/food industry become motivated, can appropriate environmental control be fostered. An EU reference document, currently under preparation, is intended to oblige abattoirs and by-product plants to use Best Available Techniques (BAT) for processing animal by-products.

Further Reading

Anon. (2002) Regulation (EC) No. 1774/2002 of the European Parliament and of the Council laying down health rules concerning animal by-products not intended for human consumption. *Official Journal of the European Communities* EU I. 273/1.

Anon. (2004) Safety vis-à-vis biological risk including TSEs of the application on pastureland of organic fertilizer and soil improvers. *The EFSA Journal* 40, 1–10.

Pearson, A.M. and Dotson, T.R. (eds) *Inedible Meat By-Products*. Elsevier, London.

Pepperell, R., Massanet-Nicolau, J., Allen, V.M. and Buncic, S. (2003) Potential for spread of some bacterial and protozoan pathogens via abattoir wastes disposed on agricultural land. *Food Protection Trends* 23, 21–31.

Stanfield, G. and Dale, P. (2002) *Assessment of Risk to Food Safety Associated with the Spreading of Animal Manure and Abattoir Wastes on Agricultural Land*. Final Report to the Food Standards Agency, Report No. UC6029, London.

2.5 Risk Profiling of Farms – the Example of Cysticercus in Calves

Introduction

Assessments of exposure of animals on farms to various public health hazards are needed for several purposes ranging from scientific (e.g. better understanding of their epidemiology in different farming systems) to practical (e.g. development and implementation of related control systems). Obviously, a large number of exposure assessments can be made by targeting various hazards and/or various farming systems. For consideration of post-farm control measures to be used at subsequent point(s) of the food chain (e.g. at abattoir), it is both important and useful to know whether animals coming from different farms represent higher or lower risks (i.e. their risk ranking) with respect to the particular hazard being considered. In the space available in this book, it is not possible to consider assessments of animals' exposure to different hazards at different types of farms. Instead, principles of such on-farm exposure assessments will be described using a framework example of risk profiling of farms with respect to exposure of calves to *Taenia saginata* cysticercus. The example is taken from a publicly available document (Anon., 2004), to which the author of this book significantly contributed.

Consideration of risk factors contributing to *T. saginata* cysticercus infection of veal calves

Water supply for animals

Cattle can acquire *T. saginata* cysticercosis infection through drinking water contaminated with viable eggs of the parasite. Obviously, water from open sources (e.g. rivers, lakes) which are known to receive untreated sewage discharges (possibly from multiple sources) and physically and/or chemically treated waters pose increased and decreased risks, respectively, of being contaminated with the eggs. In geographic areas exposed to flooding, even at farms normally having a good water supply, the water may become contaminated with *T. saginata* eggs from the floodwater.

Use of organic wastes as fertilizers

Sewage sludge frequently contains *T. saginata* eggs, but no accurate prevalence in a given area could be established due to both variability of control techniques and lack of data collection. Nevertheless, the use of sewage sludge as fertilizer can be directly correlated to cattle infection, as demonstrated for areas having high records of cysticercosis. Farm manure used as fertilizer should not contain, by itself, the eggs, but cross-contamination with *T. saginata* eggs (e.g. water during floods, human excrement, etc.) probably cannot be excluded.

Roughage types

Roughage, such as hay, silage, or crop by-products (e.g. potato by-products), originating from locations contaminated with human waste, can serve as sources for *T. saginata* eggs for cattle. In addition, even if not contaminated at harvesting, these feed components can become cross-contaminated later, during storage and/or distribution.

Farm location

As *T. saginata* proglottids are excreted in human excrement, cattle on farms near locations where high numbers of people with varying hygiene habits and of varying geographical origin aggregate (such as bus/railways stations) or are passing by (such as public countryside footpaths, train tracks) may have – directly or indirectly – a higher exposure to the infective agent.

Direct on-farm human excrement deposition

The most direct way of cattle infection with *T. saginata* eggs would be from excrements deposited by human *T. saginata* carriers on pasture, in or near livestock pens and/or other feeds used by the farm. It is difficult to judge whether frequencies of excrement deposition differ between outdoor (i.e. on grazing areas) and indoor deposition (i.e. in animal housing units), but it may be hypothesized that outdoor areas may be accessed by a wider range of people including 'unknown', whilst indoor are accessed primarily by 'known' people associated with the farm. On the other hand, due to concentration of animals, perhaps higher number of animals may be exposed to excrement from a single tapeworm carrier if they are housed indoors, rather than if kept outdoors.

Staff training and turnover

Farm employees who have received basic public health training, including awareness of the life cycle of the parasite, pose less risk as a source of the cattle infection than untrained ones. In addition, high staff turnover would represent an additional epidemiological risk and, also, may make it more difficult for the farm to maintain the needed level of training.

Calf age

It can be assumed that the chances of *T. saginata* cysticercosis infection increase with the age of animals. The main reasons include: (i) roughage feeding increases with age; and (ii) older animals generally have had more exposure time to egg-contaminated sources.

T. saginata cysticercosis monitoring/surveillance

It is likely that good information on the real prevalence/distribution of *T. saginata* cysticercosis in cattle population, where the monitoring/surveillance system is in place, results in better epidemiological situation due to better targeted, or more thoroughly applied, control measures. The lack of such information probably increases the epidemiological risks.

T. saginata taeniasis monitoring/surveillance

It is likely that good information on the real prevalence/distribution of *T. saginata* taeniasis in the human population, where the monitoring/surveillance system is in place, results in a better epidemiological situation due to better targeted, or more thoroughly applied, control measures. The lack of such information probably increases the epidemiological risks.

Evaluation of risks associated with different veal calves production systems

To conduct a full quantitative risk assessment of *T. saginata* cysticercosis in veal calves raised in different production systems, good quality data would be needed on:

1. Prevalences of the pathogen in varying animal and human populations and related environments.
2. Quantitative parameters of environmental survival (e.g. D-values) and infectivity of *T. saginata* eggs in/on different substrates and under different physicochemical conditions.
3. The effects of the regional and seasonal variations on the data under 1 and 2.
4. Quantitative participation (weighting) of each of the risk factors in the overall risk calculated.
5. Clear definitions and detailed process descriptions for a large number of different types of veal calf production systems existing across the EU.

However, as most of the required data indicated above are either lacking, or of dated/insufficient quality, and also because risk factors can be represented in a large number of different combinations in a large number of different systems, it could be concluded that a quantitative exposure assessment applicable to all differing production systems is not achievable at this stage.

Nevertheless, instead, an attempt was made to develop a general framework for semi-quantitative evaluation of *T. saginata* cysticercosis risks associated with different veal calf production systems. The approach used was based on adaptation of the principles previously used in the determination of microbial risk profiles of foods (see Chapter 7.5). First, each risk factor listed above (including its variations) was further elaborated with respect to varying scenarios posing varying levels of the risks. For a given risk factor, to each of the scenarios a risk score (e.g. using a scale of 1 to 4) can be arbitrarily allocated, reflecting the perceived relationship between probability of its occurrence and severity of the consequences if it occurred (a general example is shown in Table 2.9). Second, for each individual production system for veal calves, the total sum of scores given for all risk factors evaluated can determine the system's risk profile with respect to *T. saginata* cysticercosis infections. In a theoretical example shown in Table 2.10, three veal calf production systems, to which different scores were randomly given for the same risk factors, resulted in three different risk profiles: high-risk, medium-risk and low-risk.

Such a global grouping was useful for the purpose of this book in order to highlight the principle and the approach of how to differentiate/rank production systems with respect to the risk of *T. saginata* cysticercosis in veal calves. Again, the examples of risk profiling (Table 2.10) should not be taken as an evaluation of real-life production systems, but as an illustration of the approach. Rather, it is believed that competent authorities and/or shareholders could use a framework, based on the principles indicated here, for their own *T. saginata* cysticercosis risk profiling at individual veal calf production system level.

Potential uses of risk-profiling of veal calf production systems: an example of use for meat inspection purposes

With respect to post-mortem inspection of veal calves for *T. saginata* cysticercosis, it is believed that different approaches could be used for calves originating from different production systems having different risk profiles.

Table 2.9. Principles for semiquantitative determination of risk levels (probability versus severity scoring) for individual risk factors.

Severity of consequences[a]	Probability of occurrence				
	Frequent	Likely	Occasional	Seldom	Unlikely
Catastrophic	Very high (Score: 4)	Very high (Score: 4)	High (Score: 3)	High (Score: 3)	Medium (Score: 2)
Critical	Very high (Score: 4)	High (Score: 3)	High (Score: 3)	Medium (Score: 2)	Low (Score: 1)
Moderate	High (Score: 3)	Medium (Score: 2)	Medium (Score: 2)	Low (Score: 1)	Low (Score: 1)
Negligible	Medium (Score: 2)	Low (Score: 1)	Low (Score: 1)	Low (Score: 1)	Low (Score: 1)

[a] The expressions are from general risk assessment terminology, and are not meant to describe actual medical consequences of human taeniasis.

Table 2.10. Theoretical examples of *T. saginata* cysticercosis risk profiling of three different veal calf production systems (risk scores for each individual risk factor are given randomly to the systems).

Risk factors potentially contributing to infection of calves with *T. saginata* eggs	Risk scoring of different related scenarios	Risk profiles of different veal calf production systems: theoretical, imaginary examples		
		Example A	Example B	Example C
Water supply for animals potentially contaminated with *T. saginata* eggs	Score 4: Use of untreated surface (river/lake) water	4		
	Score 3: Use of untreated local water (e.g. wells)			
	Score 2: Use of treated local water		2	
	Score 1: Use of municipal water			1
Floods potentially spreading *T. saginata* eggs on the grazing and/or feed components' production areas	Score 4: Regularly occurring, with waters known as receiving sewage			
	Score 3: Irregularly occurring, with waters known to be receiving sewage	3		
	Score 2: Regularly or irregularly occurring with waters not receiving sewage		2	
	Score 1: No floods			1
Organic wastes potentially contaminated with *T. saginata* eggs used as fertilizers on grazing and/or feed components production areas	Score 4: Use of untreated sewage	4		
	Score 3: Use of treated sewage			
	Score 2: Use of farm manure		2	
	Score 1: No organic wastes used			1
Potential for *T. saginata* eggs contamination as related to general animal husbandry	Score 4: Animals kept mainly outdoor, grazing at multiple locations	4		
	Score 3: Animals kept combined indoor (milk-fed) and outdoor (local grazing)		3	
	Score 2: Animals kept indoor only; milk-fed with some roughage			2
	Score 1: Animals kept indoor only, milk-fed only			
Potential for *T. saginata* egg contamination of roughage	Score 4: traceability indicates origin of roughage from high-risk geographic areas			
	Score 3: Roughage used is not traceable; multi-source and multi-component roughage	3		
	Score 2: Roughage used is traceable; multi-source and multi-component roughage		2	
	Score 1: Roughage used is traceable; single-source and single-component roughage			1

Continued

Table 2.10. *Continued*

Risk factors potentially contributing to infection of calves with *T. saginata* eggs	Risk scoring of different related scenarios	Risk profiles of different veal calf production systems: theoretical, imaginary examples		
		Example A	Example B	Example C
Potential for exposure to *T. saginata* eggs as related to farm location	Score 4: Near camping sites	4		
	Score 3: Near bus/railway stations			
	Score 2: Near public footpaths		2	
	Score 1: Isolated			1
Potential for *T. saginata* egg exposure as related to calf age	Score 4: >6 months	4		
	Score 3: 3–6 months		3	
	Score 1: <3 months			1
Potential for *T. saginata* egg exposure from direct human excrement deposition	Score 4: Unknown number of people accessing grazing area			
	Score 3: Unknown number of people accessing animal housing	3		
	Score 2: Unknown number of people accessing area for feed components production		2	
	Score 1: Little human access			1
Potential for *T. saginata* egg exposure *vis-à-vis* staff-related aspects	Score 4: Staff not trained; high turnover			
	Score 3: Staff not trained; low turnover	3		
	Score 2: Staff trained; high turnover		2	
	Score 1: Staff trained; low turnover			1
T. saginata cysticercosis monitoring/surveillance in animals from the farm area	Score 4: No data available	4		
	Score 3: Irregular, with positive findings		3	
	Score 2: Regular, but infrequent, with positive findings			2
	Score 1: Regular, frequent, no positives			
T. saginata monitoring/surveillance in humans from the farm area	Score 4: No data available	4		
	Score 3: Irregular, with positive findings		3	
	Score 2: Regular, but infrequent, with positive findings			2
	Score 1: Regular, frequent, no positives			
TOTAL		40 (higher-risk profile range: 32–43)	26 (medium-risk profile range: 21–31)	14 (lower-risk profile range: 10–20)

The residual *T. saginata* public health risks arising from omitting the routine muscle incision/cutting procedure could be considered as negligible in calves coming from lower-risk profile systems, whilst reduced handling of their meat/organs would be beneficial from the perspective of reducing the microbial cross-contamination. The lower-risk category could include slaughtered calves less than 3 months old as they are likely either not to be infected (because of diet) or, if infected, the cysts would not be infective by the time of slaughter. For the lower-risk calves, detailed post-mortem inspection for cysticercosis – including tissue cutting – may not be necessary (apart from visual inspection only). This would be, generally, supported by published suggestions that traditional meat inspection procedures to detect cysticercosis have negligible impact on reducing the level of public health risk in the country where *T. saginata* cysticercosis infection of cattle is low.

For veal calves coming from a medium-risk profile production system, the residual *T. saginata* public health risks arising from omitting the cutting procedure may be higher than negligible but still not very high. Still, reduction of handling of meat/organs would have desirable effects on reduction of microbial cross-contamination of meat. For such calves, omitting the inspection cutting procedure could still be possible, if combined with a statistically valid batch-based testing (using a validated pathogen's antigen-based blood test) of a representative number of animals before slaughter (either on-farm or during ante-mortem at abattoir) showing negative results.

For veal calves coming from a high-risk profile system, the residual *T. saginata* public health risks arising from omitting incision-based cysticercosis inspection at post-mortem could be higher than acceptable, so routine physical inspection should remain until full validation of sufficiently sensitive methods for *T. saginata* antigen detection has occurred. There are indications that sensitivity of such an Ag-ELISA method (see Chapter 2.2 above) is much higher (around 10-fold) than the meat incision–inspection method, but the sensitivity of the former may be reduced when very low numbers of cysts are present. Nevertheless, the current muscle-cutting–visual-inspection procedure could be replaced by such alternative methods if proven to be sensitive enough and validated for veal calves.

The risk profile-based assessments of individual farm production systems, such as in this example for veal calf farms, should be updated regularly, periodically and when any change in the system occurs, to detect an increase in exposure should it occur.

Further Reading

Anon. (2000) *Opinion of the Scientific Committee on Veterinary Measures Relating to Public Health on the Control of taeniasis/cysticercosis in man and animals*. The European Commission, Consumer Health and Protection Directorate-General, Brussels.

Anon. (2004) Opinion of the Scientific Panel on Biological Hazards on 'the risk assessment of a simplified meat inspection for the presence of Cysticercosis cysts in veal calves kept under specific management conditions'. *The EFSA Journal* 176, 1–40.

II Hygiene of Meat Production – Processing and Meat Inspection

3 Meat Industry

3.1 Trends in the Organization of the Meat Industry

JEFFREY WOOD

Introduction

In this chapter we consider the organization of the UK meat industry against the background of EU and world meat production. International trade in meat is increasing, driven by the differentials in production costs between countries. The UK has high production costs in comparison, for example, with Brazil and Thailand, who currently supply significant amounts of poultry meat to the UK market.

Production costs of pig meat in different countries are illustrated in Fig. 3.1. These are influenced by factors such as average feed and land prices, which are high in UK, and the costs of compliance with legislation – for example, controls over nitrogen pollution, which are high in Japan. There is a general trend for production costs to be high in UK, which puts British producers at a disadvantage.

UK, EU and World Meat Production

Data for the volume of meat production in UK and other countries are shown in Table 3.1. The USA is the world's major beef-producing country, producing 65% more than all the EU countries together. China produces more than double the amount of sheep and pig meat than the EU countries and the USA double the amount of poultry meat. Within the EU, the UK is the major sheep producer and is high on the list of poultry producers. In 1990, the UK produced 990,000 tonnes of beef. The BSE crisis is primarily responsible for reducing this to the present 700,000 tonnes.

In the world generally, the production of meat is increasing to meet demand. Poultry and pork production is increasing faster than that of the other meats and this is occurring in intensive rather than in extensive production systems. In Europe, legislation is encouraging more extensive meat production.

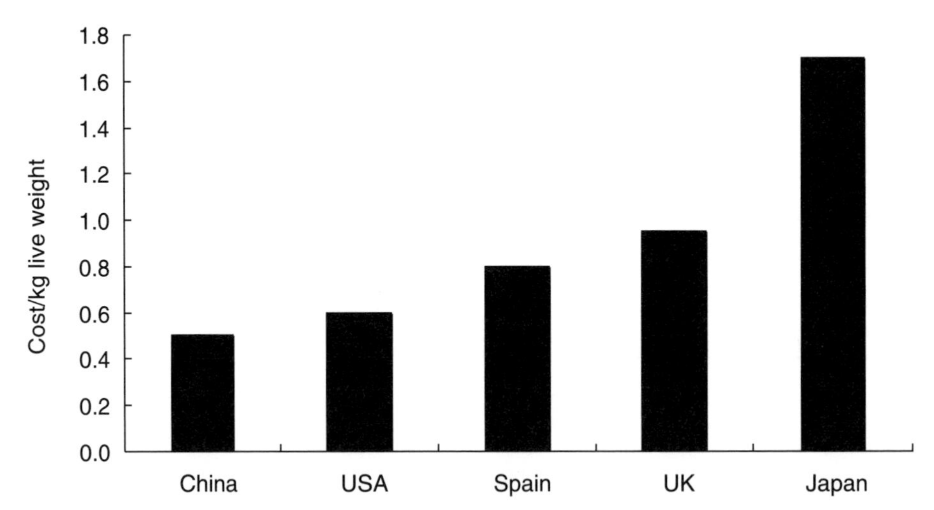

Fig. 3.1. Actual production costs of pig meat in various countries, 2003 (£ sterling/kg live weight) (from UK Meat and Livestock Commission).

Table 3.1. Total meat production in different countries (1000 tonnes) (data taken from UK Meat and Livestock Commission).

Meat species	Highest world	EU (15 countries, pre-2004)	UK	Highest EU
Beef and veal	USA 12,311	7,445	700	France 1,755
Sheep and goat	China 2,654	1,149	392	UK 392
Pig meat	China 43,053	17,606	901	Germany 3,864
Poultry	USA 16,471	8,802	1,526	France 2,255

Meat consumption patterns

Countries differ in meat consumption as in meat production patterns. Figures for the UK and the average for the EU countries are shown in Fig. 3.2. Total meat consumption is lower in the UK, particularly for pig meat. This partly reflects the many forms, fresh and processed, in which pig meat products are consumed in other EU countries. Although the average EU consumption of pig meat is currently 43 kg, it is 66 kg in Spain and 64 kg in Denmark.

There are many factors influencing meat consumption other than price and availability. Some of the important ones in the UK include the popularity of high-protein rather than of high-carbohydrate foods (e.g. Dr Atkins diet), vegetarianism, food safety scares (especially BSE), animal

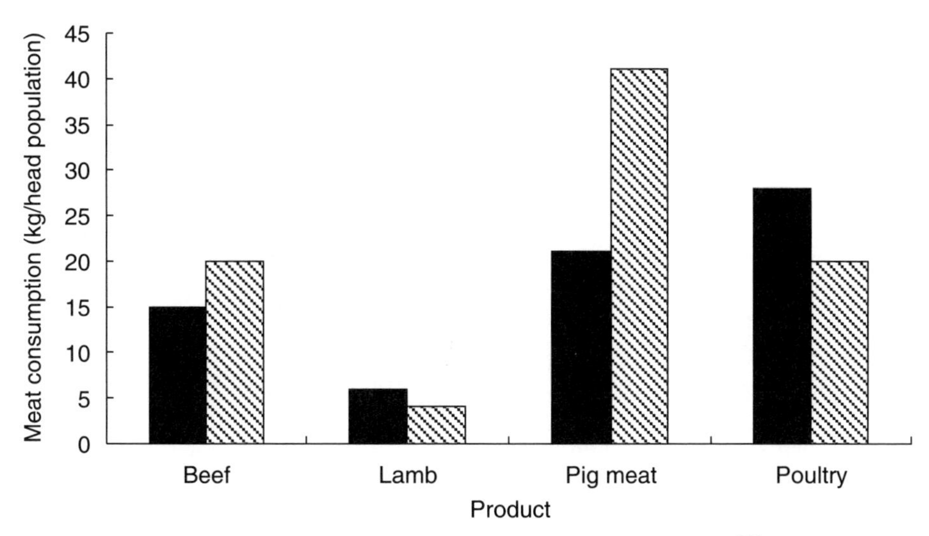

Fig. 3.2. Meat consumption by species in the UK (■) and EU (average, ▨). Data taken from the UK Meat and Livestock Commission, 2000).

welfare issues (e.g. intensification) and nutritional value (red meats high in saturated fat). For such diverse reasons, meat consumption patterns change over time. Consumption trends in the UK between 1900 and 2000 are shown in Fig. 3.3. Meat consumption rose dramatically after the Second World War, especially for poultry meat. Over time, beef has become less popular than poultry meat and suffered a major fall during the BSE crisis. However, beef consumption in the UK is now well above the pre-BSE level.

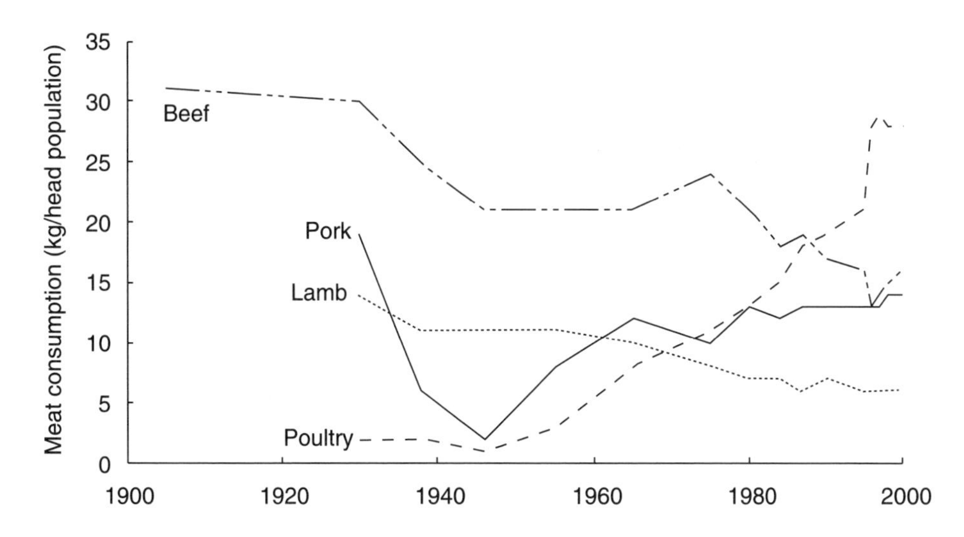

Fig. 3.3. UK meat consumption, 1900–2000 (from various sources including Eurostat and the UK Meat and Livestock Commission).

Organization of meat industries

The meat industry in a typical country such as the UK consists of many individual producers who supply the raw material, far fewer processors who transform this into fresh meat and meat products, an even smaller number of retailers who distribute and sell to consumers and finally, large numbers of consumers. The model shown in Table 3.2 is very dynamic and constantly changing. In the UK, the number of individual livestock farms and farmers has declined greatly as we have changed from being a rural to an industrial society and beyond, and continues to decline (Table 3.3). Processors need sufficient scale to operate sufficiently and their contraction has been even more marked than that of producers (Table 3.4). Retailing in many developed countries is falling into fewer and fewer hands, and supermarkets have taken over from butchers as the major retailers of meat (Fig. 3.4). The major supermarket retailers, such as Walmart in the USA, Carrefour in France and Tesco in the UK, operate globally and have a policy of low prices. They are in a strong position to influence prices paid to processors and indirectly to producers. In some countries, perhaps

Table 3.2. Typical meat industry organization in the UK.

Industry member	Relative size	Relationship with other industry members
Producers	Large numbers	Not well integrated with other groups in the meat chain
Processors	Recent reduction in numbers has led to larger abattoirs with bigger throughputs	Strategic links with retailers
Retailers	Small group	Strong position Global sourcing Trusted by consumers
Consumers	Large numbers	Fickle Price-conscious

Table 3.3. Numbers of UK livestock holdings (data taken from UK National Census).

		Year	
Species	Animal type	1990	2003
Cattle	All	142,000	107,000
	Beef cattle	73,000	60,000
Sheep	All	94,000	86,000
	Breeding ewes	90,000	78,000
Pig	All	17,100	12,600
	Breeding pigs	10,000	5,800

Table 3.4. Company share of UK pig slaughter, 1998–2002 (data taken from UK Meat and Livestock Commission).

Year	Total number of pigs slaughtered	% slaughtered through top ten companies	% slaughtered through top five companies
1998	14 m	71	55
2002	10 m	80	60

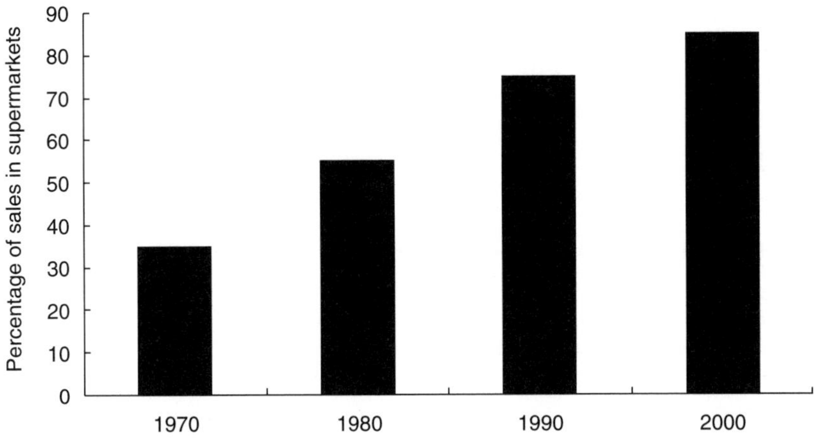

Fig. 3.4. Percentage of retail food sales in supermarkets, 1970–2000 (from UK Meat and Livestock Commission).

particularly in the UK, these 'partners in the meat supply chain' have acted separately, with little active cooperation between them. In others, a higher degree of integration has developed. For example in Denmark, the companies who dominate pig processing and manufacturing are owned by producers as part of a cooperative arrangement. Danish Crown now controls 90% of pig processing in Denmark.

Importance of adding value, developing new markets and Farm Assurance schemes

When producers have no financial involvement in processing and adding value to their raw material, they are vulnerable to the price changes resulting from cheaper imports. There is now great interest in ways of them becoming involved further along the supply chain. Producers can share in the added value generated beyond the farm gate through:

1. Collective arrangements with other producers to supply a standard animal type to processors linked to a particular retailer. Examples are Tesco Producer clubs, Waitrose Lamb contracts, ABP-Sainsburys.
2. Local arrangements between producer and abattoir, linked to Farmers Markets, Farm Shops or traditional butchers.

3. Regional products, e.g. Somerset Levels Organic Meat Producers, Herdwick Lamb.

Producing the right type of animal/carcass for a particular retailer as a member of a 'producer club' is likely to lead to a higher price and a more secure future than selling speculatively through the live animal auction market, where prices fluctuate much more. Some producers may link up with a local abattoir to supply specialist butchers with products likely to appeal to consumers, such as grass-fed local breeds. The Traditional Breeds Meat Marketing Company markets traditional British breeds of cattle, sheep and pigs in this way.

A recent development is the formation of Farm Assurance schemes organized by producers. These ensure high standards of animal welfare and food safety and show consumers that meat is being properly produced.

Animal welfare standards as a point of difference in meat marketing

Animal welfare standards are of great interest to European consumers and can be used to increase the value of products. A good example is free-range rather than battery-produced eggs. In pigs, the interest in outdoor production is connected with the assumption that animal welfare is likely to be better in pigs housed outdoors. The Royal Society for the Prevention of Cruelty to Animals (RSPCA) initiated the Freedom Foods scheme, which emphasizes animal welfare in the marketing of meat. As with other issues affecting consumer preferences, the extent to which people are prepared to pay significantly higher prices for higher animal welfare standards is debatable.

Organic meat production

The market for organic produce in the UK and other countries is growing rapidly at present. Until recently, organic meat was not widely available, but now demand in the UK is outstripping supplies. In 2002, 38% of organic meat was imported from abroad, although low prices were one reason for this. Nevertheless, the price paid for organic meat is likely to be higher than that for the conventional product (Fig. 3.5).

Selling direct or via live auction markets

Involvement of producers with activities further along the supply chain is leading to more direct marketing, i.e. straight to an abattoir/processor rather than via the auction market. Direct marketing is also probably advantageous for animal welfare, since the practice of trading groups of animals leads to stresses of various kinds. In pigs, over 99% of UK animals

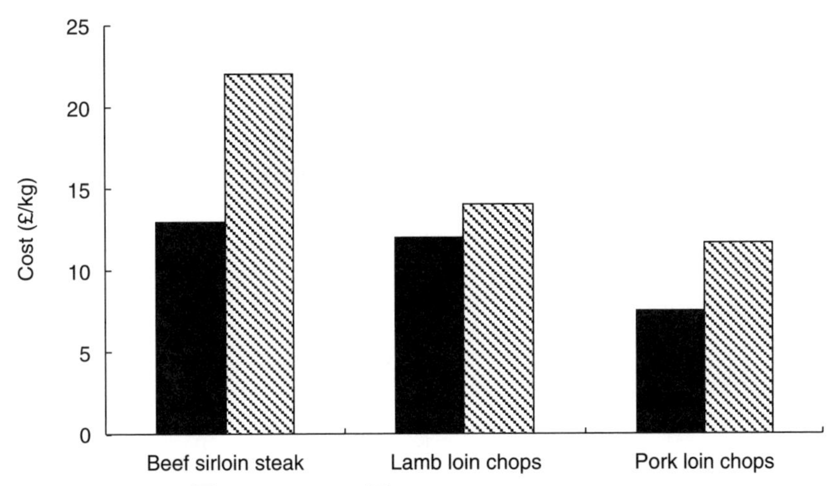

Fig. 3.5. Conventional (■) and organic (▨) UK meat prices (data taken from UK Meat and Livestock Commission, 2003a).

are sold direct to processors and this has been the case for many years. In cattle, about 20% are currently sold live through auction markets, down from 37% in 2000. Higher numbers of sheep are sold through auction markets, since integrated arrangements with processors and retailers are less developed than for other species.

The processed and food service sectors

The meat processing companies illustrated in Table 3.2 are involved mainly in fresh meat slaughtering, primary butchery and the supply of cuts and joints to retailers. However, an increasing trend is for them to be involved in further processing, including the production of ready meals. This area is also the province of specialist food manufacturing companies such as Northern Foods. Processed meats and ready meals supply the increasing demand for meals prepared simply and quickly (convenience food). People today are less prepared to spend the time required to cook a traditional 'meat and two veg' meal, especially during the week. An advantage of processed meats to the supply chain as a whole is their higher value. The market for processed beef (for example) has a much higher value per kg than has fresh beef (Table 3.5) and is growing more rapidly. In 2000 and 2003, the retail market for fresh beef remained constant but that for fresh processed beef increased by 17%. Even more marked were the increases in the food service sector, reflecting an increase in the number of meals eaten outside the home. For example, between 2000 and 2003, food service sales of beef increased by 56% and 52% for the fresh/frozen and processed sectors, respectively.

Table 3.5. Weight and value of different markets for beef, 2003 (data taken from UK Meat and Livestock Commission).

	Weight (1000 tonnes)	Value (£m)
Retail fresh/frozen	491	1900
Retail processed	317	1900
Food service fresh/frozen	244	900
Food service processed	117	700

Conclusions

This chapter shows that the UK meat industry, in common with meat industries in other countries, is changing to reflect the shift in consumer preferences and the globalization of meat production driven by low production costs in some countries. A direct result of globalization is lower prices.

Contraction in the numbers of meat producers (farmers), processors and retail outlets has coincided with a large increase in their size, especially for processors and retailers.

Animal welfare and food safety are of great importance to consumers and perceptions about those issues affect consumption. The BSE episode caused an immediate decline in beef consumption, although this has now recovered to pre-BSE levels. The meat industry is responding in various positive ways to these challenges. Producers who are involved in some part of the 'added value' stages of meat production beyond the farm gate are in a better position than those who rely on the standard market price. Farm shops and farmers markets involving slaughtering by small abattoirs in localities are one way to add value. Production of particular kinds of animals (e.g. breeds) fed special diets in an integrated arrangement between a processor and retailer is another. This ensures a reliable market for the animals and sometimes a higher price. Farm Assurance schemes are a proactive response by producers to consumer's concerns. These guarantee high standards of animal welfare and food safety. Other trends are towards organic meat production and meat meals that can be prepared more quickly.

References

UK Meat and Livestock Commission (2003a) *Meat Demand Trends*. Milton Keynes, UK.
UK Meat and Livestock Commission (2003b) *Pig Yearbook*. Milton Keynes, UK.

3.2 Construction of Abattoirs

Introduction

Designing and constructing abattoirs involves a team of specialist architects, engineers and construction personnel, amongst others. The main function of the Official Veterinary Surgeon is normally regarded as being to audit the abattoir, post-construction. At this stage, problems which were not anticipated when abattoir structure was built may be highlighted. However, preferably, Official Veterinary Surgeons should provide professional advice encompassing the principles of hygienic meat production and the best methods to achieve this, even during the planning stages. Aspects to be addressed during planning include location, provision of services, layout, materials and equipment.

Location

Location is the first consideration during planning for abattoir construction. Land section size required for abattoirs, depending on their capacity, is approximately: 1–2 acres for small abattoirs (slaughtering >30,000 animal units per year), 2–4 acres for medium abattoirs (>50,000/year) and 4–6 acres for large abattoirs (>100,000/year). In the UK, one animal unit equals one adult bovine, two pigs, three calves or five sheep/goats.

The abattoir must not, itself, contaminate the environment. Odour emissions must be anticipated using a worst-case scenario with the prevailing winds. Odour emissions will probably cause more nuisance during summer, as the ambient temperature is higher and local inhabitants live and work more frequently outdoors or have open windows. Urban populations may be less tolerant to animal-related odours than are agricultural populations. Traffic density and flow in the area must be studied; sufficient road capacity must be available. Noise will need careful consideration, as early-morning noise from stock and/or trucks will occur.

The abattoir itself must be protected from contamination from the surrounding environment; industrial zones may contain spatial or temporal pockets with high air pollution levels, where safe meat production could be compromised. Pest control is a requirement not just in abattoirs, but in the surrounds as well. Abattoirs should not be sited in flood-prone areas, because of risks from contamination of the abattoir itself and/or its water supply, additionally because effluent discharge is likely to be simple- and more cost-effective in non-flood zones.

Water supply

The availability of potable water required for abattoir operation must be ensured, as large volumes are necessary: approximately 10,000 litres per tonne of final carcass, although this depends on the technology used. Effluent-based liquid wastes are to be removed via drainage networks into the sewerage system, or into in-plant treatment areas (lagoons, sedimentation ponds, etc.), so suitable facilities must be provided. Solid wastes include inedible tissues, gut contents, lairage waste and bedding, which must be stored in suitable on-site areas before disposal.

Animal transport

Animals are transported to the abattoir by various vehicles and then unloaded; for details on animal transport see Chapter 4.1. At the site, a vehicle cleaning/disinfection station must be provided for sanitation of vehicles before they leave the premises.

Lairage

Within the buildings, the lairage capacity must be sufficient to hold at least one day's supply of livestock, in case the production line has to be stopped. Once stock is on the premises, it cannot be normally returned to the farm. The lairage should allow recovery of animals from transport stress, normal animal behaviour and interaction, and also effective ante-mortem inspection by the Official Veterinary Surgeon. On average, bovines require 2.3 to 2.8 m^2 pen space per animal; bacon pigs (light) require 0.6 m^2; while heavy pigs, sheep and calves require 0.7 to 0.8 m^2 per animal. Animals must be able to eat, drink, lie down and move comfortably, thus meeting their welfare needs. Space must be available for droving and sorting of animals, and for cleaning. Sharp corners should be avoided within the lairage area. An isolation pen with separate drainage must be provided within the lairage area to separate unwell stock or suspect stock that require in-depth inspection. The lairage area is classified as dirty, and must be physically separated from the slaughter line.

Stunning/killing

The stunning box and equipment is tailored for each animal species; provision of suitable constraints facilitates best stunning practice. Stunned animals must be rapidly bled and shackled, fulfilling animal welfare requirements (see Chapter 5.1). Blood is usually collected using contained drainage or a receptacle, but special equipment (hollow knives connected with tubing to a sealed tank) is required if blood is intended for human consumption. The stunning box must be physically separated from the carcass dressing area.

Slaughterline

The layout of each abattoir depends primarily on the flow of operations. During construction planning, the consultant Official Veterinary Surgeon must have knowledge of the hygienic flow of operations for each species to be slaughtered. Within the slaughterline for each species, different operations must be physically separated into clean and dirty areas, and this must be extended to include staff and airflow. The guiding principle is that edible tissue, or paths of their movement, should not cross any dirty area. The only individual to move between clean and dirty areas is the Official Veterinary Surgeon, who may conduct both ante-mortem and post-mortem inspection; but this include between-areas sanitation. Within clean areas, there is a requirement for any dirty materials (e.g. digestive tract) to be removed from the space as quickly as possible.

The design of the carcass dressing area depends primarily on the animal species to be slaughtered and the technology selected. Floor/wall intersections should not be 90°, as right-angle joints are difficult to clean and sanitize effectively, but should be smoothly arced. Surfaces coming into contact with edible tissues must be capable of being sterilized; this is achieved normally by hot water (at 82°C), effectively killing most vegetative bacteria, but not spores and prions. Planning for multi-species abattoirs must allow separate lines for each species to be slaughtered. Separation is ideally physical, with completely separate lines and equipment. Nonetheless, species separation can be improvised in smaller abattoirs by temporal separation of slaughter for different animal species. Separate containers for edible and non-edible tissues are required within the slaughterhall, and these must be dedicated and easily identifiable. Separate rooms must be provided for gut separation and processing. At each workstation along the slaughterline, appropriately located washing stations and knife sterilizers must be provided.

Meat inspection

Adequate facilities for meat inspection must be provided, including means of approaching carcasses and organs during inspection, as well as appropriate facilities, including good lighting, washing stations, knife sterilizers, separate room for retained meat, office, etc. Lighting, measured at 0.9–1.5 m height, should be ≥540 lux at the inspection points, ≥200 lux in work rooms, and ≥110 lux in other rooms.

Meat refrigeration

The chill capacity must be related to the slaughter capacity of the plant, and must be sufficient to lower the temperature within the specified time. Chilling of meat is primarily conducted to limit bacterial growth, but also to facilitate normal post-mortal processes in the meat. Naturally, some of the bacteria which contaminate meat may be pathogenic, so effective meat chilling (carcasses ≤7°C, offal ≤3°C) is required to limit their proliferation. The layout of the chillers is critical, since positioning of rails must allow carcass separation, while positioning of the blowers must ensure the air is circulated evenly throughout the room. In a full chiller, all carcasses must be effectively and evenly chilled, and their surfaces dried. During chilling, it is essential to avoid condensation on the carcass surfaces, as it can enable bacteria to grow. Also, condensate from chiller/blower and rail lubricants must not drip on carcasses. In addition, the chiller doors must be effectively sealed. Keeping the doors closed and sealed helps maintenance of correct temperature, and also reduces moisture condensation from warm outside air on the carcass surfaces.

Meat cutting/boning

The meat-cutting and deboning areas involve extensive meat handling and resulting microbial cross-contamination. Therefore, meat leaving these areas carries higher levels of bacteria than meat in the preceding chiller areas. The temperature in meat-cutting areas should be (≤12°C) low in order to control bacterial proliferation. However, it is not practical to debone meat in a room much below 12°C, due to chill stress of the workers and loss of their manipulative abilities. Also, in cold rooms of 4°C and below, nasal discharges from personnel can be more frequent/prolific. Because each piece of meat contacts many surfaces (conveyor belts, cutting boards), these must be designed to allow effective cleaning and sanitation. Butchery and wrapping areas must be separate from storage room for packaging materials, as they are a source of bacterial contamination.

Materials and equipment

Materials and equipment used in the abattoir should be considered from the point of view of controlling contamination. Materials should be as durable as possible and be capable of being cleaned and sanitized effectively. However, a frequent drawback of such materials is that they tend to be more expensive than other available choices. Both materials and equipment should have smooth, impermeable surfaces. Concrete, tiles or modern, composite moulded plastic walling is often used. Surfaces should not be subject to cracking, and should have as few joints as possible. Cracked surfaces and joints are difficult to clean effectively, which will make later dirt removal and sanitation difficult. Floors of lairages and slaughterhalls must be easily drained, so that pooling of water and liquid wastes does not occur, with a gradient of not less than 1 in 50. Drains should be covered with screens (holes of 4–6 mm diameter) and located at the rate of at least one per 40 m^2.

In general, equipment used within abattoirs should be considered by the same principles as materials and surfaces (discussed above). Equipment must be composed of smooth materials; rough materials are more likely to be harbour organic matter and microorganisms. Abattoir equipment is mostly manufactured from stainless steel or other non-oxidizing metal alloys. Machinery must be easy to dismantle, enabling cleaning and sanitation of all parts. Water from wash stations should not drain onto floors as this is conducive to the spread of contamination, but must be ducted directly into the sewerage system. Separate and identifiable equipment is required for inedible and condemned animal parts/tissues.

Further Reading

Anon. (1984) *A Guide to Construction, Equipment and Layout.* USDA–FSIS, Agricultural Handbook No. 570, Washington, DC.

Anon. (2004) *Good Practices for Meat Industry.* FAO Animal Production and Health Manual. FAO, Rome.

3.3 Water Quality and Sanitation in the Food Industry

Alison Small

This chapter aims to outline controls on the hygienic quality of water used within the food industry, and then to examine the processes involved in managing cleansing and sanitation operations in food premises.

Water Quality

As is well known, water is a colourless liquid at atmospheric pressure, between the temperatures of 0°C and 100°C. In liquid form it is partially ionized into hydrogen (H^+) and hydroxyl (OH^-) ions. Natural water contains many dissolved substances and minute particles in suspension. Water for human consumption can be obtained from a number of sources, for example a natural spring, a reservoir, a well or a borehole. Public water supplies undergo a process of purification, which may involve filtration, the addition of certain permitted antimicrobial chemicals – for example fluoride – distillation or ozone treatment (which primarily aims to eliminate *Cryptosporidia*). After purification, the water is delivered through a closed system of pipes, to prevent recontamination, to the point of use. After use, waste water is collected through the waste water drainage or sewerage system to a treatment plant. There, it undergoes a system of sedimentation, filtration and digestion to reduce the biological oxygen demand of the effluent, and to render it safe to be returned to the environment.

Water to be used for drinking and within the food industry must be potable (drinkable, from the Latin '*potabilis*' or '*potare*' – to drink), and must achieve certain standards to be considered such. These standards are laid down in national and community legislation, and cover the organoleptic, physical and chemical qualities of the water, as well as the microbiological status and the absence of undesirable and toxic compounds. All water supplies must be regularly monitored to ensure that they meet the requirements of potability. In the UK, this may be carried out by the water supply company in the case of public water supplies, or by the local authority in the case of private water supplies.

Water systems in food premises

In food-producing premises, all workstations should be provided with sufficient clean, wholesome water to allow personnel to satisfactorily clean themselves and their equipment whenever necessary. Potable water should be used for nearly all purposes, but certain functions, such as fire-fighting or the production of steam, or within cooling towers, may use water from sources that are not monitored, or may not be potable. If such water is used in a food premises, the outlets for such water should be clearly marked, to prevent its being used on food, hands or equipment, and the circulation system for such water should be designed in such a way that there is no risk of contamination of potable water. From henceforth in this chapter, reference to water should be taken to mean potable water.

The distribution system for water should be closed, to prevent contamination, and constructed of materials that will not corrode or taint the water. Blind ends on disused side-branches should not be present, as these are likely to hold stagnant water, where microbial contamination may persist. Within a food premises, the hygiene of the water system should be monitored on a regular basis. The manager of the business should keep a water distribution plan (Fig. 3.6) showing the water outlets, and also designated sampling points, which will each be sampled in rotation, ideally on a monthly basis. Carefully chosen sampling points are essential in both verifying the suitability of the water used in the premises and in locating the origin of hygiene failures.

Water sampling and analysis

When the distribution system is sampled, the correct technique is vital to prevent contamination of the sample, and also to ensure that the sample represents the contents of the distribution system, and not just the cleanliness of the outlet. Ideally, special sampler taps should be fitted at the sampling points, which should be adjacent to water outlets. Where special sampling taps are fitted, they can be heat-sterilized using a hand-held blow-torch after external dirt and grease have been removed. After heat sterilization, the tap should be opened and run to waste for 2–3 minutes before collection of the sample. Where the sample is to be taken from a standard water outlet, for example a tap or hose, heat sterilization cannot be used as this would destroy the rubber or plastic washers within the outlet. In this case, after removing external dirt and grease, the outlet should be sterilized by the application of a 1:10 solution of commercial

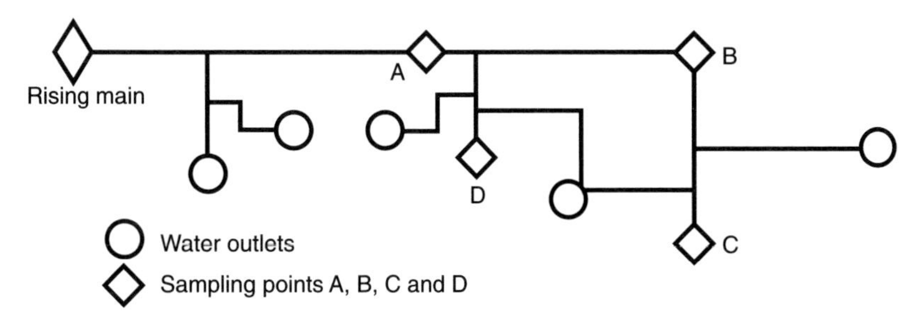

Fig. 3.6. Example of water distribution plan for food premises, showing rising main, water outlets and sampling points.

hypochlorite (giving a concentration of 1% free chlorine). This solution must be left for 2–3 minutes to achieve full sterilization of the outlet, and then the water must be allowed to run to waste for 5 minutes, to rinse off any residual chlorine which would affect the analysis of the sample, before the sample is collected. The sample should be collected without splashing (which could result in contamination of the sample) into a sterile bottle containing sodium thiosulphate. This chemical is added to neutralize chlorine, which may be present in the water, if the supply has been chlorinated, or may be a residue of chemical sterilization of the outlet. It is important to neutralize chlorine, as it will interfere with microbial growth and give falsely low counts.

The sample should be analysed in accordance with the legislation, and this would include determination of Total Viable Count of bacteria (TVC) at 22°C and with 72 h incubation, TVC at 37°C over 48 h incubation, and coliform count (an indication of faecal contamination). Other analyses, which may be carried out less frequently, for example annually, should include *Escherichia coli*, *Streptococcus faecalis* and sulphite-reducing *Clostridia* species, all of which are further indicators of faecal contamination.

Targets for water analysis

The TVC in water will fluctuate throughout the year, and a chart of the values obtained should be kept to show the normal trend for the plant. One would expect TVC at 22°C to be <100 colony-forming units per millilitre (cfu/ml), and TVC at 37°C to be <10 cfu/ml most months. Once the background trend for the plant is known, the monthly result can be compared with this, and action taken if a count greater than twice the expected level is obtained. The outlet in question, and the outlet immediately before it in the distribution system, should be resampled, and these samples analysed for the full range of criteria, including *E. coli*, *S. faecalis* and sulphite-reducing *Clostridia*. The most common cause of failure in TVC is contamination of the outlet sampled, either due to insufficient decontamination prior to taking the sample, or often to microbial contamination being harboured in perished rubber washers.

The level of coliforms in water should never be >3 cfu in 100 ml, and the target should be <1 cfu in 100 ml. If two consecutive samples are positive for coliforms, action should be taken to sanitize the water distribution system. When testing for *E. coli* and *S. faecalis*, the result should always be <1 cfu in 100 ml, and for sulphite-reducing *Clostridia* <1 cfu in 20 ml. If the water sample fails to meet any of these criteria, it should be considered that the water distribution system has suffered faecal contamination, and food production should cease until the system has been sanitized. A full investigation should be carried out to identify the source of contamination and measures put into place to prevent recurrence. The water should be sampled and analysed more frequently until it is considered that the risk of further contamination has been rectified.

To sanitize a water distribution system, the system may be flushed with a proprietary sanitizing agent, or with copious fresh, clean water (dilution being 'the solution to pollution'). Water entering the system may be subjected to ultra-violet light treatment, or be chlorinated to reduce its microbial load. Chlorine is often added to public water supplies at 0.1–0.2 ppm, as free chlorine ions are an active biocide. Further chlorination of water at the food premises may raise the chlorine concentration to 0.5 ppm or above; however, in some countries, e.g. in the EU, hyperchlorination of water (to levels greater than 0.5 ppm) has been outlawed. When water has been chlorinated, it is advisable to test the chlorine level on a regular basis to ensure it remains within the desired limits. Proprietary test kits are available for such monitoring procedures.

Sanitation in Food Premises

Various terms are used when describing sanitation procedures in the food industry, and for clarity, these require definition. 'Cleaning' means the physical removal of soil, e.g. dirt, food residue or grease. 'Disinfection' is the reduction of pathogenic (disease-causing) microorganisms to safe levels. In scientific circles, disinfection means the reduction in microbial numbers by a factor of 100,000. A disinfectant is a chemical that is lethal to microbes, and in the food industry, the term 'sanitizer' is synonymous. To achieve 'sterilization', the treatment must ensure total elimination of all microorganisms.

Sanitation of food premises is carried out for a number of reasons, not only to satisfy legal requirements. By reducing the numbers of microorganisms in the food production environment, the risk of food poisoning and spoilage is reduced. Removal of physical soil reduces the risk of foreign body contamination of the food and also assists in maintaining the equipment in good working order and in preventing blockages and corrosion. Dirty premises with food residues remaining on the floor and equipment are an unsafe, unpleasant working environment, and vermin infestations may occur, which in turn contribute to microbial and foreign body contamination of the food produced. A clean, bright working environment is conducive to health and safety and happy workers, and leaves a good impression on visiting customers and officials.

The premises manager has a very important role in sanitation of the premises, even though he may not physically participate in the visible procedure of cleaning. The manager needs to know and understand the requirements of the relevant legislation and also principles of food microbiology, including spoilage and food poisoning organisms, in order to fully appreciate the importance of premises sanitation. The manager must balance the aims of running a profitable business with the needs of hygiene, and must plan and implement a sanitation programme that prevents food contamination and pest infestation. When considering sanitation, the manager must provide sufficient staff, services and equipment to carry out the procedure. He must ensure that the personnel are trained in correct and safe use of the equipment, and the equipment is suitable for the job. For example, brushes with long handles may be required to reach the high-level areas, or different-coloured equipment may be used in different parts of the premises to prevent cross-contamination. The provision of services such as hot water, drainage or electricity must also be taken into account when selecting the method and equipment for cleaning procedures. Most importantly, the nature of the premises and equipment to be cleaned must be considered, both to ensure effective cleaning and to prevent damage being caused by the cleaning operation itself.

Instructions to personnel should be clear and simple, and laid down as a formal procedure that is monitored on a regular basis. These instructions often take the form of a 'Cleaning Schedule', against which the performance of the cleaning team is audited. It is the premises manager's responsibility to ensure that a cleaning schedule is prepared, is communicated to the cleaning team, and is reviewed in response to cleaning failures or alterations in the premises or production, and at regular intervals. The manager should be aware that it is not sufficient merely to give a copy of the cleaning schedule to the cleaning team and to expect its contents to be adhered to, but that each member of the team should be trained and updated with any changes to the cleaning schedule. Literacy problems, time constraints, paper overload and apathy all contribute to personnel not reading and understanding written instructions, so care should be taken to demonstrate procedures and discuss the process. Often, when personnel understand the reason why a particular procedure is required, that procedure will be carried out with far more dedication than if the procedure seems pointless. A major part of the manager's role in personnel management is staff motivation, and this can only be achieved if the manager shows commitment to high standards.

The manager must also be aware of the sources of the costs of cleaning. As a rough guide, labour, or personnel costs, will comprise up to 70% of the overall cost of cleaning, equipment and chemicals a further 20%, and services (water, drainage, electricity) the remainder.

The Cleaning Schedule

The Cleaning Schedule should be a user-friendly document, containing detailed instructions for the sanitation of the premises. It should include safety information on all procedures and chemicals used, and should also detail a system for the monitoring and control of the sanitation procedure. The Schedule should detail what is to be cleaned, by whom, when and how it should be cleaned. When drawing up a Cleaning Schedule, the manager needs to take into account the construction and layout of the plant, and the time required to clean a particular area or piece of equipment. The cleaning process should progress in a logical manner, so that there is no risk of re-contamination of previously cleaned items. For example, if the floor was cleaned before the walls, then the dirty water and residue from the walls would flow onto the floor, making it dirty once more. The manager should also take into account the existing cleaning routines in use in the premises, as these have often developed over time into a form that makes the task easier or quicker for the cleaning team. Good points in the existing routine may be retained, but care must be taken to ensure that the cleaning procedure is effective. The Cleaning Schedule should detail all the chemical agents to be used during the cleaning process, and their correct use, including safety information, dilution instructions and method of application. It is important also to include a prescribed system of audit and review, detailing the persons responsible for each task, and exactly how often the area or item should be cleaned, inspected or sampled. To audit the cleaning process, regular visual inspections should be carried out, supplemented by microbiological sampling of equipment, particularly of food contact equipment. It is also important, however, to sample items that are not in contact with foods, as the entire premises should be cleaned to an equal standard. As a guideline level, Total Viable Count on cleaned surfaces prior to production beginning should be no more than 100 cfu/cm^2, and there should be no evidence of faecal contamination, which may be demonstrated by analysing the sample for Enterobacteriaceae.

The sanitation process

Cleaning involves systematic application of energy to a surface in order to remove soil. This energy can consist of thermal energy – such as the use of hot water or steam, chemical energy – from detergents and disinfectants, and kinetic energy – the product of manual labour, mechanical cleaning tools or water turbulence within pipes and containers. A cleaning process will normally begin with a pre-clean phase, where visible debris is removed manually, perhaps using a brush or squeegee. Next is the cleaning phase proper. Manual cleaning, using hand-held tools, is often used for smaller pieces of equipment, which may have to be dismantled prior to cleaning. Neutral or near-neutral detergents are used due to the close proximity of the operator, for safety reasons. Detergents with greater acidity or alkalinity are used in cleaning operations set a little more remote from the worker. These compounds, which may form a foam or gel, are sprayed onto large areas of the premises using special apparatus, such as a pressure lance, and are ideal for cleaning areas where access is restricted. The foaming nature of such detergents improve contact between the detergent and the surface, whilst gel detergents adhere even more closely to the surface, giving a prolonged contact time during which the chemical cleaning process takes place. The detergent may be mixed with hot water in order to benefit from thermal energy effects as well.

After the cleaning phase, which would include sufficient contact time for any chemical agents used to be fully effective, the equipment and surfaces are rinsed with potable water. A disinfection phase may then begin, where a sanitizer is applied to the surfaces and equipment. After the required contact time, the sanitizer may then be rinsed off with potable water. Some food-safe chemicals, however, are designed to remain on the surface and do not require rinsing.

Water turbulence as a form of kinetic energy cleaning is commonly used in the dairy industry, and is often combined with thermal energy (very hot water) and chemical compounds. The cleaning effected here is carried out by a Clean-In-Place (CIP) system, where the cleaning solution is automatically circulated at high velocity through the pipes and containers of the production line. Highly acidic or highly alkaline detergents may be used, as the system is closed, allowing no access by personnel, and the flow rate of the solution is critical to ensure that there is sufficient turbulence in the system to effect cleaning (Fig. 3.7). Here, as in water distribution systems, blind-ended junctions on pipes can be bypassed by the cleaning solution, and contaminated food residue may remain. As a general rule, if there is a blind branch on the pipe, its height should be no more than three times the diameter of the main pipe, and where blind branches occur on bends, the cleaning solution should be directed into the branch at high velocity to ensure adequate cleaning.

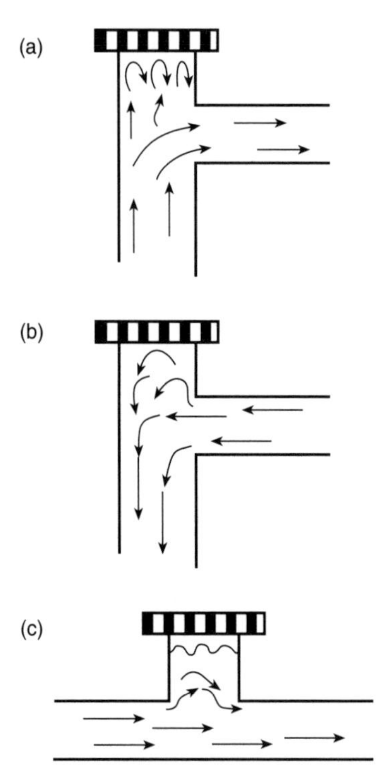

Fig. 3.7. Water flow effects of internal cleaning of pipes. (a) Where flow is directed at a branch, turbulence is high and cleaning is good; (b) where flow curves past a branch, turbulence in the branch is low and cleaning is poor; and (c) where flow passes a perpendicular branch, turbulence is very low and cleaning very poor. If the branch is three times longer than the diameter of the pipe, air will be trapped in the blind end, and the cleaning fluid will not even contact the surfaces.

Detergents

There are a number of different classes of detergent, with differing properties. Desireable characteristics of detergents to be used in food premises include being non-tainting, non-toxic and non-corrosive. They should be effective when used at low temperatures and at low concentrations, for operator safety, and should easily be rinsed off when the cleaning process is completed. It should be a simple measure to detect residues of the chemical to prevent tainting of the food, and the run-off waste effluent should be biodegradable and not harmful to the environment. The product used, however, should be sufficiently stable that its efficacy remains for a sufficient period of time to ensure sanitation before the compound degrades, and the product should be cost-effective for use in business.

Detergents are often described in terms of their surfactancy (ability to reduce the surface tension of the solution to improve wetting of the surface to be cleaned), dispersion (ability to break up particles of dirt or grease) and suspension (ability to keep the particles afloat within the rinse water so that they are removed from the surface). In general, a detergent molecule has a hydrophilic end and a hydrophobic end. When the detergent solution contacts oil- or fat-based residues on a surface, the hydrophobic portion buries itself in the residue, leaving the hydrophilic tail within the water of the detergent solution. As the detergent molecules squeeze into the residue, the residue is divided up into globules, the surfaces of which are covered in the hydrophilic tails of the detergent molecules (Fig. 3.8). These globules of residue are then lifted off the surface being cleaned, into suspension and can be rinsed off.

Commonly used chemicals in the food industry include halogen-based compounds, quaternary ammonium compounds, amphoteric compounds and acids or alkalis.

Halogen-based compounds

Halogen-based compounds release free chlorine radicals as the active agent, which react with the cell wall constituents of food residues and microorganisms. They are non-tainting, biodegrade into non-toxic compounds, and can be detected using a simple chemical test kit. However, the solution has limited stability, and is quickly inactivated in the presence of organic material, e.g. food residues. Some halogen-based compounds release iodine rather than chlorine, but these are more corrosive, and are more likely to cause tainting of foods.

Quarternary ammonium compounds

Quaternary ammonium compounds are effective at neutral pH, so are suitable for use with manual cleaning procedures. They act by damaging the cytoplasmic membrane of cells in the residue. They are non-toxic, can

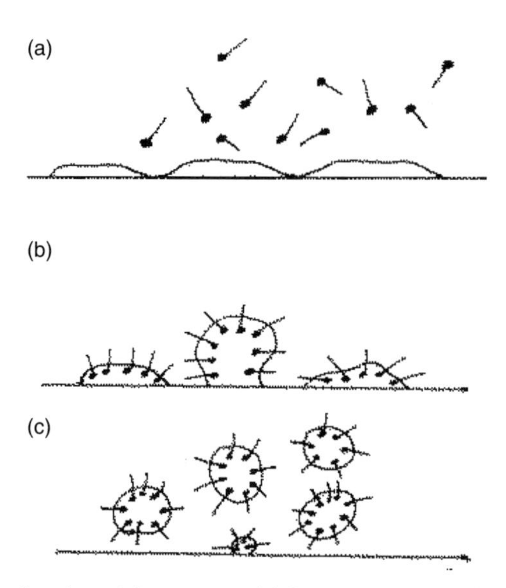

Fig. 3.8. Mechanism of action of detergents. (a) Detergent molecules in solution are applied to the greasy surface; (b) the hydrophobic pole of the detergent molecules becomes buried in the grease; and (c) this pulls the grease off the surface and into suspension.

be detected using a chemical test kit, and most are biodegradable. However, they may cause tainting of foods, and are inactivated in the presence of organic material, and also by excessive lime in hard water.

Amphoteric compounds

Amphoteric compounds contain long-chain substituted amino acids, and are unaffected by the mineral content of the water used. They are non-tainting, stable but biodegradable, and have low toxicity. They can be detected chemically, and are compatible with other classes of detergent and sanitizer, but they require a long contact time to complete their function.

Acids and alkalis

Acids and alkalis have long been used in cleaning products, and they act by oxidizing the proteins in the cells of the residue or in microorganisms. They are non-toxic and non-tainting, and although corrosive in concentrate form, when used at the correct dilution are not. Acids and alkalis can be detected chemically, are fairly stable, and are biodegradable. They should never be used in conjunction with halogen-based compounds as this would result in the liberation of chlorine gas, which is highly toxic.

Activity of disinfectants and sanitizers against microorganisms is often used in the sales literature for the compound. Most of these data are gathered through laboratory experiments, and often indicate the activity of the compound *in vitro*, against pure cultures of a particular organism. However, when used in the field, the compound is often inactivated by organic material present on the surface to be cleaned, and the reduction in microbial numbers reduced from the expected 100,000-fold to only 100-fold or 1000-fold.

Further Reading

Denier, S.P. and Hugo, W.B. (1991) *Mechanisms of Action of Chemical Biocides*. Blackwell, Oxford.

Denier, S.P., Gorman, S.P. and Sussman, M. (1993) *Microbial Biofilus: Formation and Control*. Blackwell, Oxford.

4 Pre-slaughter Phase

4.1 Farm-to-Abattoir Phase

PAUL WARRISS

Introduction

Practically all the animals that we produce must eventually be slaughtered, even if their primary value to man has not been as a source of meat. In the UK we slaughter every year about 900 million poultry, 10 million pigs, 15 million sheep and 2 million cattle. Getting these from farm to abattoir forms the first link in the chain of meat production and one that is both important and, to some degree, contentious. It is important because how it is done can influence carcass and lean meat quality, and contentious because the processes of handling and transport provide many opportunities for the animal's welfare to be compromised. In fact, quality and welfare are closely linked. Improvements in one are often associated with improvements in the other.

Animals can spend a long time getting from the farm to the slaughter plant. Additionally, they may spend time held in lairage, which can prolong this potentially stressful period, and many are sold, not directly, but indirectly through live auction markets. About 60% of cattle and 70% of sheep in the UK pass through markets. This practice increases the overall number of journeys. The period is stressful because it involves removal of animals from their home environment and holding in unfamiliar surroundings, food and water deprivation, exposure to noise, strange smells, vibration and changes of velocity, extremes of temperature, the breakdown of social groupings, close confinement and sometimes overcrowding. The longer that animals are exposed to these stressors the greater the chance that their welfare is compromised and that carcass and meat quality are reduced.

Journey times are likely to have increased because of changes in the structure of the slaughtering industry. The number of red meat slaughter plants in 2000 was less than one-third of those operating 20 years previously, and these plants were generally bigger. Overall, nearly 50% of red meat animals are now killed in plants with throughputs greater than

100,000 animals per year, and the average throughput of these plants is nearly 200,000 per year. There are therefore fewer local abattoirs and the remaining larger plants operate at higher line speeds. Faster processing requires moving animals more quickly and this is likely to be more stressful.

Effects on welfare and quality

A number of quality problems attributable to pre-slaughter handling can be recognized and these generally also reflect poor welfare. Animals may die, they may suffer trauma such as bruises or broken bones, long periods without food may reduce carcass yield, deprivation of water may cause dehydration, and stress may produce poor quality of the lean meat. In particular, short-term (acute) stress may stimulate glycolysis immediately post-mortem and produce PSE (pale, soft, exudative) meat, and long-term (chronic) stress may deplete muscle glycogen levels and produce DFD (dark, firm, dry) meat. The transport of animals can spread disease, which has implications for both welfare and quality, and may compromise traceability if systems for animal identification are less than perfect. Effective traceability, so that the exact origin and provenance of each piece of meat sold at retail are known, is central to the quality control of hygiene and safety.

Legislative control of transport and animal handling procedures

In the UK the handling of animals during the period from farm to slaughter is currently controlled by four main pieces of legislation. Transport is governed by The Welfare of Animals (Transport) Order 1997, handling in markets by The Welfare of Animals at Markets Order 1990, and handling at the abattoir by The Welfare of Animals (Slaughter or Killing) Regulations 1995 and The Fresh Meat (Hygiene and Inspection) Regulations 1995. UK legislation reflects EU Directives, so in general terms European legislation is harmonized. The general provisions of The Welfare of Animals (Transport) Order 1997 make it an offence to cause injury or unnecessary suffering or to transport unfit animals. Transporters must be authorized by the appropriate Government Minister, animal handlers must be competent (as demonstrated by training or experience) and all journeys must have appropriate documentation. The Order prescribes amongst other things, maximum journey times, space requirements and feeding and watering intervals. Although legislation is always subject to change the general principles embodied in it are unlikely to. In general, if there is change, it tends to be in the direction of stronger protection for the welfare of animals. For example, there is currently much pressure to reduce maximum permitted journey times.

Fitness to travel

Animals that are ill, infirm or fatigued (unless only slightly affected and where the intended journey is unlikely to cause them unnecessary suffering) are unfit to be transported. Transport is prohibited in pregnant animals (likely to give birth, or within 48 h of birth) or new-born animals in which the navel has not completely healed. Animals must be able to be loaded without using force and be able to bear weight on all four legs. Examples of unfit animals include animals suffering pain (which is likely to be made worse by transport), animals with fractures or severe wounds, animals with prolapses and lame animals.

The Welfare of Animals (Transport) Order 1997 (Section 6) allows an unfit animal to be transported to the nearest available place of slaughter if the animal is not likely to be subject to unnecessary suffering by reason of its unfitness. The Fresh Meat (Hygiene and Inspection) Regulations 1995 (Part V, 17(2)(a)–(b)) require that the animal be accompanied by a written declaration by the animal's owner, or person in charge of it, which is handed to the Inspector or OVS (Official Veterinary Surgeon) on arrival at the slaughterhouse, and which contains the information prescribed in Schedule 18 of the Regulations. This is often referred to as the 'Schedule 18 declaration' and includes declarations regarding the animal's identity, medicinal treatment it has received and signs of disease or injury exhibited. The decision of whether an animal is fit to travel is that of the owner. The Declaration does not have to be signed by a veterinarian. If a person certifies that an animal is fit to travel, but the Inspector or OVS at the abattoir thinks it was not, the person is open to prosecution because the animal is likely to have been caused unnecessary suffering.

Stocking densities in transit

There are commercial pressures to increase stocking densities. The more animals that can be carried on a transport vehicle, the less the average cost of transport per animal. The legislation prescribes appropriate space allowances. In general, animals should have enough space to lie down. For example, the loading density for pigs weighing around 100 kg should not exceed 235 kg/m^2, equivalent to 0.425 m^2/100 kg live weight. This is about the space needed by a pig to lie down in sternal recumbency. The legislation points out that in hot weather the space allowance may need to be increased by up to 20%. The reason for this is that pigs are very sensitive to overheating in hot weather and at high stocking densities they may be unable to cool themselves effectively. In the worst case they will die. Transporting cattle at high stocking densities has also been shown to increase levels of bruising.

Mortality in transit

Death of an animal is the ultimate compromise of its welfare and results in total loss of value. The problem affects mainly pigs and poultry; ruminants are generally more resilient. This is largely because of their different heat loss strategies. Pigs can only lose heat effectively by wallowing. In the UK pig deaths in transit (DOAs – dead on arrival) are particularly a problem above average daily temperatures of about 18°C. This means that the number of deaths in transit is higher in the summer months. Mortality is also higher on longer journeys and in genotypes of pig that show greater stress susceptibility. Stress susceptibility in pigs is associated with the so-called Halothane gene (Hal+). The gene is present at relatively high frequencies in some breeds, notably the Belgian Pietrain, some strains of Landrace and meat-type hybrids, and is closely linked to genes that promote leanness and muscularity, so carcasses from these breeds have little fat and show desirable high conformation. Overall, the average mortalities in transit in the UK are about 0.1% for pigs and 0.02% for sheep. These contrast with the much higher level (0.2%) found in broiler chickens.

Methods used to handle animals

Animals need to be moved from and into pens, along races and passageways and on to vehicles. Vehicles must have their own unloading system. Usually this is formed from the tailboard, which acts as an external ramp, and internal ramps to access the higher decks in multi-tiered transporters. Animals find negotiating steep (>20° to the horizontal) ramps difficult. In particular, pigs do not climb or descend ramps very easily or willingly. Some transporters are therefore fitted with hydraulic platform lifts instead of ramps. The legislation prescribes maximum angles for vehicle ramps: 29° for external and 33° for internal ramps. These are, however, far steeper than is realistic.

There are recommended ways of handling animals, in particular making use of their natural behaviour patterns. For example, sheep have a well-developed, strong following behaviour. The legislation prescribes that no excessive force may be used to move animals and there must be no lifting or dragging by the horns, legs, tail or fleece. Animals must not be hit with sticks. The use of electric goads is strictly limited: they may be used only on the hindquarters of cattle over 6 months old, or on adult pigs which are refusing to move forward when there is space for them to do so. The shocks must be for no longer than 2 seconds and successive shocks must be adequately spaced out.

Poor handling can lead to animals slipping and falling and bumping into obstacles. This results in bruising or internal haemorrhages. By analogy with human experience, bruising is painful and therefore has welfare implications. It also damages the appearance of a carcass and may therefore lead to downgrading. Extensive bruising may require trimming, leading to weight loss and therefore direct economic loss. Bruising is always higher in the carcasses from animals sold via live auction markets than in those sent directly from the farm to slaughter, partly because the handling they receive is often poorer and partly because they must be handled more.

Segregation of animals in transit

Some animals are naturally incompatible: if mixed they fight, leading to injury. A particular and common problem is fighting caused by the mixing of pigs that have been reared in separate pens. This is stressful to them and leads to unsightly lacerations on the carcass and poorer lean meat quality. The problem is commoner in entire males (boars) compared with gilts or castrates. Mixed groups of young bulls will also fight, leading to bruising and reduced meat quality. The Legislation specifies various animals that must be segregated during transport to prevent serious injury or suffering, including bulls over 10 months old unless reared in compatible groups or accustomed to one another. Mixing of horned and unhorned cattle is generally proscribed and certainly not recommended.

Deprivation of food and water

Some period of food withdrawal before slaughter is desirable to reduce gut contents and therefore the chances of contamination of the carcass at evisceration if the distended gut is accidentally cut or broken. Pigs do not travel well on a full stomach, and mortality is higher in pigs fed too soon before loading. However, water should be available to animals at all practicable times. Long periods without food reduce live weights and carcass yields, a loss referred to as 'shrinkage' in North America. They also lead to hunger and hence poor welfare. A compromise therefore needs to be struck between the benefits and disadvantages of longer and shorter pre-slaughter fasting times.

PSE and DFD meat

PSE meat occurs in pigs. The meat is very pale, soft in texture (in the raw state) and exudative, meaning that it is wet in appearance and loses a lot of drip on cutting and during storage. The condition is caused by acute stress at slaughter, which speeds up the metabolism of the muscles, specifically glycolysis, immediately post-mortem. The resulting rapid acidification, at a time when the carcass is still hot, denatures some of the muscle proteins so that they lose bound water, leading to the characteristic changes seen subsequently. A major cause of PSE is the stress associated with moving them through race-restrainer systems immediately before they are stunned if this is carried out thoughtlessly or with excessive coercion. However, even when handled carefully at slaughter, stress-susceptible pigs tend to produce a high frequency of carcasses that show PSE meat.

DFD meat can occur in all species. In cattle it is often referred to as Dark Cutting Beef (DCB). The meat is very dark in colour, firm in texture and dry or even sticky to the touch. DFD is caused by chronic stress pre-slaughter that depletes muscle glycogen levels. This limits the degree of glycolysis, and therefore acidification, post-mortem. DFD meat is therefore characterized by a high ultimate pH, so it tends to be prone to spoilage, partly because this high pH promotes bacterial growth, and partly because the deficiency of glycogen and other carbohydrates encourages the growth of bacteria that break down nitrogen-containing compounds such as proteins. This produces very unpleasant putrefactive smells. The high pH means that the proteins do not denature and retain their high water-holding capacity, so the meat surface is dry. Examples of stresses that cause DFD are prolonged food deprivation, transport fatigue and the fighting that often occurs between unfamiliar animals, especially pigs and young bulls.

Very occasionally, pig carcasses apparently show both PSE and normal, DFD and normal, or PSE and DFD characteristics in adjacent parts of the musculature. This is referred to as 'two-toning'. It is difficult to explain in physiological terms but probably reflects differences in the inherent biochemistry of different muscles and how actively they have been used in the animal. So, red muscles, which have more oxidative fibres, tend to be prone to DFD and white muscles, which have a more glycolytic metabolism, are more susceptible to PSE.

Both PSE and DFD meat are discriminated against by consumers and have poor eating quality as well as appearance. They also both reflect poor animal welfare because they result from stress.

The spread of disease

The movement of animals from farm to slaughter has obvious implications for the spread of disease, particularly if they pass through one or more auction markets in the process. The stresses associated with handling and transport may additionally increase the animal's susceptibility to infection by compromising the function of its immune system. When animals are held in lairage there is also the danger of rapid cross-infection of healthy individuals from infected ones by pathogens such as salmonellae. The spread of disease between animals may well compromise their welfare, and the spread of pathogens potentially compromises meat hygiene, and therefore quality.

Further Reading

Mcnally, P.W. and Warriss, P.D. (1996) Prevalence of carcass bruising and skin-marking between cattle bought from different live auction markets. *Veterinary Record* 140, 231–232.

Warriss, P.D. (1992) *Animal Welfare – Handling Animals Before Slaughter and the Consequences for Welfare and Product Quality*. Meat Focus International, July 1992, CAB International, Wallingford, UK, pp. 135–138.

Warriss, P.D. (1994a) Ante-mortem handling of pigs. In: Cole, D.J.A., Wiseman, J. and Varley, M.A. (eds) *Principles of Pig Science*. University of Nottingham Press, Nottingham, UK, pp. 425–432.

Warriss, P.D. (1994b) Ante-mortem factors influencing the yield and quality of meat from farm animals. In: Jones, S.D.M. (ed.) *Quality and Grading of Carcass of Meat Animals*. CRC Press Inc., Boca Raton, Florida, pp. 1–15.

Warriss, P.D. (1995) The welfare of animals during transport. In: Raw, M.-E. and Parkinson, T.J. (eds) *The Veterinary Annual*, vol. 36. Blackwell Scientific Publications, Oxford, UK, pp. 73–85.

Warriss, P.D. (1998a) Choosing appropriate space allowances for slaughter pigs transported by road: a review. *Veterinary Record* 142, 449–454.

Warriss, P.D. (1998b) The welfare of slaughter pigs during transport. *Animal Welfare* 7, 365–381.

Warriss, P.D. (2000) *Meat Science: an Introductory Text*. CAB International, Wallingford, UK, 312 pp.

Warriss, P.D. (2003) Optimal lairage times for slaughter pigs. *Veterinary Record* 153, 170–176.

Weeks, C.A., Mcnally, P.W. and Warriss, P.D. (2002) Influence of the design of facilities at auction markets and animal handling procedures on bruising in cattle. *Veterinary Record* 150, 743–748.

4.2 Food Chain Information (FCI)

The Role of FCI

Based on appropriate and detailed information on pre-history of animals intended for slaughter, as well as on ante-mortem inspection findings, they can be categorized into suspect animal (posing a higher public health risk) and non-suspect animal (posing a lower risk) groups before arriving at the abattoir – or at least before slaughter. Such pre-history information should comprise all relevant data from birth, through all stages of rearing and up to the day of slaughter, and is called 'Food Chain Information' (FCI).

The higher- and lower-risk animal groups should be handled separately (during transport, lairaging and slaughter/dressing) so as to avoid cross-contamination of the latter from the former. During ante-mortem inspection at the abattoir, the initial FCI-based categorization of the animals into the two risk categories should again be re-evaluated in the light of any relevant findings. In cases where animals pre-categorized into the low-risk group (based on FCI) show any abnormalities potentially relevant for public health, they should be moved into the higher-risk category. With respect to post-mortem inspection (see Chapter 6), all higher-risk animals, understandably, would require detailed examination – including laboratory testing if needed, whilst lower-risk animals could be subjected to a simplified inspection system.

Main elements of FCI

Animal production systems can be divided into so-called 'integrated' and 'non-integrated' systems. Integrated animal production systems have recently been defined by relevant expert groups (Anon., 2004), and the criteria can be divided into two main groups: (i) they must operate by using Good Farming Practice (GFP), Good Hygiene Practice (GHP) and Hazard Analysis and Critical Control Points principles; and (ii) they must have quality assurance systems in place ensuring control over, and information availability about, aspects indicated below.

Identification, movement and traceability

Systems must be in place to record animal movements and to identify animals individually. Problems with individual identification exist particularly with sheep, but are expected to be resolved in the near future. Movement records must include a residency period to qualify for Farm Assurance status (see later). Currently, in the UK, this is 90 days for beef and 60 days for lamb. Generally, animals with higher movement frequencies should be considered as posing higher epidemiological risk.

Epidemiological intelligence

Monitoring and surveillance programmes provide data on existence and relevant changes in disease prevalences and zoonotic agents in animals. Epidemiological intelligence to be used for FCI includes any relevant baseline information and/or risk assessments available. The EU Directive 2003/99/EC on monitoring zoonoses and zoonotic agents at all points along the food chain became mandatory for all EU member states in June 2004. The exchange of relevant information is two-way, originating from each member state, having been digested by the EU and then distributed to relevant veterinarians and other public heath officials in all EU member states. In addition to locally available epidemiological intelligence information, these EU-managed data will be very relevant for FCI purposes.

Farm animal management

Relevant information must be gathered from each farm supplying animals, enabling proper analysis of the risks presented by the livestock. Naturally, animals must be well managed to good standards of husbandry and welfare by competent stockmen. Farm production data must be analysed properly and cover a wide scope of livestock production practices, including the frequency of herd or flock inspection, management and treatment of stock, surgical operations, dehorning and disbudding treatments, the management of neonate animals, the use of exposed grazing areas and dog control.

Environment and hygiene management

There must be on-farm systems to prevent pollution of the environment and potential re-cycling of hazards via the environment back to the animals. Naturally, this must involve detailed analysis of animal waste (slurry, dirty water, farmyard manure, etc.) storage, treatment and disposal. Methods and associated appropriate records for casualty stock disposal and isolation facilities for sick animals must be assessed. The cleanliness of stock at marketing should be known, as should methods and associated appropriate records for dog worming and sheep dip disposal. Overall farm biosecurity (e.g. movement of animals, people and vehicles, vermin) plays an important role in protecting public health.

Animal feed composition, storage and use

Animals must be fed appropriate feed which has been stored correctly. Contaminants and residues in animal feeds can ultimately be found in meat derived from stock which has eaten contaminated feeds. Therefore, knowledge of feed suppliers, feed composition and declarations, feed transport systems and whether the feeds have been examined for public health hazards must be obtained and analysed. Attention must be paid to the biosecurity of feeds stored on-farm, since pathogen-free feeds can become contaminated via contact with vermin, wild birds or insects if stored inappropriately on-farm.

Housing and handling facilities

Facilities must be adequate to provide safe housing, sufficient for the handling of stock. The structure and size, lighting and electrical installations and cleaning routine should be considered.

Production parameters

Good production parameters (e.g. growth rate, feed conversion rate and similar) normally indicate general good health and welfare of the animals.

Farm quality assurance in the FCI context

Many quality assurance schemes operate in different countries. One example is the Assured British Meat (ABM) scheme, which will be used here. ABM has around 23,000 members producing cattle or sheep; around 75% of cattle and 60% of sheep slaughtered in the UK come from ABM-assured farms. ABM membership effectively is an 'unwritten' condition for success on the market, since large retailers will only purchase meat from abattoirs slaughtering animals from ABM-assured farms. In practice, the ABM scheme involves independent on-farm inspections (10% of inspections are unannounced). A negative inspection results in loss of certification, which must be re-applied for. Naturally, the farm business stands the cost incurred.

The ABM scheme has numerous farm quality assurance standards, including (as at 2004):

- animal identification and movement: 3 standards;
- farm management: 20 standards;
- management of the environment and hygiene: 8 standards;
- animal feed (composition, quality, storage): 9 standards;
- animal husbandry conditions: 10 standards; and
- medications and veterinary treatment: 12 standards.

These standards are available from the ABM scheme directly, or from their website, and are being continually updated.

Herd health plans

Herd health plans, and related data, are one of the most relevant considerations form the FCI perspective.

Medicines and veterinary treatment

Medicines and treatments, posing a risk from residues in edible tissues, must be administered in an appropriate manner and all relevant records kept. Medicines must be used appropriately, with proper respect of withdrawal periods and safe, environmentally friendly storage and disposal.

Operative aspects of the food chain information (FCI) system, in the context of meat inspection

Operative aspects of the FCI are still under development, with the main points being considered and approved from practical, regulatory and public health aspects. Operators must deliver the necessary FCI to the Official Veterinary Surgeon (OVS), preferably through an information technology (computer) system. The FCI should be received 24 h before anticipated delivery of the animals. This is necessary to avoid unnecessary transport of animals which would not otherwise be accepted for slaughter. If FCI is not received from the holding or farm, the animals should not be accepted on the abattoir premises, so withholding of FCI will have serious consequences.

Exceptions to the standard provision of FCI may apply if appropriate data have already been provided through a recognized, validated and audited Farm Quality Assurance scheme. Some small farmers may not be able to provide appropriately detailed FCI: their position is currently under discussion. Any information relevant to public health must be relayed to the OVS at least 24 h before ante-mortem inspection, in addition to the FCI.

If no FCI is available the OVS must be informed; only the OVS can permit slaughter of animals without FCI. In such case, final judgement on fitness of the meat must be pending and the meat must be stored separately.

If FCI is available, but not provided sufficiently in advance (24 h), the animals must be killed separately, since the risks to public health they represent cannot be appropriately determined. If storage space is unavailable, meat slaughtered without suitable analysis of FCI could be even declared unfit for human consumption.

FCI should flow not just from farm to abattoir, but also as feedback from abattoir back to the farm of animal origin. Post-mortem inspection data, as part of FCI, will provide very valuable information about animal health.

In addition, FCI can help to modernize meat inspection (refer to later chapters) in which public health hazards are controlled – but physical meat inspection handling (palpation, incision) is reduced so as to reduce microbial cross-contamination.

The following responsibilities are envisaged for those involved in FCI and subsequently modernized meat inspection:

1. Official Veterinary Surgeons
   - use FCI to categorize animals according to the public health risk they pose;
   - carry out ante-mortem inspection;
   - assess animal welfare;
   - supervise post-mortem inspection;
   - assess and audit GHP- and HACCP-based systems within the abattoir;
   - take samples as necessary for laboratory examination; and
   - BSE/TSE controls (e.g. SRM).
2. OVS Auxiliaries (trained)
   - Carry out post-mortem inspection in the presence of OVS (except in small or poultry abattoirs).
3. Abattoir staff (trained)
   - Staff should have the same duties as OVS Auxiliaries, but only within entirely integrated systems (primarily pork or poultry).

Further Reading

ABM (2005) www.abm.org.uk (accessed November 2005).

Anon. (2000) Opinion of the scientific committee on veterinary measures relating to public health on revision of meat inspection procedures. European Commission, Health and Consumer Protection Directorate-General, Brussels.

Anon. (2001) Opinion of the scientific committee on veterinary measures relating to public health on identification of species/categories of meat-producing animals in integrated production systems where meat inspection may be revised. European Commission, Health and Consumer Protection Directorate-General, Brussels.

Anon. (2003) Directive on the Monitoring of Zoonoses and Zoonotic Agents. *Official Journal of the European Union* L325, 31–40.

Anon. (2004) Regulation (EC) No. 854/2004 of the European Parliament and of the Council laying down specific rules for the organisation of official controls on products of animal origin intended for human consumption. *Official Journal of the European Union* L139, 206–319.

Johnston, A.M. (2000) HACCP and farm production. In: Brown, M. (ed.) *HACCP in the Meat Industry*. Woodhead Publishing Ltd, Cambridge, UK.

Maunsell, B. and Bolton, D.J. (2004) *Guidelines for Food Safety Management on Farms*. Teagasc – The National Food Centre, Dublin.

4.3 Ante-mortem Inspection

ALISON SMALL

Introduction

This chapter outlines the process of pre-slaughter inspection and evaluation of animals presented for processing for human consumption.

The roles of the veterinarian at the pre-slaughter point include protecting the public from food-borne disease and zoonoses, protecting the slaughter staff from zoonoses, protecting animal health through surveillance for serious and Notifiable Disease, and also protecting animal welfare through monitoring transport conditions, ensuring fatigued animals are allowed sufficient rest, separating bulls from heifers, polled animals from horned animals, and taking appropriate action regarding injured and infirm animals. Ante-mortem inspection aims to sort animals into three broad categories: those that can progress to slaughter normally; those that must be removed from the food chain; and those that need further, detailed post-mortem examination or require to be processed separately from the normal kill. The ante-mortem inspection should take into consideration information gathered from the holding of origin, as well as a visual assessment of the animal in motion and at rest during the 24 h period just prior to slaughter.

The ante-mortem inspection must be carried out under adequate natural or artificial light, and is an important part of the process involved in the production of wholesome, safe meat. As well as providing an assessment of the welfare status of the animal, it is an excellent opportunity for Notifiable Disease surveillance. However, its main aims are to gather clinical information which will assist in the final judgement of the resultant carcass, and to remove from the slaughterhall animals which should not be processed for human consumption. Ante-mortem inspection of the casualty animal often extends to clinical examination of the subject, in order to formulate a considered opinion on the fitness of that animal for human consumption. An animal that has been presented to the veterinarian already dead cannot be subjected to ante-mortem inspection, so cannot be processed for human consumption

Certain conditions, such as clinical tuberculosis, septicaemia or Bovine Spongiform Encephalopathy (BSE), automatically render the carcass unfit for human consumption. If an animal exhibits clinical signs of any of these conditions, it will fail the ante-mortem inspection. Animals containing residues of pharmaceutical agents also may not enter the human food chain. When the veterinarian carries out the ante-mortem inspection, it is important to bear in mind the clinical history of the animal, and also the health status of the farm of origin. It is also important that the details of the inspection or examination are recorded and that these records accompany the body to the abattoir, as they are very useful in the final judgement of the resultant carcass. If a body arrives at the abattoir with insufficient information to allow this final judgement, it may be rejected as high risk.

Another major consideration during the ante-mortem inspection is the issue of microbiological hazards. The major issue in the production of wholesome, safe meat at the present time is food-borne disease, caused by organisms such as *Salmonella* species, *Campylobacter* species, *Listeria* species and pathogenic and toxigenic strains of *Escherichia coli*. These organisms are carried asymptomatically in the intestines of livestock, and excreted in faeces. As animals age, they are more likely to have encountered these organisms, and as such, the prevalence in older stock is greater than in younger stock. Stress also increases the shedding of these organisms in the faeces, so a stressed animal, for example a casualty animal, is more likely to be shedding the organisms, and thus poses a high risk to its associated carcass, and to the carcasses of other animals processed at the same time as the carrier animal.

In order to protect the slaughterhall environment, and the carcasses therein, animals that are excessively dirty are not permitted to be processed for human consumption. The UK Meat Hygiene Service (MHS) uses a five-point system of scoring of livestock cleanliness, in which 1 is show-condition cleanliness, dry animal and 2 is a dry animal with small amounts of adherent bedding. Animals of scores 3, 4 and 5, with increasing dirtiness and wetness are rejected at ante-mortem inspection, and must be cleaned prior to being presented once more for ante-mortem inspection (Figs 4.1, 4.2).

The Casualty Animal

Within livestock practice, the casualty animal often poses challenges in the form of a complex decision-making process. Often, the producer has already made the first decision, that the animal is to be destroyed rather than treated, before the veterinarian is summoned. The veterinarian then has a duty both to that animal, on welfare grounds – to prevent its continued suffering, and also to the producer – to provide sound advice on the remainder of the process. Poor advice could lead to increased or unnecessary cost to the producer, or to failures to protect public health and animal welfare. There are two main classes of casualty animal, those that are fit to transport and those that are not. The veterinarian must assist the producer to rapidly decide in which class of casualty the animal belongs, following a decision-making process such as that outlined in Fig. 4.3, and act accordingly. Any delay will impact upon the welfare of the animal concerned. When the outcome of the decision has been reached, there is then a duty to ensure that the animal is destroyed without undue delay, in a manner that is humane and appropriate to the circumstances and to the species.

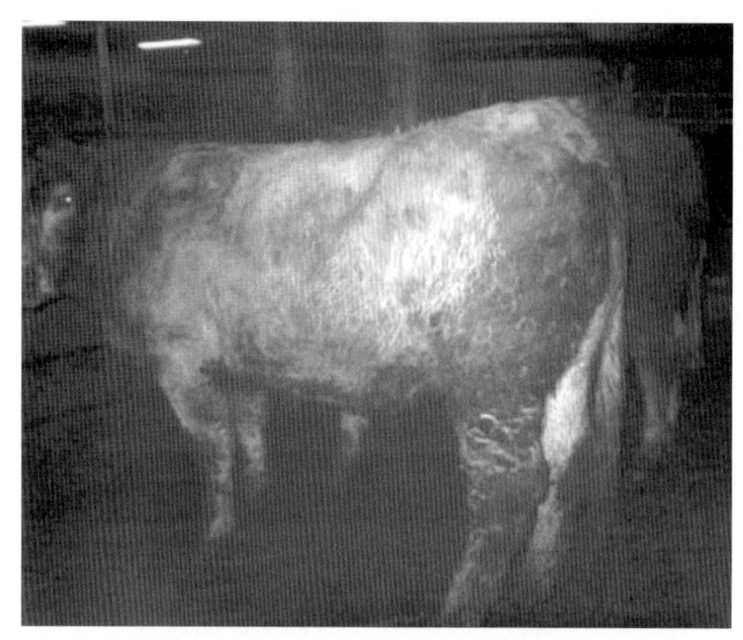

Fig. 4.1. Bovine animal which will require cleaning before slaughter. Note heavy tag on hind quarters and belly.

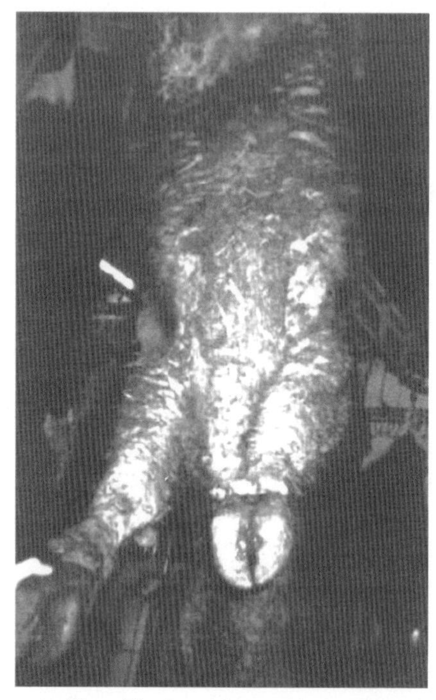

Fig. 4.2. Dirty bovine presented for skinning. Heavy tag on brisket and belly will make skinning difficult to perform hygienically. The dried faecal matter and bedding will also damage workers' hands and knives.

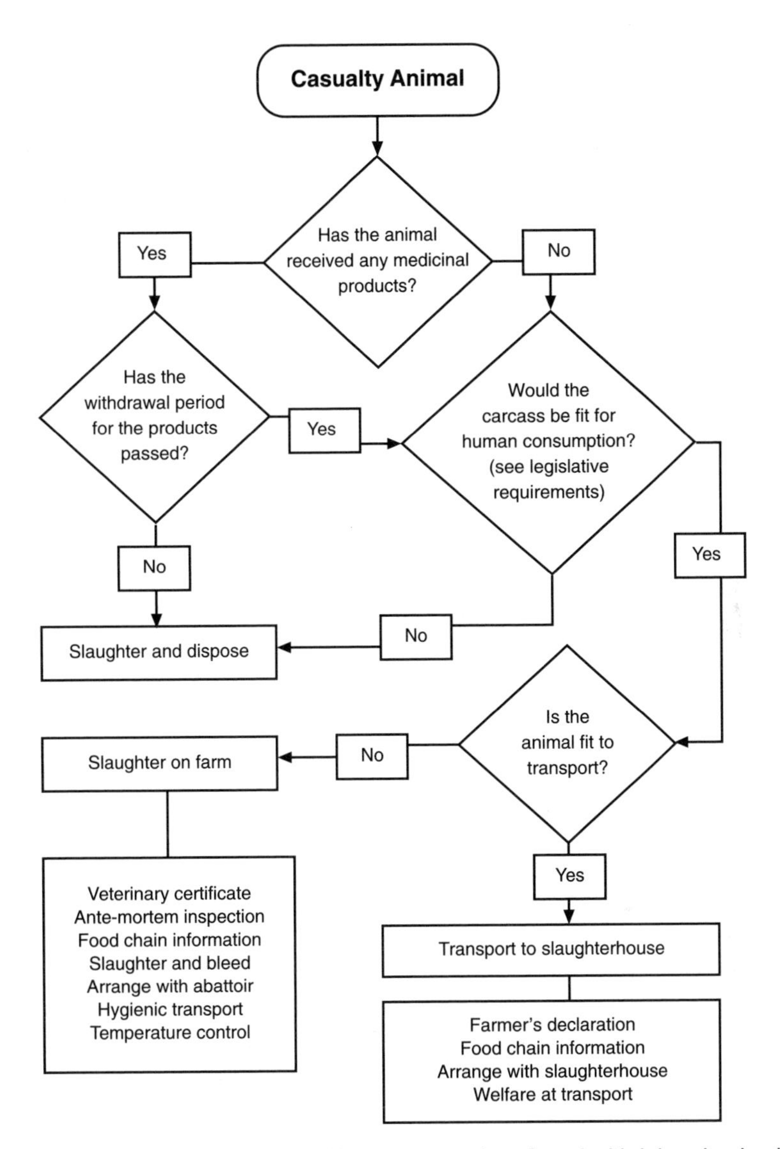

Fig. 4.3. The veterinarian's decision-making process when faced with injured animals destined for slaughter.

The decision

Fitness to transport

Animals that are ill, infirm or fatigued are considered to be unfit to transport, unless the condition of the animal is such that unnecessary suffering will not be caused by the journey. Similarly, animals which are very close to parturition, or have given birth within the previous 24 h, are not fit to transport, and neither are neonates, in whom the navel is not completely healed, nor infant animals incapable of feeding themselves. It may be argued that an animal could be transported direct to the nearest available place of slaughter or treatment, but only if the animal would be unlikely to be subject to unnecessary suffering by transportation in its condition.

The decision as to whether or not an animal is fit to transport can be very difficult, and needs to take into account the nature of the animal's condition, the form of transport available and the distance to be travelled. The animal must be able to walk unaided into the transport container, and be transported in such a way that does not allow the animal to experience any suffering. It is better practice from a welfare point of view to slaughter the animal on-farm than to subject it to the rigours of transportation.

Fitness for consumption

A casualty animal may be processed for human consumption provided that it has been slaughtered as a result of an accident, or because it was suffering from a serious physiological or functional disorder. If the animal is to be processed for human consumption, it must first pass a veterinary ante-mortem inspection. In the case of animals transported to the slaughterhouse, this inspection is carried out by the Official Veterinary Surgeon at the slaughterhouse. When faced with casualty livestock, the attending veterinarian is in a position to advise the producer on the animal's likelihood of passing that inspection. If the animal would be rejected at ante-mortem inspection at the slaughterhouse, there is little point in transporting the animal to the slaughterhouse. Where an animal is deemed unfit to transport, and is to be slaughtered on-farm, it is the duty of the attending veterinarian to carry out that ante-mortem inspection. If the animal does not pass this inspection, there is little point transporting the body to the slaughterhouse.

Economic considerations

Unfortunately, the majority of animals presented to the veterinarian as casualty animals are of low economic value. Occasionally, traumatic injury to an animal close to slaughter weight produces an animal of inherently greater value, but the majority are animals at the end of their productive life, or animals that for any number of reasons have not attained slaughter weight. The casualty process then adds costs, further reducing the value of the resultant carcass. As well as the obvious costs generated from the veterinary attendance, slaughter fees and haulage, there will be loss of any part of the carcass that is rejected as unfit for human consumption.

Many abattoirs do not accept casualty animals, as the processing often involves greater manpower and time than that in processing healthy animals, and often the abattoir may not have an outlet for sale of the resultant meat. An abattoir may be willing to process the carcass for the producer's own consumption, but there is often a fee for this service, and also fees for disposal of unfit and inedible tissues. If the animal is deemed unsuitable for processing on arrival at the abattoir, e.g. if it is excessively dirty, or had been suffering from a disease condition which confers automatic rejection, the entire carcass will be disposed of, and the cost of disposal passed back to the producer. These costs can be quite significant.

Certain animals may require diagnostic tests carried out on the carcass prior to being released for human consumption. For example, casualty cattle over the age of 24 months must have the brainstem removed and tested for BSE. The cost of this test may be passed back to the producer, and also costs of disposal if the carcass must subsequently be rejected. Similarly, if there is suspicion that the carcass may contain residues of pharmaceutical agents, tissues may be screened. This process carries high costs and can continue for a protracted period of time, during which the carcass must be stored. This storage may require the carcass to be boned, boxed and frozen, and again, these costs may be passed back to the producer.

The outcomes

The animal is not destined for human consumption

The animal that is deemed unsuitable for processing for whatever reason should be euthanased without delay to prevent further suffering. In the case of a bovine over the age of 24 months, the brainstem integrity must be maintained to allow BSE testing, so pithing should not be carried out. The body is now an animal by-product and should be disposed of accordingly, via an approved collection service or knackery. If the carcass is destined for animal consumption, such as to a registered Hunt Kennel, chemical euthanasia should not be used. Full records must be kept of the route of disposal, including individual identification of the animal. Cattle passports must be completed to show the death of the animal, and returned to the competent authority.

The animal is fit for consumption

An animal that is to be processed for human consumption must be slaughtered and bled using an approved method. This slaughter must be carried out either by the attending veterinarian or by a licensed slaughterperson. The animal or body must be individually identified, and be accompanied to the abattoir by the appropriate documentation and as much clinical history as possible. It is possible that in the absence of sufficient clinical history, the carcass may be rejected as 'high risk'. In the case of cattle, the cattle passport must accompany the animal or body.

In the case of the animal that is fit to transport, the occupier of the abattoir must be contacted and given notice of the intention to send a casualty animal, so that arrangements can be made to ensure that the animal is processed without delay, avoiding unnecessary suffering.

Where the animal is not fit to be transported, it must be slaughtered on-farm, having undergone veterinary ante-mortem inspection. These animals again must be positively identified, and must be accompanied by appropriate documentation, including a certificate of ante-mortem inspection and clinical history. Slaughter of the animal must be carried out within 24 h of the ante-mortem inspection, but the veterinarian has a duty to prevent unnecessary suffering, and may slaughter the animal there and then. Note that the technique of pithing may not be used in animals destined for human consumption. The producer certifies that the withdrawal period of any therapeutic agents used has elapsed, and the licensed slaughterperson certifies that the animal was slaughtered and bled in an approved manner. The slaughtered and bled body of the animal undergoes no further dressing, and is transported to the abattoir under hygienic conditions. This transportation must be completed within 1 hour of slaughter, unless the vehicle is refrigerated to between 0°C and 4°C

Biosecurity Issues

Any movement of animals, vehicles and animal products onto or off a holding carries risks to animal health. Consideration should be given to the fact that fallen stock collection vehicles may move from farm to farm, carrying out multiple pick-ups. It may be desirable to move the body of a casualty animal to a designated collection point, where vehicles and personnel can easily be decontaminated. For welfare reasons, the animal in life may not be able to be moved, and slaughter may be carried out remote from the designated collection point.

5 Slaughter and Dressing

5.1 Humane Slaughter

STEVE WOTTON

When any animal is slaughtered for food, it is important for ethical reasons that the methodology employed does not inflict pain. Researchers have demonstrated a relationship between the degree of pre-slaughter stress and carcass and meat quality, with increasing levels of stress resulting in decreasing levels of quality. Stunning prior to slaughter by exsanguination was introduced for mammals in the UK in the 1920s. The concept of 'stunning' in relation to an animal means any process that causes immediate loss of consciousness, which lasts until death (The Welfare of Animals (Slaughter or Killing) Regulations – DEFRA, 1995). It is essential that once an animal is stunned it is slaughtered as quickly as possible to prevent recovery before or during the bleeding process. A number of systems are specifically designed to kill the animal at the point of stun and following these methods exsanguination simply voids the carcass of blood.

Mechanical Stunning Methods

Mechanical stunning employs a percussive blow to produce brain dysfunction through the induction of a concussed state. The stun can be recoverable, e.g. as in a boxer's 'knock-out blow', or irrecoverable if extensive trauma to brain tissue is produced. The importance of the role of the skull in the induction of concussion is recognized in UK legislation (DEFRA, 1995) where the stun must be produced without fracture to the skull when using a non-penetrative blow. With mechanical stunning it is difficult to calculate exactly the forces acting on the head. However, the energy of the mechanical stunning system can be measured.

$$\text{Kinetic Energy (Joules)} = 0.5 \times mv^2 \quad (1)$$

where m = mass of the bolt (kg) and v = velocity (m/s).

The relationship between velocity, mass and the resulting energy produced is such that a change in the weight of the bolt produces a very small change in the energy of the mechanical system compared to changing the velocity of the bolt. Taking an average bolt extension of 7 cm and an average velocity of 50 m/s, the extension phase takes approximately 1.2–1.5 ms, in those guns that are fully buffered, and the bolt returns into the gun almost as fast as it is projected out. The physical trauma to the brain produced by penetrating captive bolt guns may prevent recovery; however, the application of a captive bolt gun is classified as a stunning method because the trajectory of the bolt – and hence the area of the brain that is traumatized – cannot be guaranteed, and some animals will recover following mechanical stunning. Therefore, it is important that the stun-to-stick interval is kept to a minimum and that the welfare of the animal is monitored throughout the whole process.

Recommended shooting positions

Sheep

When a captive bolt is used with sheep the target area is the highest central point of the head, aiming straight down towards the angle of the jaw. Adjustments are necessary when shooting horned animals to ensure accuracy and penetration. With horned sheep and goats the position is further back, behind the ridge between the horns on the midline and aiming towards the base of the tongue. The horned animals must be bled within 15 s of the shot to prevent recovery.

Pigs

In young pigs, i.e. pork and bacon weight, the shot position is at a point 2 cm above the rear margin of the eyes, on the midline and aiming towards the tail. In larger boars and sows the skull has a more 'dished' conformation, which has to be taken into account when positioning the captive bolt pistol. Shot position for adult pigs is at a point 5 cm caudal to a line joining the rear margin of the eyes slightly to one side of the midline. It is recommended that electrical stunning be used for adult pigs, because of the bone and sinus development.

Cattle

Cattle should be shot at the cross-point of two imaginary lines from the rear corners of the eyes to the opposite horn buds. In the event of an ineffective stun, the back-up gun should be repositioned 1 cm caudal and 1 cm lateral to the ideal position. With non-penetrative captive bolt stunning the shot position is 2 cm above that used for a penetrative captive bolt.

Recognizing the effectiveness of a captive bolt or concussion stunner

Signs of an effective captive bolt stun

Following an effective captive bolt stun the animal should immediately collapse, become rigid with its forelimbs extended and hindlegs tucked under the abdomen. The eyes should have a fixed and glazed appearance. There should be no positive corneal reflex and no rhythmic breathing (brainstem reflexes). Heart action, however, does not stop but continues for some time (3–4 min). If bolt penetration occurred there may be enough physical damage to make recovery impossible.

Signs of an ineffective captive bolt stun

When an ineffective stun occurs, the animal's eye tends to be rolled down, and instead of having a fixed glazed appearance the animal will show a positive eye reflex and can be observed to be breathing rhythmically. In the worst cases the animal may not collapse at all, or if it does so at the outset, it may get back on its feet. Ineffective captive bolt stunning can be caused by incorrect positioning or problems associated with the stunning equipment, for example poor maintenance, incorrect cartridge, etc.

Electrical Stunning Methods

The application to red meat animals of alternating electrical currents (AC) of sufficient magnitude will produce epileptiform activity in the brain. This is analogous to a human being undergoing a 'tonic/clonic' epileptic fit. During this fit an epileptic human is always unconscious, therefore a similar brain condition in animals is analogous to a stunned state. The production of epileptiform activity in the brain may not be immediate (>200 ms) however, but the application of high-amplitude AC to brain tissue will inhibit normal neuronal function for the duration of current application, thus bridging a possible delay between the start of current application and the initiation of epileptiform activity. The criteria for an 'immediate' stun are therefore assured.

Cook (1993) demonstrated that epileptiform activity is generated in the brain through the over-stimulation of nerve endings by the stunning current. The 'over-excitation' stimulates the release of two neurotransmitters (glutamate and aspartate), which at very high levels of production result in epileptiform activity in the brain. Thus a threshold is reached which, once exceeded, produces brain dysfunction and unconsciousness. This simplified view of what is physiologically a complex series of events does help to explain the results of Anil (1991) and Daly (1990) (Table 5.1).

The start of the recovery process can be identified by the return of rhythmic breathing movements (brainstem reflex), which returns when the epileptiform activity in the brain subsides. The times given in Table 5.1

Table 5.1. Time to recovery of rhythmic breathing movements following electrical stunning with low or high voltage. (Adapted from Anil, 1991 and Daly, 1990).

Species	Stun duration (s)	Time to recovery of breathing (s)	
		Low voltage	High voltage
Sheep	3	30	27
	7	30	31
Pig	3	43	46
	7	45	46

are from the start of the current application. Neither an increase in the stun duration from 3 to 7 s, nor an increase in applied voltage had any effect on the duration of unconsciousness produced by the stun. The results suggest that in both sheep and pigs unconsciousness is produced very quickly after the start of current application and that, provided sufficient current is applied, this period of unconsciousness is unaffected by prolonged application (across the range evaluated) or by increased current amplitude.

The recommended minimum current to stun is given in the Table 5.2. Low-frequency (50 Hz) electrical current can be used to initiate a cardiac arrest through ventricular fibrillation. Therefore, stunning systems that include the heart in the electrical pathway between the electrodes, e.g. head-to-back, will promote the start of death to the point of stun and therefore should be promoted.

Recent research has shown that the impedance of a live pig's head is predominantly a function of the stunning voltage, and decreases non-linearly with increasing voltage. These results suggest that voltage may be a more significant parameter in the production of an effective pre-slaughter electrical stun than was previously thought. In particular, the applied voltage should be in excess of the threshold necessary to break down the initial high impedance, to promote effective and immediate stunning.

Table 5.2. Head-only minimum currents to stun for red meat species.

Species	Minimum current to stun (amps)
Pigs	1.3
Sheep/goats	1.0
Lambs/kids	0.6
Calves	1.0
Cattle	1.2

How to recognize an effective stun when using electricity

1. The tonic phase starts from the onset of current application when the whole body of the animal will become rigid, rhythmic breathing will stop and the eyes may roll. The head becomes raised and the hind legs are flexed under the body. The forelegs may initially be flexed but then usually straighten out. This is the tonic phase, which usually lasts for about 10–12 s.
2. The clonic phase immediately follows the tonic phase and can be recognized by the presence of uncontrollable involuntary motor activity, i.e. kicking, which generally lasts between about 20 and 45 s. Eye roll or flicker and salivation are also often seen during the clonic phase. Termination of the clonic phase will lead to the return of rhythmic breathing and the subsequent recovery in an unbled animal.

The one exception to the above symptoms can be observed following electrical cardiac arrest stunning of cattle, when rhythmic breathing, as a result of residual brainstem activity, can occur in a cortically dead animal.

Carbon Dioxide Killing

Carbon dioxide is used for killing pigs in the UK, and more widely in Europe and America as a stunning, but not necessarily as a killing, method. UK legislation states that pigs may be killed at a slaughterhouse by exposure to a carbon dioxide gas mixture in a chamber provided for the purpose (DEFRA, 1995). CO_2 is an acidic gas that will dissolve in water or saliva to form an acidic substance. The gas is also absorbed through the lungs, where it enters the blood system and is carried in a readily available form. Once in the blood the CO_2 compound will cross into the fluid (CSF) bathing the spinal cord and the brain, where it increases the acidity (measured in pH units). When the pH is lowered from its normal value of 7.4 to 7.1 the animal will begin to lose consciousness. If the exposure continues, the pH will drop further and below pH 6.8 the animal will enter a stage of deep anaesthesia followed by death.

Concern has been expressed about the humaneness of the induction of anaesthesia with CO_2 in all species. Raj and Gregory (1996) showed that pigs would avoid high concentrations of CO_2, to the extent that they would not enter an atmosphere of CO_2 for a reward of chopped apples, even when fasted for 24 hours. When the CO_2 was replaced by an atmosphere containing the inert gas argon, with less than 2% oxygen, the pigs entered, fed and were stunned, recovered and voluntarily repeated the process. The researchers demonstrated that the use of an anoxic atmosphere, produced by an inert gas, to kill pigs was not stressful. Similar results have been obtained with poultry and fish. Anoxic killing using either argon or nitrogen is seen as a more humane method of slaughter, provided animals are killed in the modified atmosphere. However, because recovery from anoxia is very rapid, animals need to be exposed for sufficient time to kill them rather than just to stun them.

Carbon dioxide is pungent to inhale at high concentrations and is a potent respiratory stimulant that can cause hyperventilation prior to loss of consciousness. The time to loss of consciousness, based on the time to loss of somatosensory evoked potentials, could be as long as 38 s following exposure to 80–90% CO_2. Therefore, on welfare grounds, the use of high concentrations of carbon dioxide to stun or kill pigs remains controversial.

Mammalian Stunning and Slaughter

In a commercial slaughterhouse, pre-slaughter stunning is followed by exsanguination to produce the death of the animal. The majority of stunning systems do not kill, e.g. head-only electrical stunning, but simply render the animal unconscious for a sufficient period to allow the animal to die following the severance of major blood vessels. In the laboratory, death can be defined as the irreversible breakdown of the central nervous system (CNS). Brain failure or death can be diagnosed through the production of an isoelectric EEG or, objectively, through the irreversible failure of specific neural pathways.

The visual pathway is a basic pathway with perhaps only a single synapse between the retina and visual cortex. Photic stimulation of the retina with a strobe can be measured in the visual cortex with EEG or ECoG electrodes. Signal averaging techniques permit the identification of the visually evoked response (VER) and through the use of a system of moving averages the time to loss of brain responsiveness to visual stimuli can be identified.

The times shown in Table 5.3 are the average values for each sticking method in sheep. The different sticking methods were carried out under full anaesthesia and their accuracy was verified at the end of each recording session. A bilateral neck cut severing both carotid arteries and both jugular veins resulted in the fastest time to loss of brain responsiveness (14 s). Taken in isolation, this method could be considered as the most humane of the four methods tested; however, as we shall see later, these results should not be viewed in isolation. An inaccurate stick that might miss the vessels on one side of the neck prolongs the time to brain death by a factor of five. However, if the carotids are missed altogether the time is extended to nearly 5 minutes. Cardiac arrest produced an average time of 28 s but also promoted the start of death to the point of stun, presenting a distinct welfare advantage over the other methods.

Table 5.3. Sheep: time to loss of brain responsiveness. (From Gregory and Wotton, 1984a.)

Sticking method	Number of sheep	Time to loss of brain responsiveness (s)
Both carotid arteries and both jugular veins	20	14
One carotid artery and one jugular vein	8	70
Neither carotid artery and both jugular veins	8	298
Electrically induced cardiac arrest	8	28

With pigs the usual method of sticking is a thoracic stick, which severs the major vessels of the brachiocephalic trunk very close to the heart. For pigs there was no significant difference between a chest stick and cardiac arrest. The animals die due to a lack of oxygen reaching the neural tissues of the brain. This is achieved either by voiding the blood from the carcass through the sticking wound or by electrically stopping the heart and therefore halting the circulation.

When to stick

Effective head-only electrical stunning has been shown to result in a minimum time to return of rhythmic breathing (symptomatic of the start of recovery) of 37 s with pigs. On average, a pig will take 19 s to reach brain death following sticking. However the maximum time was 22 s. Given that sticking would result in a maximum of 22 s to 'kill' the pig, in practice this limits the maximum stun to stick interval to 37–22 = 15 s (Anil *et al.*, 1997).

The calf showed little difference from sheep and pigs, demonstrating an average time to loss of brain responsiveness of 17 s when both carotid arteries and jugular veins were severed during sticking (Gregory and Wotton, 1984b; Table 5.4).

Shechita in adult cattle resulted in the severance of both carotid arteries and both jugular veins. However, the average time to loss of brain responsiveness was 55 s, which was significantly greater than that observed in the other species. The range of times was also seen to vary greatly (20–102 s) (Daly *et al.*, 1988). This can be explained by considering the anatomy of blood vessels in the neck of cattle compared to those of sheep and pigs. In sheep and pigs, the vertebral artery has no direct connection with the brain, whereas in cattle it corresponds directly. Therefore, after severance of the main blood vessels in the neck of cattle this artery can still supply blood to the head. The delayed loss of brain function is also exacerbated by the formation of carotid balloons. This phenomenon was described by Anil *et al.* (1995 a,b), who examined the relationships between the blood flow through the carotid and vertebral arteries and brain function in calves during slaughter. They concluded that brain function can be sustained following severance of both carotid arteries and both jugular veins in the neck of calves, due to the occlusion of the severed

Table 5.4. Pigs: time to loss of brain responsiveness. (From Wotton and Gregory, 1986.)

Procedure used	Number of pigs	Time to loss of brain responsiveness (s)
Chest stick	8	18 ± 3
Cardiac arrest	8	19 ± 2

caudal ends of the carotid artery. When the carotid artery is severed at sticking, occasionally the muscle wall retracts within the connective tissue sheath and the sheath forms a blood-filled balloon, which quickly clots, thereby occluding the cut vessel and impeding blood loss. A solution to the problem is the use of a thoracic stick with both calves and adult cattle. If the blood vessels inside the chest close to the heart are severed, then blood cannot flow through the vertebral artery to the brain.

Poultry Stunning and Slaughter

Good practice in the poultry lairage and during shackling requires continual monitoring by personnel responsible for bird welfare. Lairage conditions should take into account ambient temperature, humidity and the general condition of birds arriving at the processing plant. Bird activity within and outside the transport containers should be kept to a minimum. Flapping, for example on the shackle line, will increase downgrading and reduce the effectiveness of electrical waterbath stunning. The shackling procedure itself combined with bird inversion has been shown to be painful to birds, therefore the time birds are shackled before stunning should be kept to a minimum (12 s for chicken and 25 s for turkeys). By minimizing this period, the welfare of the birds can be more easily maintained in the event of a line breakdown, in that there will be less birds to remove or, preferably, stun/kill with a back-up device. Research has demonstrated that there are doubts as to the welfare aspects of decapitation and neck dislocation, which has led to the development of an alternative killing system for use in the casualty slaughter of poultry (Hewitt, 2000). A pneumatically powered percussive device has been developed for use either as a back-up to the killer or for the dispatch of shackled birds in the event of a line breakdown. It is hoped that both neck dislocation and decapitation will be phased out.

Electrical stunning

Pre-stun shocks

The turkey can be used as a prime example of the welfare problem of pre-stun shocks, as the average incidence of pre-stun shocks in a survey of turkey plants was found to be 45% (range 0–87%). The prevalence of shocks in turkeys is exacerbated by the anatomy of the bird. Turkeys have wings that hang lower than their heads when the bird is inverted and suspended on a shackle line. This means that their wings will enter the 'live' water first and the bird will receive a pre-stun shock. It is also important that the water does not overflow at the entrance ramp, creating a wet route through which live contact can be made, otherwise birds will receive a painful pre-stun shock on the way into the bath. This is particularly a problem at slow line speeds and with badly designed waterbath entrances. Contact with a 'live' ramp will induce painful muscle contractions, which may result in birds flying the stunner or making and breaking contact throughout the stunner length. Waterbath entry ramp design and manipulation can be the solution for plants by holding back the bird at the top of the ramp for sufficient time to ensure that they swing down into the 'live' water in a fast, clean entry.

Electrical stunning equipment

Electrical stunning is the most commonly applied stunning method by the poultry industry. Birds are electrically stunned in waterbath stunners where the water is 'live' and the stunning current flows through the head (brain) and body of the bird to ground through an earthed shackle. Sufficient electrical current must penetrate the brain to induce a stunned state that will enable the bird to remain unconscious until it is dead either through cardiac arrest, induced at the point of stun, or by exsanguination.

Commonly, electrical stunners apply mains frequency (50 Hz) alternating current (AC) of sinusoidal waveform. A 50 Hz sinewave is one of the optimum frequencies and waveforms for inducing cardiac arrest though ventricular fibrillation. In addition to the induction of brain dysfunction, the applied voltage will also stimulate muscles to contract. This muscle stimulation is brought about in three ways: first, through direct muscle stimulation; second, through stimulation of the motor cortex in the brain; and third, through the stimulation of motor nerves in the periphery. The direct muscle stimulation can result in muscle haemorrhages and broken bones and this has led the industry to apply higher frequencies, which have a reduced effect on muscle stimulation.

Methods for assessing effective electrical stunning

Laboratory methods:

1. The method of EEG assessment is not without certain limitations; for example, it has failed to provide unequivocal indication of the state of unconsciousness as produced by sleep or anaesthesia.
2. Somatosensory-evoked responses (SERs) represent a basic level of response, which can be used to investigate the patency of a nervous pathway. The presence of an evoked response does not necessarily indicate consciousness, as they occur in conscious and anaesthetised animals (Gregory and Wotton, 1983). However, the abolition of SERs does indicate a profound loss of consciousness in poultry.
3. The return of rhythmic breathing has been used extensively in red meat species and poultry to indicate the start of the recovery process. The presence of rhythmic breathing indicates that the brain stem and spinal cord are still functioning. It is not a proof of consciousness, but indicates the need for further tests to establish whether the birds are conscious.

In the processing plant:

1. The use of rhythmic breathing assessment is a basic method that can be used in the processing plant to determine the effectiveness of a stunning system. If the bird has been stunned effectively, rhythmic breathing will not resume for about 8 s or more from the bird's exit from the waterbath. Looking for signs of rhythmic breathing is not a valid test of consciousness and/or death if the spinal cord has been broken or severed by neck cutting.

Effect of stunning current on efficacy of stun

The use of SERs has allowed researchers to measure the effect of increasing current amplitude on the effectiveness of electrical waterbath stunning. The abolition of the SER suggested that 120 mA should be the minimum recommended current level per bird. Measurement of whether a treatment can abolish a multisynaptic response is an objective method; however, it can be argued that it gives a very conservative answer, whereas the return of neck tension more closely follows the bird's recovery. These results, taken together with the subjective results using the return of neck tension, produced a recommendation for a minimum current of 105 mA per bird for chickens when an AC voltage is applied. Recent research combining EEG analysis by Fast Fourier Analysis and SER abolition has suggested a minimum rms AC of 100 mA per bird for 100 and 200 Hz, and that the current should be increased for frequencies above 400 Hz.

The poultry industry has adopted waterbath stunning using a high-frequency pulsed DC waveform with a 25–30% duty cycle, because of the improvements in carcass and meat quality that they can achieve. In addition, the use of low-frequency AC stunners at the minimum current to stun (105 mA per bird) will result in some birds receiving less than the minimum current, due to variation in impedance between birds whereas, with high-frequency pulsed DC stunners, three or four times the minimum current can be applied i.e. 40–50 mA per bird, and all birds should receive more than the minimum recommended current.

Slaughter

It is important that the correct blood vessels are severed and that the cut is made as quickly as possible following electrical waterbath stunning. When 105 mA is applied per bird at 50 Hz, about 90% of birds will be killed in the stunner (ventricular fibrillation). However, it is still important that the neck-cutting procedure is accurate. When higher frequencies are applied, the majority of the birds will survive the stunning treatment. The death process starts from the severance of major blood vessels when insufficient oxygenated blood reaches the brain. It is essential that both carotid arteries are severed at neck cutting to ensure the birds do not recover. An additional advantage can be achieved if heads can be removed by the killer for immediate maceration, which is a solution to the welfare concern over: (i) neck cutting procedures; (ii) the duration of unconsciousness produced by the electrical stun; and (iii) misinterpretation of normal post-kill bird movement.

References

Anil, M.H. (1991) Studies on the return of physical reflexes in pigs following electrical stunning. *Meat Science* 30, 13–21.

Anil, M.H., McKinstry, J.L., Wotton, S.B. and Gregory, N.G. (1995a) Welfare of calves – 1. Investigations into some aspects of calf slaughter. *Meat Science* 41, 101–112.

Anil, M.H., McKinstry, J.L., Gregory, N.G., Wotton, S.B. and Symonds, H. (1995b) Welfare of Calves – 2. Increase in vertebral artery blood flow following exsanguination by neck sticking and evaluation of chest sticking as an alternative slaughter method. *Meat Science* 41(2), 113–123.

Anil, M.H., McKinstry, J.L. and Wotton, S.B. (1997) Electrical stunning and slaughter of pigs. *Fleischwirtschaft* 77(5), 473–476.

Cook, C.J. (1993) A guide to better electrical stunning. *Meat Focus International* (March), 128–131.

Daly, C.C. (1990) Stunning and slaughter an overview – meat quality from gate to plate. Proceedings of a two-day course organized by the Meat Technology Service, Division of Meat Animal Science, University of Bristol, Langford, UK.

Daly, C.C., Kalweit, E. and Ellendorf, F. (1988) Cortical function in cattle during slaughter: conventional captive bolt stunning followed by exsanguination compared with shechita slaughter. *Veterinary Record* 122, 325–329.

DEFRA (1995) The Welfare of Animals (Slaughter or Killing) Regulations. Statutory Instruments No. 731, HMSO, London.

Gregory, N.G. and Wotton, S.B. (1983) Studies on the central nervous system: visually evoked cortical responses in sheep. *Research in Veterinary Science* 34, 315–319.

Gregory, N.G. and Wotton, S.B. (1984a) Sheep slaughtering procedures. 2. Time to loss of brain responsiveness after exsanguination or cardiac arrest. *British Veterinary Journal* 140, 354–360.

Gregory, N.G. and Wotton, S.B. (1984b) Time to loss of brain responsiveness following exsanguination in calves. *Research in Veterinary Science* 37, 141–143.

Hewitt, L. (2000) The development of a novel device for humanely dispatching casualty poultry. PhD thesis, University of Bristol, UK.

Raj, A.B.M. and Gregory, N.G. (1996) Welfare implications of the gas stunning of pigs 2. Stress of induction of anaesthesia. *Animal Welfare* 5, 71–78.

Wotton, S.B. and Gregory, N.G. (1986) Pig slaughtering procedures: time to loss of brain responsiveness after exsanguination or cardiac arrest. *Research in Veterinary Science* 40, 148–151.

5.2 Hygiene of Slaughter – Cattle

The general flow of operations during cattle slaughter and dressing is illustrated in Fig. 5.1.

General Hygiene Requirements

Staff

Staff working in abattoirs must be adequately trained, with training records suitably maintained. Suitable health records must be maintained for all persons working or visiting abattoirs, including veterinary science students, abattoir workers and veterinarians. Health must be assessed on the basis of transmissible diseases, and the issue of whether workers are healthy carriers of food-borne pathogens (e.g. *Salmonella,* viruses). Naturally, employees must not work when ill, and should undergo regular medical checks. In addition, staff should not work if immunocompromised, as this status could put them at risk from infectious agents from the livestock/meat.

Hair nets, beard covers, knives, steels, lockers, aprons, smocks, boots, etc. should be maintained and handled in a clean and sanitary manner. These measures help to ensure that the meat produced is protected from direct contamination from plant personnel.

Proper changing room facilities and suitable facilities for personnel to wash and clean personal equipment must be provided. Storage lockers should be kept clean and free of dirty clothes, rags etc. Shrouds, aprons, gloves and cotton items should be placed in a marked plastic container after use. These must be washed and dried before being returned to the processing plant. Staff must wash their hands on leaving the restrooms.

Equipment

Hot water (82°C) sterilizers for knives/steels must be monitored regularly for temperature. Multiple knives must be used by each worker, to allow adequate time in the sterilizer to ensure proper microbial kill. Hot water sterilization is effective against most bacterial pathogens, but ineffective against prions.

Equipment must be cleaned and sanitized at least daily. However, the Official Veterinary Surgeon (OVS) can require that cleaning and sanitation regimes are conducted more often, as necessary. Before work commences in the morning, the OVS must inspect the premises, checking that the abattoir is ready to use, all equipment is in correct working order and that cleaning and sanitation has been conducted properly. Regular maintenance and repair of equipment must be thoroughly conducted. Belts and other meat

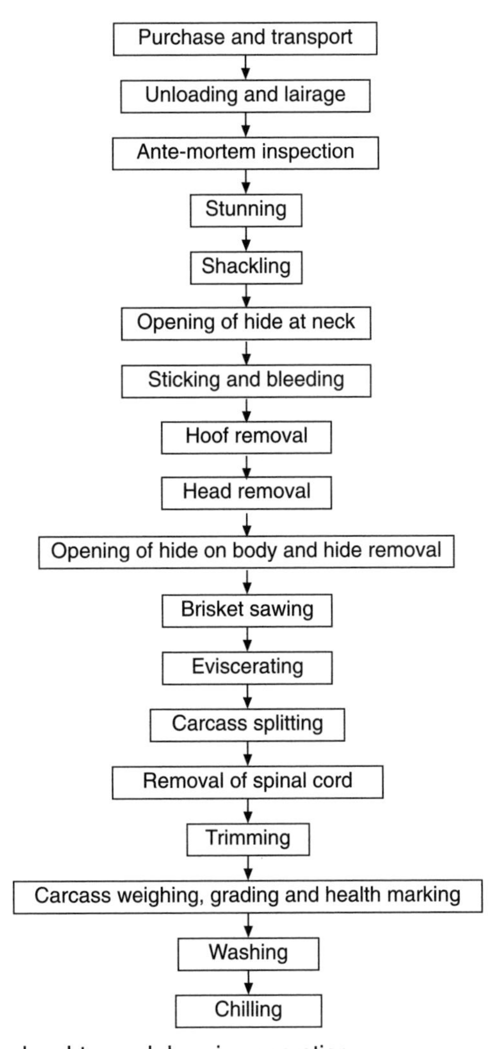

Fig. 5.1. Flow of cattle slaughter and dressing operation.

conveyance surfaces should be inspected frequently for cracks, pitting, etc., which can hamper cleaning/sanitizing. Complex equipment can experience a build-up of bone dust, meat and fat particles, which require special measures to remove. The OVS' role is to advise on the hygienic acceptability of, but not to remove, any suitable equipment being used.

Movement of personnel and equipment

As indicated in previous chapters, slaughterhouse areas are strictly divided between dirty (e.g. the lairage area) and clean (e.g. the slaughterhall) zones. Movement of all staff and equipment between clean and dirty zones should be kept to the minimum. Sinks, boot washes and clean outer garment exchange must be used at zone entrances. All staff, including the OVS, must maintain a high hygiene status.

Biosecurity

The security of buildings must be maintained, including roof integrity and door and window controls, so that ingression of pests into the premises is impossible. Active pest control must be employed for pests, including insects, rodents and wild birds. These organisms can harbour pathogens and could be significant sources of contamination, and must not be allowed access to the premises.

Hygiene of Abattoir Operations

Sources and routes of microbial contamination of meat

The main sources of microbial contamination of meat are the skin and hair of animals, the alimentary tract, the nasopharyngeal cavities and the external portion of the urogenital tract. Meat can also become contaminated from the environment, including the bacteria originating from the lairage area, from equipment on the slaughterline, from the chiller area and from the boning area. Grease, condensate, drip and cutting surfaces are possible sources of contamination. Naturally, staff are also a source of microorganisms in the slaughter environment.

Routes of microbial contamination of carcasses are numerous, but can be divided into two main groups: internal and external.

Normally sterile muscles of healthy animals can become contaminated internally, while the animal is alive, in diseased or stressed animals with bacteraemia (microorganisms in their blood). Other internal routes of contamination include penetrative stunning and/or sticking knife (see later).

External routes of contamination include all possible routes from the slaughter process during the production of dressed carcass. Such external contamination can be direct, from the animal coats to the meat, or indirectly, e.g. from animal coat – knife – meat. Other external routes of contamination are from the digestive tract during evisceration, from scald water (pigs only) and via airborne contamination within the slaughter area.

Lairage hygiene

An important principle in lairage hygiene is that animals must not increase their contamination beyond that which they have brought from the farm/transport. From the perspectives of animal welfare and meat quality, animals should relax and rest before slaughter; this would include lying down. However, if animals lie on lairage floors, their coats will become contaminated and animal coats are a significant source of meat contamination. Therefore, lairage floors should be kept as clean as possible. Flooring should be solid, non-slip and suitably sloped to adequate drains. Slatted floors can be effective, but difficulties in removing manure and conducting disinfection can occur – unless slats are movable (e.g. for sheep and pigs). Clean straw bedding is provided for sheep, but usually no bedding for cattle. The lairaging duration should be kept as short as possible, as long as animal welfare requirements are satisfied. From a meat hygiene perspective, the most desirable situation includes short transport times with animals unloaded rapidly and slaughtered immediately. Excessively long retention periods make lairage cleaning more difficult. The longer animals are held prior to slaughter the greater the build-up of infection, e.g. *Salmonella* in pigs and calves.

Clean livestock policies may be in place, as indicated in Chapter 4.3, and excessively dirty stock should not be accepted for slaughter. However, if appropriate, they may be held until last, and slaughtered after processing of clean animals is complete at the end of the day. Alternatively, they could be clipped and/or washed. Clipping of dirty hair improves the visible cleanliness of hide, but it may carry a risk of between-animal cross-contamination via non-sterilized clipping equipment and related staff. Animal washing also can remove visible dirt, but not the microbiological load. If animals are washed, they must be subsequently dried; hide–carcass transfer of microorganisms is higher if the hide is wet.

Hygiene of stunning

The action of mechanical (captive-bolt) stunning of cattle is recommended from the animal welfare point of view. It quickly produces significant damage to the brain and blood vessels and renders the animal unconscious. However, particles of central nervous tissue (CNS) in the form of emboli can then enter the circulatory system whilst the heart is still beating, and be distributed into the edible tissues. In the case of BSE-infected animals, or animals infected with other microbial agents, this may represent a risk to the human food chain. In addition, penetrating captive-bolt pistols could create the opportunity for cross-contamination between different animals via the bolt. Merely cleaning the captive bolt itself using antimicrobial wipes, as required by current legislation, cannot eliminate prions if present on the bolt. Furthermore, with penetrating captive bolt stunning, leakage of liquid from the hole in the front of the forehead can lead to contamination of the hide and the environment with CNS material, so the hole must be plugged immediately after stunning. For all these reasons, recent expert opinion (see references), recommends that mechanical stunning of cattle be appropriately modified to prevent occurrence of CNS embolism, or to be replaced by other stunning methods (e.g. electrical).

Hygiene of sticking (bleeding)

Two knives must be used during sticking to prevent internal contamination. The first knife is used to cut the skin, and it becomes contaminated from the skin. If blood vessels were severed with the same knife – whilst the heart is still beating – microorganisms would enter the circulatory system and be distributed into edible tissues. Therefore, the second sterilized knife is used to sever the blood vessels. Knives must be exchanged regularly and sterilized as frequently as possible.

Hygiene of skinning and depilation: cattle, sheep, goats, horses and deer

Dehiding is a critical process and must be controlled to reduce carcass contamination. A small initial cut is made in the hide using a sterile knife, in the normal manner, to open the skin. Thereafter, a sterilized knife is used in spear-cut fashion, cutting from inside to outside with the blade upwards, so avoiding transfer of any microorganisms on the animal's coat to the meat tissue underneath.

The workers' hands must consistently remain in the same place and must not be alternated. The 'clean' hand holding the knife is in contact with the meat, while the 'dirty' hand holds the animal's dirty coat. For manual dehiding, it is normal for two workers to process one animal, each person working one side of the carcass only. This reduces the risk that they will swap hands during the dehiding process. Ideally, the person working on the right side of the carcass is left-handed, and vice versa.

Dehiding usually starts from the free hind leg, which is skinned first, followed by the hindquarters. The skinned leg is then shackled to the rail, and the process switches to the other leg before proceeding to the hind quarters. Tail skinning should be conducted as quickly as possible, because an unskinned tail can flick or easily press onto the carcass: the area around the anus is heavily contaminated. To control spread of this contamination, an inside-out plastic bag is used as a glove. The rectum and anus area is grasped, then released from the surrounding tissue with a knife cut. The bag is then inverted over the released rectum, and sealed, either by tying or using a rubber ring. Another practice is to use a hook to fix the anus, release it and tie it up, although this is less hygienic than bagging the anus. Genitals are removed as far back as possible, and the opening of urethra should be covered with the bag covering the anus.

The next step is usually to cut the midline of the carcass: the process can start either from the ventral side of the animal (e.g. brisket) or from the dorsal side (e.g. back). The latter method, starting on the cleaner area of the animal may have advantages, because hide on brisket is the more contaminated. In-rolling must be prevented as the freed skin will contaminate the carcass if it makes contact. After the front legs are skinned, the best practice is to remove the cut surface, which is presumed to be contaminated. Hides must be freed from front legs, either abdomen or back, and hind legs, before any mechanical de-hiding can be used. Hide pullers are very desirable, although the hygiene achieved depends largely on machine design. *Downwards-pullers* are most desirable, as dirt falls downwards onto the floor, and not on to skinned areas of the carcass, and the dirt is effectively covered by the hide itself during the process. However, there is a danger of recoiling and flicking dirt onto the carcass at the last moment when the skin is released from the head. *Upwards-pullers* require the carcass to be fixed before pulling, increasing the risk of contamination. Also, dirt contained in the hide is carried above skinned areas of the carcass, producing the risk of it spilling onto the carcass. *Side-pullers* produce a lot of tension in the skin, and the large surface of skin freed increases the risk of inrolling, dust and aerosols, so these machines are less desirable.

The udder should be separated from the carcass and removed without spillage of milk on the meat, as it usually contains pathogenic bacteria.

Skinning of the head starts with removal of the horns, using sterilized equipment. Then all skin, including cattle muzzles, eyelids and poll skin, must be removed. Subsequently, the head is separated from the carcass. The head is usually heavily contaminated, particularly in the oral and nasal cavities. The animal may have been eating immediately prior to slaughter, so food may be trapped in the mouth. The head must be rinsed properly, and in many countries is considered an edible part. However, in the UK, the head is specified as risk material (SRM; BSE controls), and apart from the tongue (without any tonsil remains on it), does not contain any other edible tissue. It is important that the tonsils are not cut during tongue release, as they harbour many bacteria and could contain prions.

Overall, meat contamination from hide during skinning must be reduced by applying hygienic practices, but an additional approach is to decontaminate hide after the animal is bled (i.e. is dead) but before the start of skinning (see references). This can be carried either as decontamination of selected sites on the hide (e.g. along the lines of initial skinning cuts) or as whole-carcass decontamination. Hide decontamination treatments can be based on heat (e.g. steam or hot water) or on chemicals (e.g. acids, sanitizers, dehairing agents). Compared with meat (i.e. final carcass) decontamination, pre-skinning hide decontamination is a more preventative approach. The latter also has the advantage that hide is an inedible tissue, so its decontamination does not carry risks of leaving chemical residues in meat. Presently, hide decontamination is not used on a wide scale in the EU, but it is routinely used in a number of commercial abattoirs in the USA.

Hygiene of evisceration

After skinning, evisceration is another critical process posing risks of carcass contamination. According to current legislation, evisceration must be completed not later than 45 minutes after slaughter, or not later than 30 minutes after ritual slaughter. In the case of emergency slaughter, evisceration must be completed within 3 h of slaughter.

Abdominal cavity

The oesophagus is released from the trachea and tied very close to the rumen with a rubber band, using a special tool ('rodding' of the oesophagus), to prevent leakage of ruminal contents. Leakage from the rectum is prevented by 'bagging' of the anus; this was done during skinning. The abdominal cavity is opened by spear cutting with a round-tipped knife, to reduce the risks of puncturing the intestines and contaminating the carcass. The whole alimentary tract is removed from the abdominal cavity in one piece. As the rumen can be used for human consumption, a controlled method of separating it from the SRM intestines must be in place; leakage is prevented by tying the duodenum at two places, and cutting between, before separation of rumen from intestines. Immediately after evisceration the alimentary tract, including the inedible organs ('green offal'), must be transported to a separate room, where it is further handled. The spleen is removed with the rumen, to which it is connected, and then separated. The liver remains in the abdominal cavity connected to the diaphragm. The kidneys remain connected to the carcass.

Thoracic cavity

After opening the thoracic cavity by cutting through the middle of the sternum using a sterilized saw, the edible organs ('red offal'), consisting of the lungs, heart, and liver connected by the diaphragm, are normally removed in one piece.

Hygiene of carcass splitting and subsequent processing

Splitting of the carcass is usually carried out by cutting through the middle of vertebral column using saws, but by taking care to leave the spinal cord undamaged. The saws must be washed and sterilized between animals. As the spinal cord is a specified risk material, and may contain large amounts of prions in infected animals, it is immediately and completely removed (SRM). It would be best practice not to split carcasses down the central line but to remove the unopened vertebral column, together with associated dorsal root ganglia. In most cases, however, such practice is not used because some of the most valuable cuts of muscle are located along the vertebral column.

Washing of carcasses and offals

Carcasses are washed at the evisceration point to rinse off blood before clotting occurs and, again, after completion of the final inspection. After splitting, cattle carcasses are washed to rinse off bone particles/dust. Generally, cattle carcasses should be washed as little as possible, because microbial contamination cannot be removed – but may even be spread and re-distributed – by washing. Rather, any patches of contamination should be removed by trimming, using a sterilized knife.

Carcass chilling

Carcasses must be chilled ≤7°C, and red offal to ≤3°C. The offal tissues contain larger numbers of bacteria, and their structure and physicochemical properties make them a more suitable substrate for microorganisms. During chilling, meat must not be cross-contaminated via contact with walls or floors. Free air circulation must be provided around each carcass, which should not touch any others; contacts between carcasses lead to insufficient chilling of related surfaces and also mediate cross-contamination. Contamination by dripping from rail dirt/grease and from evaporators must also be prevented.

Cutting and boning

Cutting and boning is usually conducted after chilling, although the technique of before-chilling boning ('hot boning') may be used. The environmental temperature in the cutting/boning rooms is ≤12°C, as significant cross-contamination occurs during the process. Boning of chilled meat may have some advantages: (i) pathogens which originally contaminate a carcass are usually mesophilic, so are suppressed during chilling; and (ii) muscles are in rigor after chilling and firmer, so the boning process is then easier to conduct than before chilling. Hygienic hot boning is achievable, but may need to be conducted in specialized plants and requires specialized staff. Cut/de-boned meat is certified, packed in a separate room and shipped.

Hygiene of dressing of other species

Farmed game

The slaughter, dressing and inspection of farmed game is subject to the same arrangements and practices at abattoirs as other correlated domestic species; e.g. farmed deer are handled similarly to cattle. However, sometimes routine ante-mortem inspection and slaughter of game on-farm is permissible, i.e. in a licensed game-handling facility. In that case, the bodies must be promptly transported to the abattoir, where dressing is conducted at a separate time from other species. Subsequently, the abattoir must be thoroughly cleaned and disinfected.

Horses

Arrangements and procedures for slaughter and dressing of horses at abattoirs, and related hygiene considerations, are similar to those for cattle. One difference is the splitting of the head longitudinally through the middle, in order to enable exposure of nasal cavity surfaces to inspection for glanders.

Correlation of all parts of the animal

Throughout the slaughter and dressing process, all separated parts and the carcass must be appropriately correlated until meat inspection is completed.

BSE control measures

Specified risk material (SRM) must be removed during the dressing of animal and disposed off appropriately; for details see Chapter 6.3.

Dispatch

Carcasses and meat must be hygienically transported in clean, refrigerated vehicles. One potential problem is that hanging carcasses naturally swing and touch each other during transport, which leads to significant cross-contamination.

Further Reading

Anon. (2004a) *Good Practices for Meat Industry*. FAO Animal Production and Health Manual, FAO, Rome.

Anon. (2004b) *Meat Hygiene Service: Operational Manual* (Vols 1 and 2). The UK Food Standard Agency, Meat Hygiene Service, London.

Gracey, J., Collins, D.S. and Huey, R. (1999) *Meat Hygiene*. W.B. Saunders Company Ltd., London.

5.3 Hygiene of Slaughter – Sheep

The general flow of operations during sheep slaughter and dressing is illustrated in Fig. 5.2.

General Hygiene Requirements

The same principles and practices of hygiene during slaughter and dressing described for cattle are also applicable to sheep, so these will not be repeated in this chapter. However, there are also some specifics related to sheep/goat slaughter and dressing, and these are mentioned below.

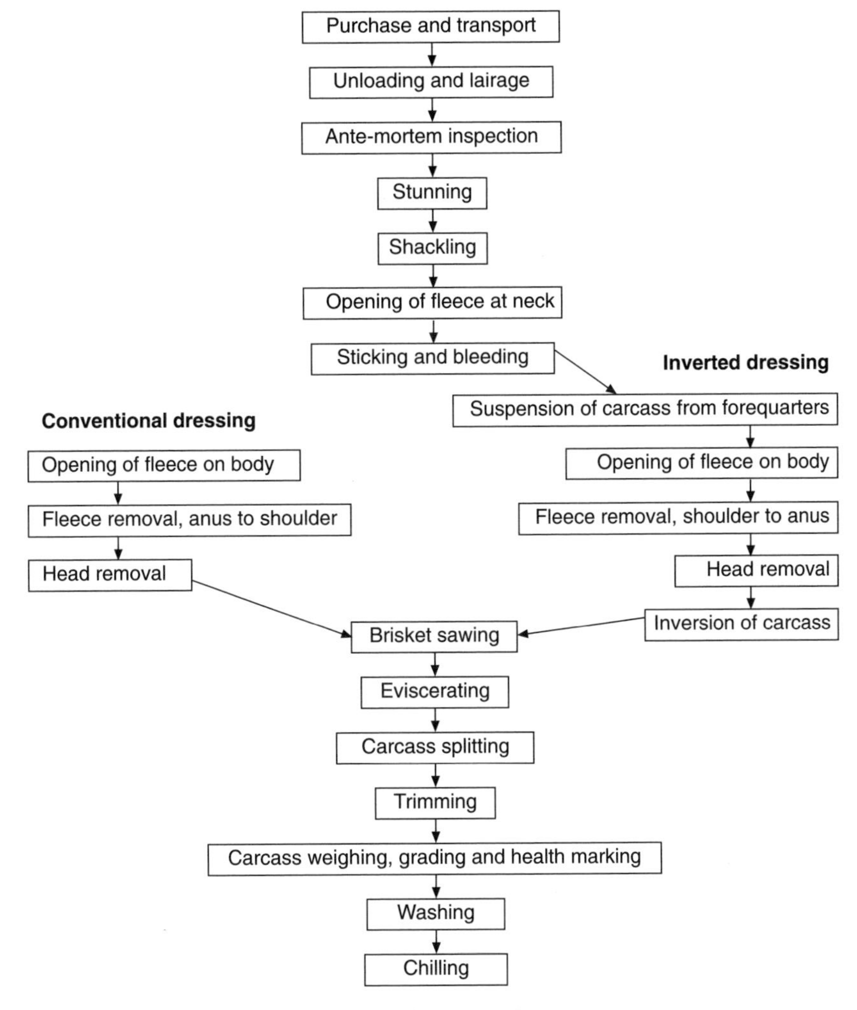

Fig. 5.2. Flow of sheep slaughter and dressing operations.

Hygiene of abattoir operations

Stunning

The electrical stunning method is most commonly used for stunning sheep. Head-only stunning results in the animal losing consciousness, but the heart remains beating. Head-to-chest stunning stops the animal's heart, resulting in death. Either of these stunning methods are acceptable. Penetrative captive-bolt stunning may also be used, but this carries the same risks as it does for cattle: dissemination of CNS embolism via the blood system to edible tissues, as well as cross-contamination from leakages from the stun hole. These are unacceptable from the public health perspective, although BSE has not yet been found in sheep – but has been in goats.

Sticking/bleeding

The two-knife system must be used for the sticking procedure, with sterile knives being used. Sheep with longer wool may present a greater risk of meat contamination, so shearing of sheep before slaughter – preferably on-farm – is beneficial.

Skinning

There are two basic methods for skinning (de-pelting) sheep and other small ruminants: inverted and traditional.

Inverted de-pelting commences at the cleaner parts of the animal, i.e. head and forequarters. Initial cuts are made on the front legs, along the neck and towards the brisket, and the first cut is then expanded. Punching of the fleece to initially separate it from the underlying muscle tissue occurs, which can potentially produce contamination of the meat if the operator has dirty hands. Operators should avoid swapping 'dirty' (holding fleece) and 'clean' (holding knife or punching) hands during the dressing procedures for small ruminants, in the same manner as for large ruminants. Use of crocodile clips can help stop in-rolling of the fleece. After these initial stages, skinning is completed by using various types of mechanical pelt-pullers. The inverted de-pelting system is considered to be more hygienic and to result in lower microbial loads on carcasses.

In contrast, the traditional de-pelting procedure commences the skinning procedure from the more contaminated rear end of the animal. Animals are usually shackled to the rail by their rear legs, initial cuts made at the rear legs, as well as between the legs, and the pelt is pulled downwards. This traditional de-pelting method is perceived to produce a higher risk of cross-contamination of the carcass, as the action involves pulling the dirty fleece downwards from the dirtiest part of the animal towards the cleanest parts. Modern sheep abattoirs most frequently use the inverted dressing system. However, the traditional system is still predominant in smaller abattoirs with low throughput, on farms and when sheep are slaughtered by hunters.

During sheep de-pelting, it is difficult to achieve the low contamination rates capable of being achieved during cattle de-hiding, as the animal is smaller, the fleece is longer and there is a much greater chance of fleece in-rolling and contacting the carcass. Therefore, overall, de-skinning is a 'dirtier' procedure in small ruminants than in larger ones.

De-pelting can be aided by injestion of compressed gas (air) under the skin using an inserted needle, which separates the skin from the carcass before skinning begins. This can make de-pelting easier, with less handling, and therefore more hygienic. However, there is a potential for gas de-pelting mediating cross-contamination, unless the air is filtered and the needle sterilized/changed between animals.

Heads of sheep may or may not be destined for human consumption. If the head is destined for human consumption, it is skinned; if not, it is left skin-on and removed later, subject to proper post-mortem inspection.

Evisceration

The oesophagus is released from the trachea and tied, in a manner similar to that used for cattle.

The anus is released, and the rectum is tied or bagged. Evisceration commences by cutting the abdominal walls, taking care not to puncture the guts. The whole abdominal cavity is emptied; the organs are removed in one piece.

The sternum and the thoracic cavity are opened so that the lungs, heart and, usually, liver linked with diaphragm, can be removed.

The red offal is separated from the green offal; the latter is removed and handled in a separate room outside the slaughterhall. With sheep, only the ileum need be removed as SRM. The different parts of the pluck must be separated, washed and trimmed.

Carcass washing

Lambs are normally washed between the completion of de-pelting and the beginning of evisceration. Any visible contamination on the carcass after dressing must be trimmed and not washed. However, a final wash is necessary to ensure that any remains of wool or fine hair is removed from the carcass.

Chilling

Carcasses must be chilled to ≤7°C, and edible offal to ≤3°C, adhering to the same hygienic principles as described for cattle.

BSE control measures

Specified risk material (SRM) must be removed during the dressing of an animal and disposed off appropriately; for details see Chapter 6.3.

Further Reading

Anon. (2001) *Opinion of the Scientific Committee on Veterinary Measures Relating to Public Health on Ovine Gas Depelting*. European Commission, Health and Consumer Protection Directorate-General, Brussels.

Anon. (2004a) *Good Practices for Meat Industry*. FAO Animal Production and Health Manual, FAO, Rome.

Anon. (2004b) *Meat Hygiene Service: Operational Manual* (Vols 1 and 2). The UK Food Standard Agency, Meat Hygiene Service, London.

Gracey, J., Collins, D.S. and Huey, R. (1999) *Meat Hygiene*. W.B. Saunders Company Ltd, London.

5.4 Hygiene of Slaughter – Pigs

The general flow of operations during pig slaughter and dressing is illustrated in Fig. 5.3.

General Hygiene Requirements

Pigs remain skin-on, and skin is considered to be an edible tissue. This creates significantly different hygiene considerations during slaughter and dressing compared to ruminants, the skin of which is not edible tissue. Hygiene procedures must ensure that the skin surface of pigs is as hygienic as the carcass of skinned ruminants.

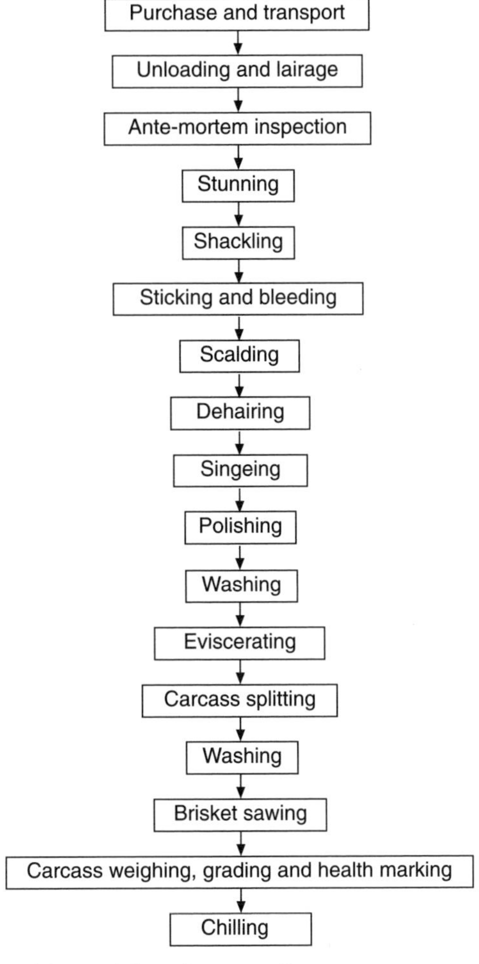

Fig. 5.3. Flow of pig slaughter and dressing operations.

Hygiene of abattoir operations

Pre-slaughter phase

On arrival at the abattoir, it is important to ensure that pigs do not become stressed. Pigs have a very sensitive nervous system, and become stressed easily. Also, they have very fragile blood vessels, and therefore can bleed and bruise easily. These stress-related aspects can have a deleterious effect on the quality of meat, more so than in case of ruminants. Therefore, the unloading, lairaging and ante-mortem inspection of pigs must be conducted with great care. During summer months, pigs may be sprayed with water. This calms them down, and can assist the process of electrical stunning by facilitating conduction of electricity. Lairage areas contain a lot of faecal material, which will easily contaminate the animals' skin if they lie down. Therefore, the lairage areas must be regularly cleaned. Passage of pigs from the lairage to the stunning area is mechanically aided in industrial, high-throughput abattoirs.

Stunning

Pig stunning can be conducted using electrical methods or with 70% CO_2 (see Chapter 5.1). With the former method, a conveyor can be used, which brings pigs individually to the stunning point. With the latter method, some animal welfare concerns have been expressed, due to a potential for pigs feeling pain when breathing carbon dioxide: CO_2 produces acid when dissolved in the blood. Mechanical stunning methods are not used for pigs.

Sticking/bleeding

The animal should be bled as quickly as possible after stunning. Sticking of pigs is not normally conducted using two knives, in contrast to the process for sticking ruminants. If blood is to be collected for human consumption, it must be collected in a closed system, using a special hollow knife with tubing connected to a dedicated container. These knives are sterilized between animals, as blood is very sensitive to spoilage, and can support growth of bacterial pathogens. Bleeding takes approximately 6 minutes, and sufficient bleeding time must be enforced to ensure live pigs are not sent into the scalding tank.

Scalding

Scalding is treatment of the skin with hot water, approximately 60–62°C. The water temperature is important, as too low a temperature will not loosen hair to facilitate its removal; and too high a temperature causes immediate denaturation of proteins at the hair root and skin, making the hair difficult to remove. Therefore, the temperature of the scalding water must be maintained and monitored. Scalding can be conducted using different techniques: (i) in a tank with submerged pigs moving horizontally through the water; (ii) by spraying with hot water in vertical position; or (iii) by treating the skin with steam. For practical reasons, the most common method in the UK is the horizontal scalding tank, although the latter two methods are considered as being more hygienic.

The hygiene of the scalding water is very relevant to the microbiological status of the carcass. Scalding dirty pigs in a scalding tank results in higher microbial contamination of the water. The water temperature (60–62°C) can kill a significant proportion of bacteria, but when dirty carcasses move through the tanks quickly, the level of incoming new bacterial contamination can be higher than the die-off. Consequently, the scalding tank water must be changed when it becomes visibly contaminated. This can be costly, in terms of heating fresh water, and because the production line must be stopped, so cleanliness of pigs is an important issue.

Contamination of the sticking wound – and even internal tissues – can occur during scalding. For this reason, the sticking wound should be as small as possible, and is always removed at a later stage during dressing.

Also, 'aspiration' of dirty tank water into the lungs can occur during submersion scalding, rendering them inedible. Naturally, this could occur if an animal is stunned but still alive (breathing) when placed into scalding water, which would represent a gross breach of animal welfare. However, this lung contamination can occur even in some dead animals, as the muscles of the elastic thorax relax, enabling water to enter the lungs. This lung contamination may be prevented by placing plugs in the animals' throat, but this has varying success. From a hygiene perspective, vertical scalding (spray) methods are more desirable, as lung contamination with scald water does not occur. However, these methods are more expensive, due to increased consumption of water and energy, greater equipment costs and more demanding maintenance.

Dehairing

Dehairing is usually done by placing scalded pigs into a dehairing machine, with horizontal rotating cylinders with rubber (or metal) fingers rubbing across the skin, which removes the bristles. The dehairing machine must be very well designed and maintained; if not, the heavy force and pressure can cause damage to loss of the skin integrity, leading to meat contamination. The dehairing machine can become very heavily contaminated as it is used on every animal, so its continuous rinsing/cleaning is desirable. Bristles removed by dehairing machine must be regularly removed and disposed of in a suitable manner.

The scalding and dehairing areas in the slaughterhouse are considered as dirty. Therefore, movement of all personnel, equipment and air from these areas to the dressing line must be restricted.

Singeing

Dehairing machines cannot remove all hair from the pig, so some hair remains, particularly at less accessible sites of the carcass. Therefore, these remaining bristles are removed by singeing. Essentially, singeing is done by placing carcasses for a short time (seconds) in a gas-flame oven with high temperatures (around 1000°C), which burns off the remaining hair. The surface colour of the skin changes during singeing to golden-brown due to the high temperature, which may be desirable for carcass quality reasons, e.g. with bacon pigs. Furthermore, singeing is an effective antimicrobial treatment for pig carcasses, and leaves the skin in an excellent hygienic status.

Scraping/polishing

Singeing leaves burnt hair on the carcass skin, which must be removed. This can be done in various ways, but usually carcasses pass through a machine with hard rotating brushes which scrub the burnt hair off. The brushes can easily become microbiologically contaminated as they are constantly in contact with a large number of carcasses. Unfortunately, this scraping/polishing process usually results in extensive microbial re-contamination of the carcasses. Therefore, the microbiological status of the post-polish skin is normally significantly worse than that of the same carcass before polishing, i.e. after singeing.

Ear and eye removal occur next, and the carcasses are normally washed between the completion of dehairing/polishing and the beginning of evisceration.

Skinning

Skinning of pigs, instead of scalding and dehairing, can be applied in some cases. The skin of older pigs may be required by the leather industry, and in this case the skin cannot be heat treated by singeing. Also, very large pigs – special breeds or older animals – may not fit into the normal slaughter line. The principles of hygiene for skinning of pigs are the same as for cattle. Again, the outside surface of the skin must not touch the underlying carcass, hands should not alternate and spear cutting must be used. Skin from the back is usually removed mechanically; some designs are more hygienic than others.

Evisceration

The cut in the middle line of the abdomen is made with a special round-tipped knife, which is much less likely to puncture the digestive tract as compared to an ordinary knife. The abdominal cavity is then opened, and the bladder and genital organs are removed, taking care not to allow urine to contaminate the meat.

All organs within the abdominal cavity are then removed in one step. Then, the sternum is cut to eviscerate the thoracic cavity, using sterilized equipment. Thoracic organs are removed and placed in trays or racked for inspection; usually, the liver stays attached to the lungs and heart via the diaphragm.

Different types of equipment are used to free fatty tissue from the abdominal cavity; understandably, these must be sterilized between carcasses.

Carcass splitting

Carcass splitting through the vertebral column is often done with automatic equipment which, again, must be cleaned and sterilized between animals. Mobile parts of equipment are always in contact with edible tissue, so sterilization must be assured to prevent between-carcass cross-contamination.

Washing

Carcasses are normally washed after polishing and before evisceration, as well as after splitting.

Carcass classification

Pigs are normally classified on-line, using a combination of several measurements. The pH is measured immediately to determine the existence of pale, soft, exudative (PSE) meat. The thickness of back fat, as well as of muscles, is also measured using electronic measuring and recording equipment. Also, after carcasses are classified, they must be marked accordingly, so the value of each pig carcass is known by the end of the slaughter line. Different carcasses are then normally diverted for different purposes, according to their value, e.g. for table meat, sausage production, bacon or ham production, etc.

Chilling, cutting and dispatch

Principles and hygiene of these processes are similar to those previously described for cattle.

Further Reading

Anon. (2004a) *Good Practices for Meat Industry*. FAO Animal Production and Health Manual. FAO, Rome.

Anon. (2004b) *Meat Hygiene Service: Operational Manual* (Vols 1 and 2). The UK Food Standard Agency, Meat Hygiene Service, London.

Gracey, J., Collins, D.S. and Huey, R. (1999) *Meat Hygiene*. W.B. Saunders Company Ltd, London.

5.5 Hygiene of Poultry Slaughter

Chicken Meat Production and Consumption in the UK

Poultry meat is the most popular meat consumed in the UK and worldwide, and has increased 100-fold over the past 50 years. In the UK, around 800,000,000 broiler chickens annually are consumed, which constitutes the largest poultry type – largely as fresh meat. Additionally, smaller numbers of spent hens and breeder birds are consumed. These latter types of poultry are normally consumed as meat products, not as fresh meat. Poultry consumption and its associated public health problems are increasing for numerous reasons, while consumption trends for other meats are steadily decreasing. The increasing popularity of poultry meat is largely due both to its simple preparation and to easy and quick cooking. Also, poultry fat is less saturated than the fat found in beef or lamb meat, which health-aware consumers may prefer. In addition, the flavour of poultry meat is very neutral, so it can be combined with numerous ingredients: it does not interfere with sensory perceptions of flavour balance in the dish when eaten.

Public health relevance of poultry meat

Poultry meats are a major source of *Campylobacter* and an important source of *Salmonella*. Poultry meat is regarded as the main source of *Campylobacter* infections in humans, although the sources of infections are not always identified. Campylobacteriosis is presently the most prevalent of foodborne bacterial pathogens, although other significant sources of this disease, including water, pets and other foods, probably also contribute to the total burden of this disease in the human population. Foodborne salmonellosis is primarily considered as being caused by poultry or poultry-derived products, including meat and meat products, eggs and dishes containing poultry and derived products as ingredients.

Poultry Slaughter and Dressing

Slaughter and dressing of poultry is highly mechanized, and has relatively simpler processing than that for ruminants and pigs. The general flow of operations during poultry slaughter and dressing is illustrated in Fig. 5.4, and will be briefly commented on in this chapter. More detailed information on poultry slaughter and dressing is available in other publications (see references).

In the UK, the hygiene and inspection of poultry meat is legislated by the Poultry meat, farm game bird meat and rabbit meat (hygiene and inspection) Regulations, 1995, providing details on procedures for

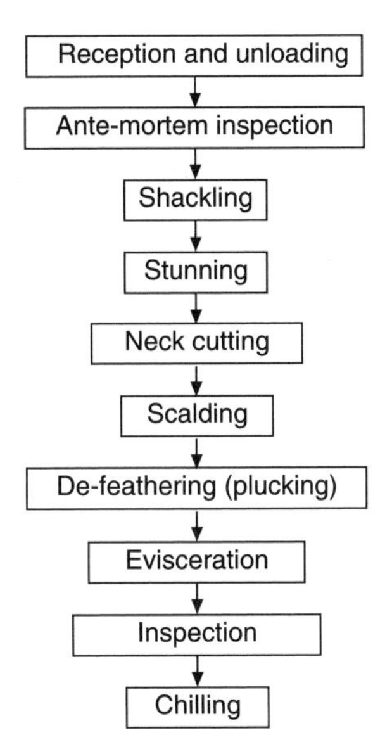

Fig. 5.4. Flow of poultry slaughter and dressing operation.

licensing poultry processing plants, ante- and post-mortem inspection, construction of premises, water supply for premises and facilities required for poultry processing facilities.

Construction of premises

In general, principles for the construction and operations of premises for poultry slaughter and dressing are similar to those for red meat abattoirs. Aspects that apply similarly to red meat and poultry abattoirs include: location, water supply, effluent/waste disposal, biosecurity, separation of clean and dirty areas, cleaning and sanitation regimes, durable and cleanable materials, staff health/hygiene requirements and related facilities, washing stations along slaughterline, meat inspection facilities including lighting, viscera processing room, detaining room for suspect carcasses, etc.

However, poultry abattoir operation significantly differs from red meat operations with respect to these two aspects: (i) lack of lairage; and (ii) specific technology and machinery used.

Transport of chickens

Broilers arrive at abattoirs in trucks, in crates stacked on multiple levels; each crate can contain up to 30 (sometimes more) birds. This normal, multiple-level stacking method of transporting provides greater opportunities for cross-contamination between birds than in the case of transport of red meat livestock. The poultry transport duration in the UK is normally around 4 hours, although some journeys may be considerably longer. However, long transport journeys are undesirable from an animal welfare perspective, as this may result in considerable stress to poultry. In the UK, normal practice with poultry is to withdraw feed before transport, in order to reduce contamination levels during transport, as well as to reduce the risk of meat contamination due to increased gut perforation during evisceration. The combination of hunger–thirst, with tight packing particularly, can be stressful for the birds during transport. Stressed poultry produce lower-quality meat than non-stressed animals, and also have increased levels of faecal shedding of food-borne pathogens; this is well documented for *Campylobacter*.

Therefore, the birds should be inspected at unloading.

Unloading and hanging

Birds are not held in lairage, but proceed directly to the hanging station, where they are picked from the crates and shackled. Diseased birds, birds showing signs of conditions causing pain, and runts, should not be shackled, but should be immediately killed.

Stunning and slaughter

On entry to the slaughterline, birds are stunned, most commonly with electricity (see Chapter 5.1). As this is an automated process, commonly with birds' heads dragged through electrically-charged water bath, it is necessary to have a back-up process for birds not stunned correctly.

Birds are usually slaughtered by mechanical neck-cutting with the head guided across a circular blade, or between two blades. In the case of mechanical slaughter, it is mandatory to have an operative manually kill any bird not slaughtered properly.

Immersion scalding

Scalding is one of the critical points in poultry processing. Scald tank water for chickens for the fresh carcass market is between 50°C and 52°C. These temperatures are too low to achieve any significant death of pathogens on the external surfaces of the carcass. Naturally, bacteria on the skin and feathers of the birds enter the scald tank along with the carcass. The scald tank processing, therefore, contributes to the spread of pathogens between all carcasses that enter the scald tank. With regard to the temperature of the tank, even relatively small increases in temperature can lead to a significantly higher death rate of pathogens in the scald tank water. However, higher scalding temperatures (e.g. 56–58°C) are used only for chickens to be frozen.

Feather removal

Feather removal is one of critical points with respect to poultry hygiene. Feather removal is a dirty process, producing aerosols which contribute to pathogen spread. A series of high-capacity machines with rubber fingers, or rotating scrapers, pluck off feathers from each carcass. The rubber fingers on the plucking machines themselves become very contaminated and can harbour large numbers of *Salmonella* and *Staphylococcus*, which combine with organic material to form biofilms. Continuous water spraying during plucking is normally used to flush out feathers.

Plucking machines are a major vector for cross-contamination of birds. Also, large amounts of aerosols are generated by the plucking procedure. The air spaces around the feather plucker are likely to be the most heavily contaminated with aerosols, followed by the areas at shackling, evisceration and chilling. Carcasses exiting the plucking area are highly contaminated.

The birds are spray-washed, the heads pulled off automatically, then the feet are also cut off automatically, and the birds are re-hung.

Evisceration

Evisceration is an important critical point; it is conducted mechanically, sometimes vacuum-aided. The highly mechanised evisceration used in modern industrial poultry plants requires careful control of machine settings, in order not to damage muscle tissues of the carcass. The fragility of poultry intestines and carcasses leads to regular breaking of the gut membranes. This produces internal contamination of the poultry carcass cavity, but also leads to cross-contamination of the machine and all subsequently in-contact carcasses. Bacteria in the protected poultry carcass cavities survive to a greater extent than do those that contaminate the surface of the bird. Washing after evisceration reduces the total microbial load, as well as the numbers of *Campylobacter*, on chicken carcasses.

Chilling

Continuous, in-line, immersion water chilling is the most common method for poultry carcasses. The carcasses move through a counter-flow current of water; finally, the meat must be $\leq 4°C$. Alternatively, carcasses can be chilled in air-chillers, particularly if intended for the fresh carcass market. At chilling, *Campylobacter* numbers reduce, but are not eliminated. Air chilling may have a greater lethal effect on *Campylobacter* than water chilling.

Carcass treatments for lower pathogen levels

Limited carcass treatments are allowed by EU legislation: chemicals and water washes containing high levels of chlorine cannot be used. Heat treatments (e.g. hot water washes) have limited antimicrobial effect: they can cause skin damage and colour deterioration of poultry meat. In the USA, irradiation is successfully used to reduce bacterial contamination of chicken carcasses, but in the EU this technology is not used. An immediate fast-freeze on carcass surfaces (crust freezing) is used in Iceland to successfully reduce *Campylobacter* numbers. Finally, forced drying is exposure of carcasses to high-temperature air for a very short time; this does not affect the sensory quality of the meat, but does reduce *Campylobacter* levels, as the organism is heat-sensitive.

Poultry slaughter and dressing: specific problems

Modern poultry abattoirs have high line speeds, processing up to 12,000 birds per hour (200 birds per minute, several birds per second). This contributes to specific slaughter and dressing hygiene problems, as the line speed makes it difficult to pay attention to individual birds. However, consumers purchase individual birds, so each unit is important from a public health point of view. Also, the high line speeds make inspection of individual carcasses very difficult. Naturally, from the producers' point of view, higher line speeds make production cheaper in terms of energy, water and staff usage.

Bird-to-bird contact during processing is frequent and unavoidable, in contrast to the situation in red meat processing. In practice, this means that one contaminated carcass can spread contamination to many other carcasses on the line.

Poultry carcasses remain whole, are not split and remain skin-on. From a microbiological perspective the skin is likely to be highly contaminated, but is edible.

Poultry slaughter and dressing use large quantities of water for carcass washing – much more than the amounts used for cattle and sheep processing. In contrast to red meat animals (e.g. cattle, sheep), trimming of contamination is not used in poultry processing because the product remains skin-on, and the line speeds are too high. Also, in the case of poultry, redistribution of microbiological contamination due to carcass washing is not an issue, because the whole carcass surface is similarly contaminated as a result of the technology and small size of chicken carcasses.

There is a very short time between the death of the bird and packing of the resultant carcass, which facilitates greater pathogen survival on the carcass surface.

Particular microbial hazards associated with raw chicken

The intensity of poultry production, both on-farm and at-slaughter, mean that cross-contamination is extremely difficult to control. In 1980, around 80% of chicken carcasses produced in the UK were contaminated with *Salmonella*. In 2001, around 5% of UK-produced retail chicken carcasses harboured *Salmonella*. This reduction in *Salmonella* prevalence on retail chicken carcasses has occurred due to on-farm measures including vaccination, better husbandry and the use of competitive exclusion and probiotics. In addition, hygiene of slaughter and dressing has improved significantly. Although retail chicken carcasses harbour lower numbers of *Salmonella* than *Campylobacter*, sufficient *Salmonella* organisms can be present to cause food-borne salmonellosis.

In the UK, the majority of housed flocks (60%) harbour *Campylobacter* at the time of their slaughter. *Campylobacter* occurs naturally in high numbers, up to 10^9 CFU per gram of chicken faeces. To date, there are no reliable on-farm control measures for *Campylobacter* in poultry. The organism has a high colonization potential in chickens, so spreads very easily between birds and flocks; it does not cause disease in the animals. Around 80–90% of chicken carcasses at retail are contaminated with this pathogen. *Campylobacter* numbers on retail carcasses can exceed 10^6 per gram, and even 10^9 per gram has been detected in a carcass rinse. Currently, the only control measure for *Campylobacter* in the poultry meat chain is proper cooking.

Poultry meat carries a significant direct and indirect risk of being a vehicle for food-borne infections. Both *Salmonella* and *Campylobacter* regularly occur on poultry meats at retail, and at infectious dose levels. For further consideration of the risks see Chapter 11.2. The main public health risk is associated with consumption of under-cooked poultry meat and cross-contamination from raw poultry to ready-to-eat foods.

Further Reading

Bremner, A. and Johnston, M. (1996) *Poultry Meat Hygiene and Inspection*. W.B. Saunders Company, London.

Jordan, F.T.W. and Pattison, M. (1996) *Poultry Diseases*. W.B. Saunders Company, London.

5.6. Meat Decontamination

Introduction

Total prevention of microbial contamination on carcasses during slaughter and dressing, even when using the best available techniques and methods, is not achievable. Although most of the microflora on carcasses are spoilage organisms, food-borne pathogens also occur. Intervention measures to reduce the numbers of pathogenic bacteria on carcasses may be employed at various stages in the meat chain, including final carcass decontamination at the end of the slaughterline. Presently, meat decontamination is not practised in the EU; the main reasons include concerns that operators may lower hygiene standards if they rely on final decontamination treatments. Currently in the EU, the only method allowed for decontamination of carcasses at slaughter is hot water; steam condensation and hot water may be authorized by the Official Veterinary Surgeon. However, in the USA, decontamination treatment at the slaughterline is mandatory.

Non-chemical decontamination treatments

The effectiveness of some non-chemical treatments is indicated in Table 5.5.

Steam Pasteurization System™

With this system, steam (105°C) is used to pasteurize the external surfaces of the carcass. The steam condenses on carcass surfaces at temperatures between 80°C and 85°C, causing only temporary deleterious colour changes from red to grey–brown. However, the carcass recovers normal red colour after chilling. The carcass surface temperature is critical, since temperatures of >85°C cause permanent discolouration, i.e. the grey–brown colour of cooked meat. However, temperatures <80°C are insufficiently effective in killing microorgnisms. Reductions of 2.5 to 3.7 logs of pathogenic bacteria (e.g. *L. monocytogenes*, *E. coli* O157, *Salmonella*) have been reported for steam pasteurization. Therefore, high numbers of bacterial pathogens cannot be totally eliminated using this procedure.

Instead of steam, hot water treatments can be used, with a similar temperature window.

Irradiation

Irradiation is currently used in the USA, primarily for minced meats and poultry, which have greater public health risks. Effective doses range from 1 to 3 kGy, but irradiation at higher doses can cause sensory (particularly colour) changes in the meat. The types of irradiation used for meat decontamination (gamma rays, X-rays) do not induce secondary radiation

Table 5.5. Effectiveness of non-chemical treatments.

Treatment	Examples of bacterial reduction (log) on meat achieved
Spot-cleaning (steam/hot water vacuuming)	Total bacterial count 1.7–2.0, coliforms 1.7–2.2
Combination of knife trimming and water spray washing (28–42°C)	Total bacterial count 1.0–1.8, *E. coli* count 1.0–1.6, coliforms 1.6
Hot water (74–83.5°C)	Total bacterial count 0.66–2.00, *E. coli*/coliform count 1.8–3.0; pathogens (*Salmonella*, *E. coli* O157, *Yersinia*, *L. monocytogenes*) 3.0
Pressurized steam on chickens (180–200°C)	Total bacterial count 1.0–3.0, *Salmonella* by 50%
Steam Pasteurization System™ (105°C)	Pathogens (*L. monocytogenes*, *E. coli* O157, *Salmonella*) 2.5–3.7, total bacterial count/coliforms 1.4
Multiple hurdle decontamination	*E. coli* 4.3
Effects of high-temperature treatments on meat quality	(i) Generally, temperatures >80°C but <85°C cause bleached, grey or 'cooked' meat appearance, to approximate depth of 0.5 mm. However, this is usually unnoticed after a few hours of chilling. (ii) Exposure to temperatures >85°C causes permanent damage to surface bloom
Irradiation: poultry (frozen 3–5 kGy; chilled 1.5–2.5 kGy)	*Salmonella* 3, *Campylobacter* >3
Irradiation: eggs (4–5 kGy)	*Salmonella* 7–8, total bacterial count 6
Irradiation: red meat (1–3 kGy)	*Salmonella* 2–3
Limitations of irradiation	Does not inactivate viruses or microbial toxins, causes sensory changes at higher doses
Ultrasound (in liquid substrates)	*Salmonella* <1–4
Electromagnetic radiation (in various substrates or on meat)	(i) Microwave: *Salmonella* 1–2 (ii) Visible light: total bacterial count 1–3 (iii) Ultra-violet: *Salmonella*, *Staphylococcus*, *Yersinia*, *Campylobacter* 0.4–3.0
Electricity (high-voltage pulsed electric field)	In fluid foods: *Staphylococcus aureus*, *E. coli* up to 6
High pressure	At 400–450 MNm^{-2}: total bacterial count 3–5

in the product (the meat does not become radioactive), although this is frequently a concern in consumer acceptance tests. Pathogen reductions of 2 to 3 logs for *Salmonella* have been obtained. However, irradiation does not inactivate viruses or pre-formed microbial toxins. On the other hand, there are concerns that irradiation may enhance fat oxidation, contributing to formation of potentially toxic free radicals, believed to be carcinogenic compounds.

Electricity (high-voltage pulsed field)

Application is limited to liquid foods, in which *Staphylococcus aureus* and *E. coli* O157 reductions of up to 6 logs were achieved. However, this method is largely experimental.

High pressure

Pressure at 400 to 450 MN/m^2 has been used in experimental conditions to reduce total bacterial counts by 3 to 5 logs. This technique would be largely restricted to liquid foods.

Chemical decontamination treatments

The effectivenes and feasibility of some chemical treatments are summarized in Table 5.6.

Acid treatments (lactic, acetic, citric, fumaric)

Weak organic acids, which are used in other areas of food processing, are normally used for acid treatments of carcasses. Salts of organic acids have only bacteriostatic effects, and do not kill bacteria to a significant extent. Acid treatments of red meat carcasses are common in the USA, and reductions of up to 4.5 logs have been reported, e.g. for *Yersinia*. However, acid treatments were found to be less effective against the more common meat-borne pathogenic bacteria including *Salmonella* and *E. coli* O157.

The antimicrobial effectiveness of acid treatments depends on numerous factors, including characteristics of the acid itself and the characteristics of the target microorganism(s). Acids are less effective against mesophillic pathogens, but can be more effective against psychrotrophs. At the time of slaughter, most of the microbial load on carcasses is comprised of mesophillic bacteria. Some pathogens appear to be more acid resistant (e.g. *E. coli* O157 and *Listeria*) than others. If not all pathogens are killed, due to differences in sensitivity between and within bacterial species, meat decontamination could result in the selection of highly resistant strains. This could potentially increase problems with their control during subsequent meat preservation/ processing stages.

Technical aspects of the acid used must be also considered. These include the issue of their impact on the environment, unless they are suitably treated before disposal.

Table 5.6. Factors affecting feasibility and effectiveness of chemical treatments.

Consideration of factors affecting antimicrobial efficacy	Practical considerations	Examples of bacterial reduction (log) on meat achieved
Acid characteristics	Technical aspects	Acids (lactic, acetic, citric, fumaric)
Concentration required	Method of application	
Solubility	Contact time required	*Salmonella*: 0.4–2.0
Dissociation at meat pH	Temperature	*E. coli* O157: 0.3–2.0
Ability to penetrate the bacterial cell	Pressure	*Listeria*: up to 2
	Target tissue characteristics	*Yersinia*: up to 4.5
Intracellular action		*Aeromonas*: up to 3.5
Specific reactions with meat compounds	Impact on the environment/equipment	Salts of organic acids
Toxicity/residues (GRAS or additive)	Recycling/neutralization	Bacteriostatic effects only
	Staff health	
	Costs	
Characteristics of target organism(s)	Consumer attitude	Non-acid chemicals
		Chlorine: *Salmonella* 1.5, *E. coli* O157 1.3
Psychrotrophic or mesophyllic nature	Meat quality aspects	Trisodium phosphate: *Salmonella* 0.9, *E. coli* O157 1.4, *Listeria* 1, *Staphylococcus* 1
	Fat discolouration	
Some pathogens particularly resistant (*E. coli* O157, *Listeria*)	Lean bleaching	
	Change of flavour/odour	
	Water-holding (drip)	
Initial microbial load	Sensory scores	Hydrogen peroxide: total bacterial count 1–3
Intra-species strain/clonal selection	Meat shelf life	Ozone solution: total bacterial counts: 1.0–2.9
Enhanced regrowth in absence of competitors		Animal dehairing by sodium sulphide/H_2O_2:
Stress-mediated resistance to subsequent treatments		*E. coli* O157 3, *Salmonella* 3, *Listeria* 3, total bacterial count 1.0–1.5
Change of virulence		

Acid treatments could also have deleterious effects on meat quality. Fat discolouration, lean bleaching and alterations in flavour and odour can occur. The water-holding (drip) characteristics can also be altered. In addition, the negative effects on meat quality can actually shorten product shelf life, instead of its expected lengthening.

Non-acidic chemical treatments

Non-acidic chemicals currently in commercial use are chlorine and trisodium phosphate. Chlorine was previously widely used in the UK poultry industry (reductions of *Salmonella* by 1.5 logs), but has been banned due to its possible reactions which can result in potentially carcinogenic compounds.

Trisodium phosphate is in current commercial use, and achieved pathogen reductions range roughly between 1 and 2 logs.

Overall considerations

Because carcasses are often contaminated with food-borne pathogens even under best hygiene conditions in commercial abattoirs, decontamination treatments may be beneficial for meat safety. However, presently available treatments only proportionally reduce the microbial load, which raises questions about positive selection for toughest microbial strains in the surviving populations. Obviously, meat decontamination should not be considered as a substitute for good overall process hygiene: the cleaner the carcass the better the decontamination effects. The role of final carcass decontamination in meat safety systems should be considered simultaneously with some other alternative or additional approaches, such as pre-skinning hide decontamination.

Further Reading

Anon. (1998) *Opinion of the Scientific Committee on Veterinary Measures Relating to Public Health on Benefits and Limitations of Antimicrobial Treatments for Poultry Carcasses*. European Commission, Consumer Health and Protection Directorate-General, Brussels.

Farkas, J. (1998) Irradiation as a method for decontaminating food. A Review. *International Journal of Food Microbiology* 44, 189–206.

James, C. (1999) Past, present and future methods of meat decontamination: update 1999. MAFF Fellowship in Food Process Engineering, University of Bristol, UK.

James, C., Goksoy, E.O. and James, S.J. (1997) Past, present and future methods of meat decontamination. MAFF Fellowship in Food Process Engineering, University of Bristol, UK.

Smulders, F.J.M. and Greer, G.G. (1998) Integrating microbial decontamination with organic acids in HACCP programmes for muscle foods: prospects and controversies. *International Journal of Food Microbiology* 44, 149–169.

6 Post-mortem Meat Inspection

6.1 Meat Inspection – General Principles

The purpose of meat inspection is to certify whether or not meat is fit for human consumption. There are no clearly written guidelines covering all situations; instead, the Official Veterinary Surgeon (OVS) has overall responsibility for the decision. In the UK, meat inspection is normally conducted by meat hygiene inspectors, who do not have a university qualification, but do have up to 2 years' formal training in higher education. Meat inspectors are supervised by the OVS or veterinarian in the plant. Meat inspectors conduct routine, technical inspection, and can approve any meat which appears to have no abnormalities. For more unclear or difficult cases, however, the responsibility passes to the OVS. This is a great responsibility with both ethical and legal implications, and with serious consequences. Therefore, each OVS must feel satisfied with own decision, and be ready for further consultation, as necessary.

Meat inspection must be conducted systematically. In the case of inspection at abattoirs, the system is normally well set up, but in other situations (e.g. on-farm), there may be no normal inspection system operating. For example, if any organs are not available for inspection, the carcass cannot be inspected thoroughly, and the meat must not be passed for human consumption. Incorrect inspection and approval of unfit meat could have extremely serious consequences for a number of people purchasing and/or consuming the product.

The technical procedures for post-mortem inspection were set up around 150 years ago, and have not changed substantially since then. The basic steps include:

1. Visual examination of the whole carcass and all organs should always be conducted first, because the inspector should not endanger his/her own health or that of other people by unnecessary handling of an animal with obvious signs of a transmissible disease. Visual inspection implies that the inspector is familiar with the normal appearance of tissues and organs, so that abnormalities can be assessed; the focus is on the size, shape and colour.

2. Palpation of the organs is routinely used, as specified for different organs/tissues in different species, to get a feeling of the 'texture' of the tissue: stickiness, softness, dryness, wetness, etc. Palpation is useful for organs or tissues with conditions that do not always produce a visible difference, e.g. arthritis.
3. Incision of organs/tissues is routinely used, but not for all organs and tissues.
4. Any additional examinations are conducted when the meat inspector or OVS considers it necessary, including taking samples for rapid (on-site) laboratory tests if needed. Further investigation is needed when any abnormalities are found, to assess their nature and extent. At this stage, incisions may be applied more extensively, to obtain the necessary information, and samples may be taken for laboratory investigation as necessary. Further investigation, over that required for routine inspection, can be costly, but this is a secondary consideration when extra assurance for protection of public health is required.

During post-mortem inspection, it is often necessary to determine whether the slaughtered animal is female or male, because some diseases are sex-linked, appearance of organs/tissues can differ between sexes, and overall size/condition of the carcass can vary with the sex. The main parameters used for sex determination on carcasses are indicated in Table 6.1.

Understandably, not every single part of the tissues/organs in the animal can be inspected for signs of abnormalities in great detail, so examination of the state of the lymph nodes may help to determine the status of the correlated body parts. The lymph node is assumed to be an indicator of the existence of pathological processes in the region from which it drains lymph; its status indicates whether there is a need to inspect the related organ/tissue directly and in greater detail. The lymph node, while reacting to harmful or infectious agents, may change appearance: become enlarged, have haemorrhages, abscesses, etc. Obviously, to use the information obtained from lymph node inspection, the inspector must be familiar with the anatomical location and physiological role of individual lymph nodes, the area from where each lymph node drains the lymph fluid and the flow of the lymph between lymph nodes (see Figs 6.1 and 6.2).

Using basic inspection techniques described above, carcasses and offal (and blood where appropriate) of all animal species are routinely examined for:

- sex and age;
- state of nutrition;
- local/general oedema;
- efficacy of bleeding;
- swelling/deformity;
- abnormal colour, odour or taste;
- condition of pleura and peritoneum;
- any other abnormality; and
- signs of specific diseases.

Table 6.1. Sex determinants in carcasses post-slaughter.

Determinant	Typical visual differences between sexes	
	Male	Female
Bovine	Bull	Cow
Shoulder and neck muscles	Massive	Smaller
Gracilis muscle shape	Rhomboid or triangular	Bean or kidney
Bulbo-cavernosus muscle	Well developed	Muscle lacking
Pelvis	Narrow, with angular floor	Wide, spacious with flat floor
External genitals	Root of penis may be attached to carcass	Visible region after removal of udder
	Bullock	Heifer
	As above, but less marked	As above, but less marked
Porcine	Boar	Gilt
Gracilis muscle shape	Rhomboid or triangular	Bean or kidney
Shoulder shape	Oval piece of cartilage over shoulder region	No cartilage
Teeth	Strong, curved canines	
External genitals	Visible region after removal of scrotum and penis. Root of penis can be seen	Large space below tail after removal of anus and vulva Abdominal incision for evisceration is straight
	Hog	
	Evidence of castration scars and removal of prepuce. Otherwise, similar in appearance to gilt	

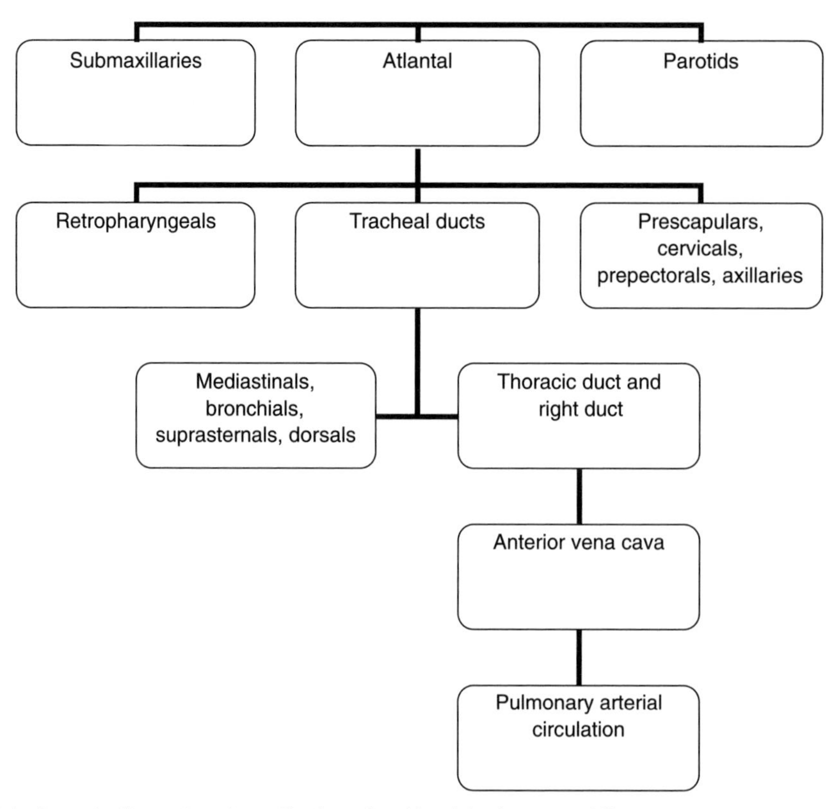

Fig. 6.1. Lymphatic system in cattle (proximal body): downward flow.

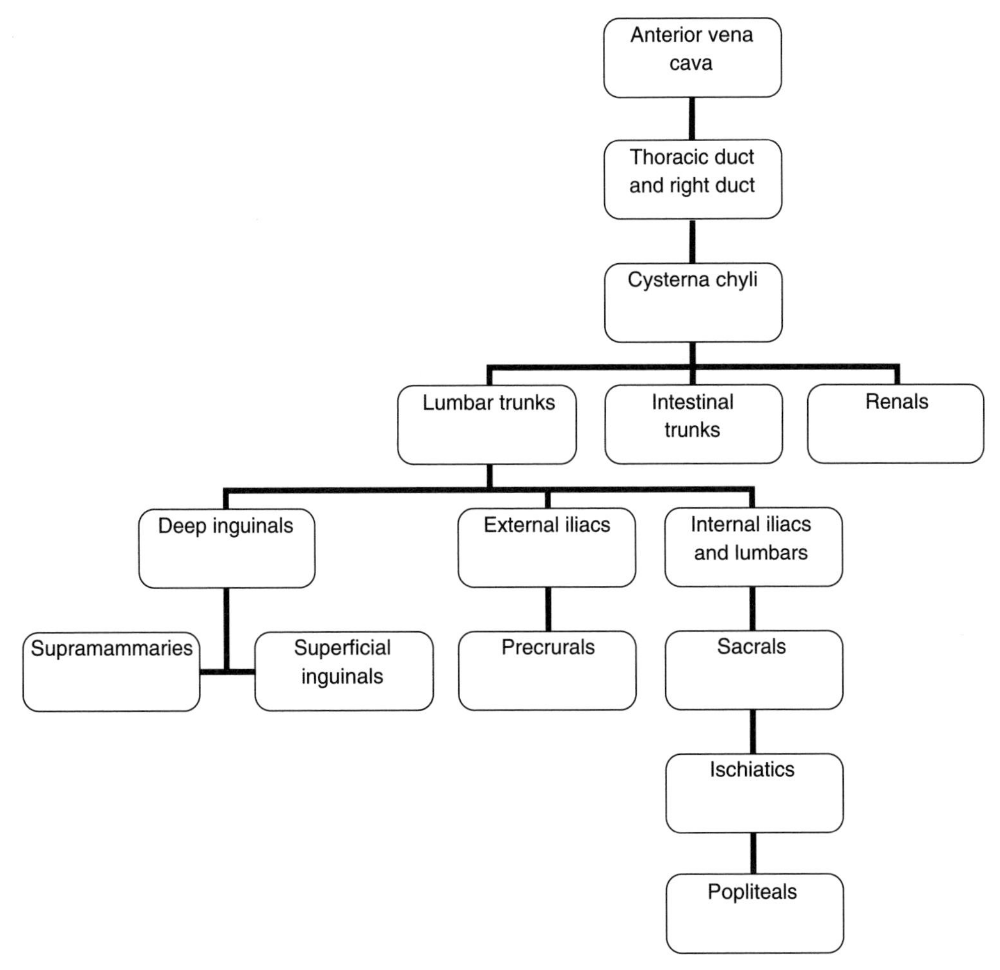

Fig. 6.2. Lymphatic system in cattle (caudal body): upward flow.

Further Reading

Wilson, A. and Wilson, W. (1998) *Practical Meat Inspection*. Blackwell, Oxford, UK.

6.2 Meat Inspection of Main Animal Species

Introduction

The currently used, routine post-mortem inspection of the main red meat animal species can be best illustrated by using the example of cattle, which is probably the most complex species from the inspection perspective. Subsequently, main comparable differences in other species can be highlighted.

Meat Inspection of Bovines >6 Months

Inspection of carcass

- Examination of the carcass visually, looking at all surfaces from all angles;
- determination of the sex of the carcass;
- examination of the joints for arthritis;
- examination of the colour of fatty and muscle tissues (both should be within the normal range) – fatty tissue yellowing can be caused by abnormal liver function, by normal ageing of the animal or by the type of feed consumed;
- examination of muscle tissue for bruising;
- inspection of visible blood vessels with care: these must be properly drained of blood;
- inspection of the abdominal cavity for signs of adherence (peritonitis);
- inspection of the thoracic cavity for signs of pleurisy or tuberculous lesions; and
- if the carcass is considered to be normal, based on the above examination, further cutting will not be required.

Inspection of kidneys

Kidneys normally remain attached to the carcass for inspection, which is conducted by visual inspection and palpation. Only if any abnormality is detected should the renal lymph nodes be cut open to detect nephritis.

Inspection of head

Visual inspection of the head from all angles. Technically, the following should be visually examined, followed by additional examination where indicated:

- mandibles for irregular shape, e.g. in the case of actinobacillosis;
- eyes for abnormal appearance or colour, e.g. yellowing caused by icterus;
- tongue for abnormal lesions, e.g. symptomatic of foot and mouth disease, and by palpation for deeper abnormalities (e.g. actinobacillosis, cysticercosis);
- incisor teeth for age; if >24 months, must be tested for BSE;
- lymph nodes, each of which exist in pairs: retropharangeal, submandibular, parotid (note: tuberculosis can be diagnosed in these lymph nodes); and
- cheek muscles: external cheek muscles are incised with two parallel cuts, and internal cheek muscles with one, to inspect for *T. saginata cystercircus*.

Inspection of lungs

- Visual inspection for pneumonia, cysts (e.g. hydatid), abscesses, tumours, etc.;
- palpation to detect any of the above within deeper tissue;
- incision and examination of bronchial, mediastinal pairs of lymph nodes (note: tuberculosis can be diagnosed in these lymph nodes); and
- incision to open trachea and lower airways to examine for inflammation and foreign contents (food, parasites, blood, etc.) or partially swallowed food.

Inspection of heart

- Visual inspection for pericarditis;
- opening of pericardial sac to examine for abnormal amount or appearance of the liquid; and
- incisions to open all chambers to examine for endocarditis, and for cysticercosis cysts in the septum.

Inspection of diaphragm

If cysticercosis has been found in the cheek muscles or in the heart, the diaphragm must also be inspected.

Inspection of liver

This organ is particularly important as a general indicator of animal health, as many abnormalities occur in the liver of sick animals:

- visual examination for degenerations, dystrophies, cysts (e.g. hydatid), abscesses, tumours, tuberculous lesions;
- palpation to detect any of the above in deeper tissue, palpation of the hepatic lymph node (and its incision if any abnormalities found); and
- incisions to open the bile ducts (along the main ducts and across the caudal lobe) to examine for liver fluke infestation.

Inspection of spleen

The spleen may be separated from, or attached to, rumen, and is examined by visual inspection and palpation for changes in colour, size (edges are normally sharp) and consistency. Splenic enlargement and/or dark colour is commonly associated with infective diseases (e.g. anthrax) and septicaemia. Note that splenic colour can differ between sexes.

Inspection of alimentary tract

Alimentary tract contents are usually inspected whilst placed in trays, and include oesophagus, rumen and large and small intestines:

- visual inspection of rumen and intestines for enteritis, etc.: salmonellosis and Johnes' disease both cause redness of the enteric tract, so may be detected by visual inspection;
- palpation of the mesenteric lymph nodes – if any abnormality is detected, these lymph nodes may be incised for further inspection; and
- palpation of oesophagus for parasitic cysts, etc.

Genital organs

These are visually inspected and palpated; they are incised only if any abnormality is detected.

Udder

The udder is examined, visually and by palpation, after it has been separated from the carcass. Although a thick fat layer may remain after udder removal, this does not indicate abnormality. Conduct a visual inspection and palpation. Mastitis is frequently caused by zoonotic agents, so care must be taken to avoid milk secretion and spillage, with possible contamination of other edible tissues. Also, tuberculous lesions may be found in the udder.

Meat Inspection of Bovines <6 Months

These young animals are inspected in a manner similar to that for adult bovine animals, with the following differences:

- cheek muscles are not incised to examine for *T. saginata cysticercus*, as the animals are considered too young to be infected with infective larvae;
- attention should be paid during inspection of the umbilical region and joints, as abnormal findings (e.g. arthritis) can be associated with salmonellosis; and
- the liver is not incised for detection of liver fluke, as these animals are considered too young for this parasite to occur.

Meat Inspection of Other Red Meat Species

Horses (solipeds), sheep/goats, pigs and farmed game are inspected in a manner similar to that for adult bovine animals, with the following differences:

Horses (solipeds)

- Head: the mucous membranes and nasal cavities/sinuses/septum are inspected after the head has been split along the median line for glanders; visual examination and palpation of other parts and incisions only if necessary;
- liver: visually inspected and palpated; incised only if necessary;
- udder: visually inspected and palpated; incised only if necessary;
- all grey horses must be examined for melanosis and melatomata, since their light pigmentation predisposes them to skin and other cancers: the attachment of one shoulder is loosened and muscles and prescapular lymph node are inspected;
- kidneys: visual examination and incision; and
- muscles: inspection for *Trichinella spiralis* (see Chapter 6.4).

Farmed deer and game

Farmed deer have similar diseases to those occurring in cattle. Therefore, inspection procedures are practically the same as those described for bovines >6 months.

Sheep/goats

Mandatory, routine inspection of sheep and goats is conducted in a manner as for bovines >6 months, except that inspection is based on visual examination and palpation. The only mandatory incision is for the hepatic bile ducts, to detect the presence of liver fluke, but other incisions can be made if necessary, i.e. in case of detected abnormalities.

Pigs

Mandatory, routine inspection of pigs is conducted in a manner as for bovines >6 months, except for:

- careful visual inspection of skin for diseases (e.g. erysipelas, swine fever) or tail biting;
- careful incision and inspection of submaxillary lymph nodes for tuberculous lesions;
- bile ducts in liver are not incised unless necessary; and
- muscle samples from the root of the diaphragm (where it is attached to the vertebral column – *Crura diaphragmatis*) are inspected for *Trichinella* infection (see Chapter 6.4).

Mandatory Provisions Where Tuberculosis is Suspected – All Species

If tuberculosis infection of an animal is suspected because of either the results of routine tuberculin testing (i.e. reactors), the epidemiological data or of the findings at ante- or post-mortem inspection, further in-depth inspection must be conducted including:

- carcass must be split and vertebrae, ribs, sternum, spinal cord and brain (where needed) are examined;
- incision and examination in detail of all major lymph nodes on the carcass and organs. The lymph nodes which are least likely to be infected must be examined first, to reduce the risk of cross-contamination; and
- careful sanitation of all knives, gloves, aprons, etc. between different areas of the carcass.

Further Reading

Anon. (2004a) *Good Practices for Meat Industry*. FAO Animal Production and Health Manual, FAO, Rome.

Anon. (2004b) *Meat Hygiene Service: Operational Manual* (Vols 1 and 2). The UK Food Standard Agency, Meat Hygiene Service, London

Gracey, J., Collins, D.S. and Huey, R. (1999) *Meat Hygiene*. W.B. Saunders Company Ltd, London.

Wilson, A. and Wilson, W. (1998) *Practical Meat Inspection*. Blackwell, Oxford, UK.

6.3 Meat Inspection – Judgement of Fitness

Deciding on fitness of meat for human consumption is a complex and serious activity, with numerous and various implications of public health; some have implications of a legal, ethical or commercial nature. The Official Veterinary Surgeon should make related decisions only when he/she is confident that the information obtained is sufficient for an appropriate decision; otherwise, he/she should seek more information (e.g. further examinations, laboratory tests, expert opinions, etc.). During the process, the Official Veterinary Surgeon should not be put, or feel, under undue pressure from interested parties.

The Judgement Process

The decision-making process should be systematic; the following questions will help to address the question of fitness of the inspected meat:

- Is there any aspect from the Food Chain Information (FCI) system relevant for the meat fitness?
- Is there any aspect from the ante-mortem inspection relevant for the meat fitness (see Fig. 6.3).

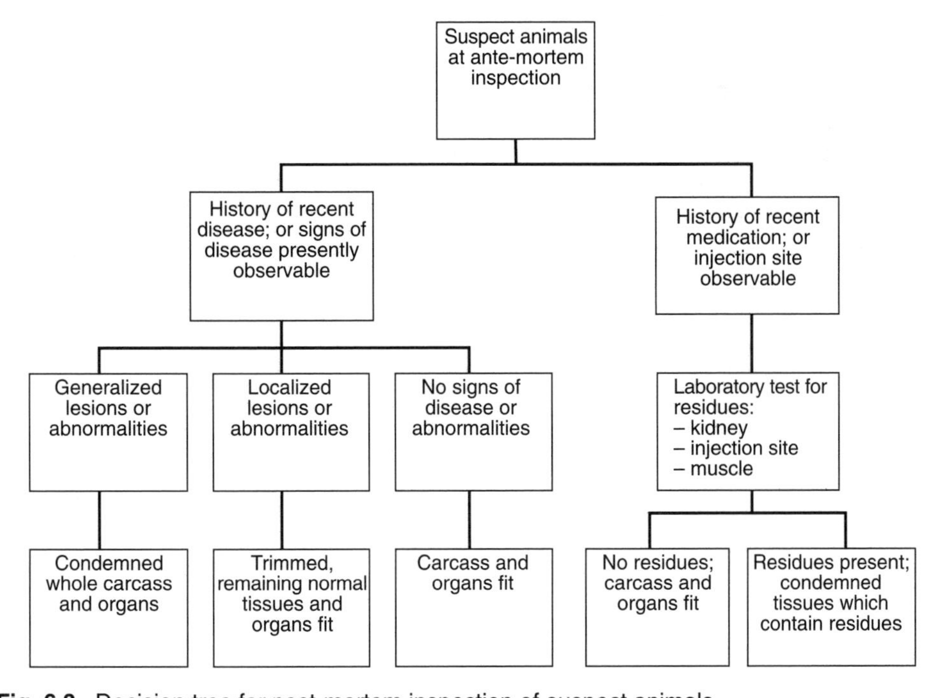

Fig. 6.3. Decision tree for post-mortem inspection of suspect animals.

- Can diseased or abnormal tissues, if found, be removed and condemned, leaving safe, edible tissues?
- Is the condition localized or generalized; is it acute or chronic? Chronic or localized disease lesions can be removed more easily than can acute or generalized lesions?
- Is there derangement of body function?
- Is the condition harmful to human health or to animal health? If the condition affects animal health, the information should be relayed to the farm of origin and/or government agencies; if the condition affects human health, it clearly must be acted on.
- Is the condition aesthetically offensive and repugnant? If yes, it is unfit although it may not represent a health risk.
- Do I feel confident with my own judgement? If not, delay the final decision.
- Is further information required? If yes, obtain help and opinion from senior colleagues, experts and laboratory tests.

Identification of conditions and judgement principles

Removal/condemnation of diseased/abnormal tissue

All abnormal organs/tissues are unfit for human consumption, regardless of the cause. Some common examples include localized abscesses in pig meat, a single hydatid cyst in liver or a bruised chicken limb. The affected parts must be removed and condemned (appropriately disposed of), while the remaining healthy normal tissues can be fit for human consumption.

Localized versus generalized and acute versus chronic

A disease process is localized when the pathological changes are in a limited area and no serious changes exist in other tissues or organs. Acute lesions are often generalized, including septicaemia, pyaemia, pyrexia and toxaemia. Recognition of these conditions requires significant knowledge and practical experience.

Derangement of body function

Derangement of body function occurs when any disease or condition has progressed to the point where an important bodily function is impaired. It affects the general physiology. This condition requires condemnation of the entire carcass, although the primary disease itself is insufficient for condemnation. Examples include obstructive uraemia, icterus, generalized oedema caused by heart failure and emaciation caused by poor teeth. In these cases, the carcass may not represent a risk to human health, but would be unacceptable to consumers.

Harmfulness to human health

There are three main categories of conditions which could seriously affect human health. First, transmissible diseases – including those caused by bacteria, viruses, parasites – and BSE are a risk to human health. Second, chemical residues – including industrial pollutants, pesticides and toxins – and residues of medicines can also be deleterious to human health. Third, contamination with food-borne pathogens can lead to development of human alimentary disease.

Offensive or repugnant

Judgement of offensive or repugnant meat is interwoven with all the previous principles. However, it is not always clearly related to public health. Condemnation in these cases is applied because the condition is aesthetically unacceptable (distasteful) to consumers. Examples include stillborn and unborn carcasses, benign tumours, dead parasites, foreign odour and spoilage.

Specific indications rendering whole carcass, offal and blood unfit for human consumption

Current UK legislation enlists the following diseases and conditions, which must result in the declaration of the meat or carcass as unfit for human consumption. Some of these conditions are not zoonotic, but declaring the meat unfit can prevent the product entering the food chain and spreading animal disease further.

Actinobacillosis (generalized) or actinomycosis (generalized)
Anaemia (advanced)
Anthrax
Blackleg
Blood from infectious conditions, or contaminated
Botulism
Brucellosis (acute)
Bruising (severe)
BSE/TSE
Caseous lymphadenitis (generalized)
Cysticercus ovis (generalized)
Decomposition (generalized)
Enteritis
Fever
Foot and mouth disease
Glanders
Jaundice
Lymphadenitis (generalized)
Malignant catarrhal fever
Mastitis (acute septic)

Melanosis (generalized)
Metritis (acute septic)
Odour, abnormal or sexual
Oedema (generalized)
Pericarditis (acute septic)
Peritonitis (acute diffuse septic)
Pleurisy (acute diffuse septic)
Pneumonia (acute septic)
Pyaemia (including joint-ill)
Rabies
Sarcocysts (generalized)
Septicaemia
Stillborn/unborn
Swine erysipelas (acute)
Swine fever
Tetanus
Toxaemia
Trichinellosis
Tuberculosis (generalized or with emaciation)
Tumours, malignant or multiple
Uraemia
Viraemia

Specific judgements for tuberculosis

When tuberculosis (TB) is detected, it must be established whether the condition is generalized (more rare) or localized (more common). There has been very little evidence for meat-borne TB infection in humans (as opposed to milk-borne) over the past 50–100 years, and only evidence appears to relate to consumption of meat from generalized infection cases. Nevertheless, consuming meat from animals which have been infected with TB is largely unappealing to consumers.

When generalized TB is detected, the whole carcass is considered as being unfit for human consumption, and must be condemned. TB is generalized if the disease is found in both lungs and elsewhere in the carcass. Also, the presence of multiple and active lesions, or if the disease is widespread in lymph nodes, indicates generalized TB. Diffuse lesions can occur on both the pleurae and peritoneum. TB is also considered generalized if active lesions are found in any two of the spleen, kidney, udder, uterus, ovary, testicle, brain or digestive tract. Congenital TB in a calf must be considered as generalized.

Localized TB is diagnosed by the presence of lesions in just part of the carcass. The infected part must be declared unfit and condemned, while the remainder of the carcass is considered edible. The head and tongue must be declared unfit if TB is detected in any related lymph node. In this case, if the lesion is inactive and is not enlarged, the lesion may be removed by the OVS, and the head can be declared fit for human consumption.

Specific judgements for BSE and unfit Specified Risk Material (SRM) in ruminants

SRMs specified by legislation are shown in Table 6.2. All SRM must be stained, stored separately from food materials and dispatched to specified licensed premises to be destroyed. Bones and mechanically separated meat are not fit for human consumption.

Specific judgements for some zoonotic parasites

- Trichinellosis (e.g. pigs, horses): unfit (see the diseases list above);
- *T. saginata* cysticersosis (bovines): if few cysts found, they are removed, and the remaining carcass is frozen at −7°C for 3 weeks or at −10°C for 2 weeks to kill any undetected larvae; if infestation is generalized, the carcass is unfit;
- *T. solium* cysticersosis (pigs): unfit;
- liver fluke: the liver is unfit for esthetical reasons, although the disease is not transmited to humans via meat;
- hydatid cysts: the organ is unfit for esthetical reasons, although the disease is not transmited to humans via meat;
- protozoan parasites (e.g. *Toxoplasma gondii*, *Sarcocystis*): obviously changed meat is unfit.

Limitations of the conventional (organoleptic) post-mortem inspection and further developments

Post-mortem inspection has been very successful in detecting classic zoonotic diseases that were prevalent at the time of its original development (mid-19th Century), but many of those are now rare or have been eradicated. On the other hand, many new hazards associated with meat have emerged in the meantime. Obviously, the nature of public health problems at post-mortem meat inspection has significantly changed over time, contributing to significant limitations of the conventional meat inspection in modern times.

Table 6.2. Specified risk materials from differing ruminant categories (UK).

Ruminant category	Specified risk material
Bovines <6 months	Thymus, intestines
Bovines >6 months	Head (excluding tongue), spinal cord, spleen, tonsils, intestines, thymus
Bovines over >24 months; must be tested for BSE	Whole carcass if not tested
Sheep/goats	Head (excluding tongue and horns), spinal cord (>12 months), tonsils, spleen, ileum
Bovines/sheep/goats of all ages	Specified solid waste collected in the drainage system

First, most of the livestock presented at modern abattoirs for slaughter are apparently clinically healthy animals. Traditional meat inspection is of relatively low efficacy in detecting public health hazards amongst this large number of apparently healthy animals. For example, less than 1% of animals show macroscopic lesions, and traditional meat inspection may be detecting only one in five of the lesions actually present in these animals. Also, there are reports that organoleptic meat inspection detects only 10% of bovines actually infected with *T. saginata* cysticercosis.

Second, the most relevant fresh meat-related public health hazards today are 'invisible' i.e. cannot be detected by traditional meat inspection. For example, *Escherichia coli* O157, *Salmonella* and *Campylobacter* are human bacterial pathogens which are typically carried by healthy animals and contaminate meat without any symptoms, but are not detectable by organoleptic post-mortem meat inspection. To make things worse, some techniques of physical examination of meat (palpation, incision) actually spread this microbial contamination within the same carcass or to other carcasses. In addition, chemical residues, including pesticides, toxins, aflatoxins, veterinary medicines and growth promotors represent public health risks that cannot be detected by traditional meat inspection. To address these shortcomings of post-mortem meat inspection, an alternative, in the form of end-product laboratory testing for microbial pathogens, has been advocated. However, end-product testing also has significant disadvantages: it is a reactive (rather than proactive) measure, requiring the product to be stored until the results are obtained; numerous samples are required to produce a statistical representation of the final product; and the testing methods are currently suboptimal and variable, and the testing results relate only to the hazards examined for, but do not guarantee overall safety of the product.

Third, most of the pathological lesions detected by traditional meat inspection are of animal health relevance, but are not necessarily of public health relevance. For example, pneumonia in pigs is caused mostly by microorganisms that cannot cause disease in humans. A second example includes some parasites (e.g. liver fluke, hydatid cysts) which can be detected by traditional meat inspection, but the meat from such carcasses does not represent a public health risk. Clearly, detection of these conditions represents important benefits for animal health (through feedback of the information from abattoirs back to the farms), but in ongoing debates questions arise as to whether these benefits are sufficient to make acceptable the increase of public health risks due to meat cross-contamination generated by these animal disease-detection procedures.

Clearly, the absence of disease symptoms and macroscopic lesions at traditional post-mortem inspection does not mean the absence of microbial or chemical public health hazards in/on meat, but the inspection procedures mediate meat contamination with microbial pathogens. Revision of traditional meat inspection is, therefore, required to improve the current situation, and in the EU a series of related scientific opinions have been produced (see Further Reading), that are expected to be incorporated into new food (meat) hygiene regulations to be introduced from 1 January 2006.

Current suggestions for improvement of traditional meat inspection procedures include the following:

1. Grouping of animals before slaughter according to level of risks they pose: lower-risk animals are those coming from integrated production systems (farms with quality assurance and providing full food-chain information – FCI).
2. Ensuring absence of public health hazards in animals through on-farm diagnostic programmes and control measures.
3. Confirming their lower-risk status by absence of any abnormalities at ante-mortem inspection.
4. Subjecting these lower-risk animals to a simplified post-mortem inspection procedure in which palpation and/or incision are largely omitted to avoid cross-contamination, unless absolutely necessary (e.g. tuberculosis detection). It is considered that in those animals public health risks from incision-mediated cross-contamination are higher than from the non-detection of certain conditions due to the omissions.
5. Removal of unfit tissues due to conditions posing no public health risk to be increasingly ensured through meat quality assurance, so to reduce overall amount of meat handling.
6. Maintaining detailed, full, physical post-mortem examination for higher-risk animals, to which the above is not applicable.
7. Controlling meat contamination from the main food-borne pathogens in healthy animals through abattoir process hygiene (e.g. GHP- and HACCP-based management systems).

Further reading

Anon. (2000) *Opinion of The Scientific Committee on Veterinary Measures Relating to Public Health on Revision of Meat Inspection Procedures*. European Commission, Health and Consumer Protection Directorate-General, Brussels.

Anon. (2001) *Opinion of The Scientific Committee on Veterinary Measures Relating to Public Health on Identification of Species/categories of Meat-Producing Animals in Integrated Production Systems Where Meat Inspection May Be Revised*. European Commission, Health and Consumer Protection Directorate-General, Brussels.

Anon. (2003) *Opinion of the Scientific Committee on Veterinary Measures Relating to Public Health on Revision of Meat Inspection in Veal Calves*. European Commission, Health and Consumer Protection Directorate-General, Brussels.

Anon. (2004a) Opinion of the Scientific Panel on Biological Hazards on Revision of Meat Inspection Procedures for Beef. *EFSA Journal* 141, 1–55.

Anon. (2004b) Opinion of the Scientific Panel on Biological Hazard on Revision of Meat Inspection Procedures for Lambs and Goats. *EFSA Journal* 54, 1–49.

Gracey, J., Collins, D.S. and Huey, R. (1999) *Meat Hygiene*. W.B. Saunders Company Ltd, London.

Wilson, A. and Wilson, W. (1998) *Practical Meat Inspection*. Blackwell, Oxford, UK.

6.4 Rapid Laboratory Tests

Introduction

Some laboratory tests may be required to obtain information additional to that derived from meat inspection. Large abattoirs can have a laboratory on-site; small operators generally do not have on-site laboratory facilities. However, many of these tests can be performed by the OVS under field conditions.

The rapid laboratory tests provide quick, field screening for presumptive positives and negatives. The judgement of carcass fitness then can be made if the owner agrees with the results. If agreement cannot be reached with the owner, further examination using more sophisticated laboratory methods must be conducted to confirm the results.

Rapid test to differentiate causes of jaundice/icterus

Yellow colouration in the tissues can originate from pigments contained in feeds (lipo-chromatosis), in which case older animals are more normally affected, and the meat is suitable for human consumption. However, this condition can also be due to jaundice, and the meat may not be suitable for human consumption. Furthermore, both causes of yellow colouration can exist in one animal. Initially, differentiation is attempted by visual examination of carcass tissues, to determine whether the yellow colouration is present in the fatty tissue only (likely from feeds) or in the connective tissues and eye whites (jaundice).

Indication: abnormal yellow colour, or its distribution, in tissues.

Procedure

- Take a 2 g sample of fat and boil with 5 ml 5% w/v NaOH for 1 min;
- cool under a tap, add 3–5 ml ether and shake; and
- allow to stand until the layers separate.

Interpretation of results

- Green to yellow colour in the aqueous (lower) layer indicates icterus;
- green to yellow colour in the solvent (upper) layer indicates the presence of carotenoid pigments, probably derived from feeds; and
- green to yellow colour in both layers indicates both icterus and feed-derived pigments are present.

Rapid test to determine the presence of anasarca/oedema in animals

Animals in poor condition may be emaciated and suffering from anasarca. Animals suffering from anasarca can be rapidly differentiated from healthy animals by examining the bone marrow. The bone marrow of healthy animals usually contains <25% water, while the bone marrow of animals with emaciation, anasarca, etc., contains >50% water.

Indication: anasarca in subcutaneous and connective tissue, or oedema accompanied by emaciation.

Procedure

- Place pieces of bone marrow (pea-sized) from a long bone in solutions of 32, 47 and 52% (v/v) ethanol.

Interpretation of results

- If the specimen floats in all three solutions, it contains <25% water and the animal is healthy but emaciated; and
- if the specimen sinks in two of the three solutions, or all three, it contains >50% water and the animal has anasarca.

Test for acetonaemia

Ketone bodies (acetone, acetoacetic acid, betahydroxybutyrate) can produce an unpleasant odour, which may be detected directly by smell alone. Acetonaemia is more prevalent in pregnant ewes, emaciated cows or cows in early lactation. These animals are usually presented for emergency slaughter, because they are showing signs of disease.

Indication: used to determine whether suspect animals have acetonaemia even if the condition cannot be detected using the sense of smell.

Procedure

- Shake 10 g diced meat in 15 ml cold water; and
- add 1 tablespoon of Rothera's reagent, shake, and leave for 5 min.

Interpretation of results

- Purple permanganate colour in the supernatant fluid indicates the animal has acetonaemia.

Test for unusual odour, e.g. boar taint

Strong, unusual odours are generally unacceptable for consumers, although they may not represent a public health risk. Androstenone and skatole can both occur in edible tissues, but the taints may be more easily detected in fatty tissues.

Indication: to determine whether meat has an unusual/abnormal odour.

Procedure

- Take sample of fat or meat and place in cold water;
- heat (covered) to boiling; repeatedly test the odour of the steam;
- remove the tissue, cut immediately and test the odour released; and
- alternatively, fry the meat and test the odour released.

Interpretation of results

- Strong odours indicate the meat may be unfit for human consumption.

Test for imperfect bleeding

Imperfect bleeding can be caused by numerous factors, including disease, stress or inappropriate handling, and can result in meat that is unfit for human consumption. Blood vessels can be full of blood; the organs may drip when removed.

Indication: to determine whether the carcass has bled out properly.

Procedure

- Take 6 g fat-free muscle, cut, place in 14 ml water, and leave to stand for 15 min;
- withdraw 0.7 ml of supernatant into an agglutination tube; and
- add 1 drop malachite green reagent, mix, add 1 drop H_2O_2, shake, allow to stand for 20 min.

Interpretation of results

- A cloudy, green colour indicates imperfect bleeding; and
- a clear, blue colour indicates proper bleeding.

Test for meat species

Meats from differing animal species usually appear quite different. However, more novelty meat species (e.g. ostrich, kangaroo, etc.) are being consumed, and some of these can be difficult to differentiate. In addition, meat products can contain meat from a variety of animal species and should be labelled as such. This rapid test for meat species can only be conducted on uncooked meat.

Indication: to determine whether uncooked meat is correctly labelled.

Procedure

- Prepare rabbit antisera against individual animal species (purchased monoclonal antibodies or purchased antisera can be used);
- cut 1 g of uncooked meat finely and shake in 2 ml 0.85% saline;
- leave for 1 h to extract antigen; decant the supernatant;
- prepare a gel diffusion test using a commerical kit; these normally come with a template for drilling wells in pre-prepared gels; place the antigen extract in one template well and antibody/antisera in another; and
- place in a moist chamber at ambient temperature for 24 h.

Interpretation of results

- A positive visible precipitation line between reservoirs indicates the meat species is present in the antigen extract.

Test for tuberculosis

Animals with tuberculosis must not enter the human food chain.

Indication: caseous necrotic lesions in lymph nodes/organs.

Procedure (Ziehl-Nielsen staining)

- Prepare an air-dried, heat-fixed slide from a typical lesion in lymph nodes or organs;
- cover the slide with carbofuchsin and heat the stain so that it steams for at least 5 min; if the stain begins to evaporate add fresh stain; remove the flame if the stain begins to boil;
- decolourize by flooding the slide with acid alcohol for 20 s; add tap water immediately to stop decolourizing;
- counter-stain with methylene blue for 60 s; rinse the smear once again and blot dry; and
- observe for acid-fast organisms under the microscope.

Interpretation of results

- Observing acid-fast rods indicates the presence of *Mycobacterium*.

Test for residues of antimicrobials

Residues of antibiotics and other antimicrobial residues in meat are unacceptable in meat. Samples of kidney tissue are always examined in suspect animals, since the kidneys metabolize most antimicrobial compounds. However, muscle tissue (e.g. diaphragm) and suspect injection sites should also be included in this test.

Indication: recent medication suspected in animals.

Procedure

- Prepare microbiological agar (pH 6, 8 and 7.4) and cool to 45–50°C;
- inoculate molten agar with a standard antimicrobial-sensitive bacterial strain from a recognized culture collection (e.g. *Bacillus subtilis* spores) using a standard concentration;
- pour plates and leave to harden;
- one of the plates should contain trimethoprim, which is synergistic with sulphonamides;
- cut wells in the agar plates with a sterile cork borer and remove the plugs with a needle;
- prepare a homogenate of the tissue (e.g. kidney, muscle) by mixing 1 g of finely cut tissue with 2 ml of 0.85% saline;
- fill a well with a standard volume of the sample homogenate and leave to pre-diffuse at 4°C for 2 h; and
- incubate at 37°C for 16–18 h.

Interpretation of results

- Measure the diameter of clear zones of inhibition of bacterial growth surrounding the well;
- inhibition zones ≥2 mm are considered positive;
- for confirmation and quantification, more sophisticated methods must be used (e.g. HPLC, gas chromatography).

Meat examination for *Trichinella*

These tests require a microscope and more complex equipment, so may require dedicated laboratory space.
1. Artificial digestion method.

Procedure

- Take tissue samples (1 g for pig, 5 g for horse) from either the pillars of the diaphragm or the tongue, masseter or intercostal muscles;
- pool the tissue samples from 100 animals and grind them using a mortar;
- place in 1–2 l of artificial digestive fluid comprising 1% (w/v) pepsin (1/10,000) and 1% (v/v) hydrochloric acid (0.12M final concentration);
- stir for 3 h at 37°C (or 0.5–1 h at 44°C) using a magnetic stirrer;
- leave to settle for 15 min;
- discard the upper 2/3 of the fluid;
- pour the remaining fluid with deposit through a 355 (177–180 is also acceptable) µm mesh screen into a conical settling glass and allow to settle for 15–20 min; if required, wash the sediment with water and repeat the settling;
- drain 125 ml into a separatory funnel and leave to settle for 10 min;

- drain 22–27 ml from the bottom layer into a Petri dish and examine microscopically for coiled *Trichinella* larvae;
- if *Trichinella* larvae are found, the test must be repeated individually on tissues from each of the animals making up the pooled sample.

2. Trichinoscope (compression) method.

This method is less sensitive than the artificial digestion method, so is not recommended; it is indicated here for historic reasons and because it may be the only method available in certain countries.

Procedure

- Take tissue samples (1 g for pig, 5 g for horse) from either the pillars of the diaphragm, or the tongue, masseter or intercostal muscles;
- cut the tissue samples into 2 × 10 mm pieces, obtaining at least 28 pieces for pig or 56 for horse;
- compress the tissue pieces between glass (compressorium) plates until they become translucent;
- examine microscopically for coiled *Trichinella* larvae (40× magnification);
- the presence of coiled larvae within an oval cyst within an individual muscle fibre is positive.

3. ELISA test: stichosyte-cell antigens, glycoproteins 45–55 kDa.

This method is primarily applied for on-farm testing and monitoring.

Procedure

- Coat the wells in 96-well microtitre plates with 100 μl of antigen in pH 9.6 buffer and leave for 60 min at 37°C or overnight at 4°C;
- repeat the buffer – at pH 7.4 – wash and dry;
- dilute pig sera (or whole blood or tissue fluids) 1/10 to 1/100 in wash buffer;
- add 100 μl diluted pig sera to the wells and incubate at ambient temperature for 30 min;
- add 100 μl of affinity-purified rabbit anti-swine IgG-peroxidase conjugate (1/1000 dilution) and incubate for 30 min;
- add 100 μl of a suitable peroxidase substrate with 0.005% hydrogen peroxide (pH 5.6–6.0);
- after 5–15 min, read the colour density of the plates at 450 nm on an automated microplate reader;
- values four times higher than normal serum control are considered as positive.

Further Reading

Gracey, J., Collins, D.S. and Huey, R. (1999) *Meat Hygiene*. W.B. Saunders Company Ltd, London.

Wilson, A. and Wilson, W. (1998) *Practical Meat Inspection*. Blackwell, Oxford, UK.

6.5 Meat Inspection – Poultry

Introduction

In contrast to red meat animal species (cattle, pigs, sheep), ante-mortem inspection of poultry is not carried out at the abattoir, but on-farm. On arrival at the abattoir, poultry are slaughtered directly from transport vehicles, without any lairaging. Nevertheless, transport conditions and related poultry welfare should be checked.

In the UK, poultry meat inspection is based on The Poultry Meat, Farmed Game Bird Meat and Rabbit Meat (Hygiene & Inspection) Regulations 1995. The Official Veterinary Surgeon is responsible for ensuring that the post-mortem inspection of poultry is carried out in accordance with the requirements. The inspection can be assisted by non-veterinarians: poultry meat hygiene inspectors (PMHIs) or plant inspection assistants (PIAs).

Meat Inspection

Poultry meat inspection is carried out immediately after slaughter, and includes primarily visual examination of:

- whole defeathered birds before evisceration; this is not a statutory requirement, but is advisable, so that obviously diseased birds can be removed from the line to prevent contamination of equipment;
- surface of the carcass, excluding the head and the feet, except where these are intended for human consumption;
- viscera, which can remain (but not necessarily) attached to the carcass – with ensured correlation between carcass and viscera being essential; and
- body cavity.

Post-mortem inspection of Effile Birds (partly eviscerated poultry), in which the non-edible intestines are removed but the edible viscera remain attached to the carcass, includes:

- inspection of 5% of birds from the batch;
- examination focuses on external surface, viscera and body cavity;
- if no abnormal conditions are found, other birds are not inspected; and
- if any anomalies are found, all birds in the batch must be inspected.

Post-mortem inspection of birds that are subject to delayed evisceration must be carried out within the 15-day period after slaughter. These birds can be eviscerated either at the abattoir, or in a cutting plant that has been specifically approved for that; the meat inspection is carried out at the place of evisceration. In the meantime, these birds must be refrigerated at a temperature of not more than 4°C.

Judgement of meat fitness

Generally, the main reasons for judgeing meat as unfit for human consumption include the finding of evidence of disease, multiple tumours, cachexia, ascites and abnormal colour (insufficient bleeding), as well as meat contamination. All these conditions can be detected by visual examination of the carcasses and the viscera. The occurrence of some abnormal conditions can vary with the seasons. For example, heat stress is common in summer, respiratory disease and ascites in winter.

Causes for meat rejection commonly include *E. coli* infections, ascites and Marek's disease. *E. coli* infections can produce a number of conditions such as colisepticaemia, cellulitis, salpingitis, egg peritonitis, coligranulom and swollen head syndrome. Ascites can be caused by hypoxia, primary liver disease or congenital cardiac defects. Marek's disease is caused by a herpes virus and can produce visceral tumours, skin tumours and nerve infiltration.

Runting/Stunting Syndrome (caused by a virus) causes very uneven growth rate in a batch. This can lead to potential welfare problems because small birds can miss the stunner. These animals should be preferably culled on-farm.

Further Reading

Bremner, A. and Johnston, M. (1996) *Poultry Meat Hygiene and Inspection*. W.B. Saunders Company Ltd, London.

Jordan, F.T.W. and Pattison, M. (1996) *Poultry Diseases*. W.B. Saunders Company Ltd, London.

6.6 Sensory Evaluation of Meat

GEOFFREY NUTE

Introduction

Consumer confidence in the safety of meat and meat products is of increasing importance, especially since the range of products available continues to increase. Consumers demand food that is of excellent eating quality, safe to eat, of high nutritional value and has an increased shelf life.

A recent study Ngapo *et al.* (2003) used focus groups in four countries (France, UK, Sweden and Denmark) to identify consumer attitudes to pig production and pork quality. UK consumers cited cleanliness of the place of purchase, unbroken packaging and healthiness as some of their criteria when purchasing pork. Interestingly, there was little or no discussion about food-borne illnesses related to the consumption of pork, probably as a result of media coverage mainly attributing microbiological spoilage to poultry products.

Decontamination of meat covers a whole range of different processes, ranging from irradiation techniques (high consumer resistance) to acid dips or sprays (low consumer awareness) (see Chapter 5.6). Microbiologists concentrate on the reduction of microorganisms in/on the meat and on the resultant improved safety of the meat. Sensory analysts concentrate on the eating quality of the meat and whether or not there are changes in the sensory attributes – and hence consumer satisfaction – as a result of applying decontamination techniques.

This chapter describes what constitutes a sensory panel and gives examples from the literature where these techniques have been documented and the sensory approach used.

Sensory Panel

In much the same way that we would check the sensitivity of an instrument, it is necessary to ascertain the sensitivity of the potential assessors. These procedures are documented in The British Standards Institution BS7667, part 1, 1993 (BSI, 1993). This standard defines the materials and methods used in the screening process, which is a way of determining whether or not a person is suitable for making sensory assessments.

The training in the first instance is not specific to a particular food product, but rather is a series of tests to ascertain the sensory acuity of the candidate.

The types of screening tests used are aimed at determining: impairment, sensory acuity and evaluation of a candidate's potential for describing and communicating sensory perceptions.

Colour vision can be checked either by a qualified optician or by sensory analysts familiar with the Ishihara test (Ishihara, 1967). Further colour discrimination tests, e.g. the 100-Hue test (Farnsworth, 1957), are used to identify the discriminational abilities of assessors. This test is different from the Ishihara test in that its prime purpose is to classify those individuals with normal colour vision into categories of superior, average and low colour discrimination.

Ageusia (lack of sensitivity to taste stimuli) and anosmia (lack of sensitivity to olfactory stimuli) are the terms used to describe the potential assessors' basic taste/odour sensitivity, or possible lack of sensitivity, at average recognition thresholds.

The taste test uses substances at known concentrations and covers the basic sensations of sweetness, acidity, bitterness, saltiness, astringency and metallic.

Odour recognition is a simple sniff test, where potential assessors are given a range of familiar odours and are required to identify them using simple descriptions.

Sensory Tests

These can be categorized into, 'difference tests', 'category tests', 'ranking and scaling tests' and 'profiling tests'. The former two groups of tests are probably the most useful when dealing with decontamination issues, and examples of their usage are given below.

Difference tests

Van der Marel *et al.* (1989) investigated the use of 1% (v/v) lactic acid treatment on the sensory quality of fresh broiler chickens. The chickens were immersed at three stages during processing, defeathering, evisceration and after air-chilling. Control birds were treated in a similar way using tap water as the immersion treatment. The carcasses were stored at 0°C for 2 days in trays. Samples of thigh and drumstick were grilled for 30 min and sub-sampled to provide sufficient samples for 12 assessors.

Each assessor received one control and one treated sample of thigh and drumstick over two sessions, respectively.

The paired comparison test (BS5929: part 2, BSI, 1982) was used where $p = 0.5$, i.e. the probability of selecting the treated sample over the control and *vice versa* is 50%.

This test is usually a directional test, where assessors are asked to state the difference in intensity of a particular sensory attribute. However, in this work the non-directional test was used, since assessors were asked which sample they preferred. Therefore, this is a two-tailed test and the expected number of choices required for a significant result at the 5% level of probability in a particular direction is 32/48. In this test 26 assessors preferred the control samples and 22 preferred the treated samples. It was concluded that using lactic acid as a decontaminant would not be a problem in terms of eating quality.

The duo–trio test (BS 5929: part 8, BSI, 1992) is statistically less powerful than the triangular test described below, and although samples are presented as a triad, one of the samples is labelled as a reference sample.

Duo–trio tests were used by Janky and Salman (1986) to investigate differences in poultry meat from carcasses that had been water-chilled or brine-chilled. After chilling, samples were either packed in ice or blast-frozen. The main objective of the trial was to determine the effect of chill-packaging with brine-chilling and its influence on texture. However, there was an inference that the brine treatment might also reduce bacterial counts, although this was not tested in this trial.

Samples were battered and breaded, then deep-fried and allowed to cool overnight. Prior to the sensory tests the batter was removed and samples cut into small pieces for distribution to the panel. Both light and dark meat were assessed. In at least half of the panels, assessors were able to distinguish between ice-packed and chill-packed products. In light meat using the brine solution there were no significant differences between the two packaging treatments. In dark meat there were significant differences between the two packaging treatments.

The authors concluded that the differences found by the sensory panel were in accordance with shear force values that showed chill-packaging produced a toughening effect on texture which was not observed in brine-chilled samples.

The triangular test method (BS5929: part 3, BSI, 1984) was used by Dickens *et al.* (1994) in a study on cooked chicken breast, to ascertain whether the immersion of chickens in an acetic acid dip (0.6%) during processing could be detected in the cooked product.

The probability of selecting the 'odd' sample is 1/3. In this test assessors are presented with three samples, two of which are identical; their task is to select the 'odd' sample on the basis of difference only. There are six possible combinations of tasting order: ABB, AAB, ABA, BAA, BBA, BAB, and these are balanced across all assessors.

Two methods of preparation were used, boil-in-the-bag (water-cooked) and oven-roast. All assessments were completed under red light to reduce appearance effects. In all, 60 triangles were presented for each preparation method. In the water-cooked samples, taking the pooled assessors' results, there were 24/60 correct identifications, and in the oven-cooked tests, 29/60 correct identifications. The requirement for a positive result requires 30/60 correct identifications, and therefore in these tests the use of an acetic acid dip would not produce significant differences in sensory quality, whilst the Enterobacteriaceae (ENT) Log_{10} counts were reduced from 4.51 to 3.80.

Category tests

Difference tests are very useful in preliminary studies, since non-significant results indicate that the samples are not perceived as different; however, when there are differences it is necessary to identify which sensory attributes are different and how they are affected by the treatments under test.

Capita *el al.* (2000) investigated the use of trisodium phosphate (TSP) dodecahydrate solutions to reduce *Salmonella* contamination in poultry meat. In this study three concentrations of TSP, 8%, 10% and 12% (w/v) were used and these were compared using chicken thighs. Nine-point hedonic category scales for colour, smell and overall acceptability (where 1 = dislike extremely and 9 = like extremely, with a central category of neither like or dislike) were used in this trial.

The consumer panel rated both raw and cooked chicken thighs at day 0 (immediately after dipping) and after 7 days' storage. At day 0 consumers found significant differences in 10% and 12% TSP samples and these differences were related to colour and smell, whereas 10% TSP samples were significantly preferred and in 12% TSP, where colour and overall acceptability were rated higher.

At 7 days' storage the colour liking of chicken samples dipped in 12% TSP were significantly lower than those treated with 8 and 10% TSP.

In cooked samples after 7 days' storage there were significant differences observed in colour, flavour and overall acceptability. The colour liking of 12% TSP samples was significantly less than for the control samples. In terms of smell there were no significant differences between treatments, but in overall acceptability the 12% TSP samples were the least preferred whilst there was no difference between the other treatments.

In this trial it was concluded that the use of TSP could have potential to sanitize chicken carcasses.

Hathcox *et al.* (1995) compared the use of TSP and lactic acid/benzoic acid on consumer acceptance of fried chicken breasts and thigh meat. 180 whole chickens were washed in either control tap water, 12% trisodium phosphate (TSP) or 0.5% lactic acid/0.05% sodium benzoate (LB). Consumer panellists evaluated raw, treated whole chickens as well as fried breast and thigh samples. Nine-point hedonic category scales were used throughout the trials. Ratings for whole raw chickens showed that there were significant differences in acceptability, colour ratings and purchase intention. At 0 days and after 7 days' storage, LB samples were rated significantly lower than TSP and control samples for all attributes.

When tasting fried chicken, consumers did not differentiate Control, TSP or LB samples for texture, flavour, moistness or overall acceptability in either breast or thigh samples. In breast acceptance LB samples were rated lower than TSP samples, but were not significantly different from control samples.

The authors concluded that 12% TSP or 0.5%/0.05% sodium benzoate solutions had potential as dips to sanitize chickens intended for frying before serving to consumers.

Griffiths *et al.* (1978) stated that poultry diets were a potential source of *Salmonellae* and could cause infection in breeding stock, either by egg transmission to their progeny or directly by infecting chicks that had been free of infection.

Methyl bromide had been used in the past to destroy bacteria, fungi and insects in soils, stored crops and some processed foods. It can also be used as a fumigant for poultry food stored in paper sacks, since methyl bromide disperses rapidly when paper sacks are exposed to air. However, there was concern that there could be a 'taint' or changes in flavour of the meat from broilers that had received feed that had been fumigated with methyl bromide. Broilers were fed on control and treated commercial diets with methyl bromide gas at 69 and 25% over the value recommended for elimination of *Salmonellae*.

Tests with both a sensory panel and a consumer panel were conducted. The sensory panel used modified category scales and were also asked to describe the flavour and odour of the samples, using a different technique from control procedure where 0 = no difference, 1 = slight difference, 2 = moderate difference and 4 = large difference. The treated samples were significantly different from the controls and the flavour descriptors indicated that the samples were, 'cabbagy', 'bloody', 'metallic', 'rancid', 'sharp' and 'onion'. The conclusion from the sensory data indicated that the treated samples were tainted.

The home consumer panel (n = 52) used a simple three-point scale of good, fair or poor. The odour and flavour of the cooked meat was assessed and rated by the cook. Other household members rated cooked chicken flavour separately. The results showed that the treated chickens had a higher percentage of poor birds and a lower percentage of good birds than the controls. The ratings given by the consumers were analysed for the frequency with which the control birds were preferred over the treated birds. This showed that in the majority of cases, the control birds were preferred.

The authors concluded that a trained sensory panel found a significant taint in the roasted meat from birds fed on fumigated food. More than 50% of consumers also rated control birds better than treated birds.

Conclusions

When considering methods of decontamination of meat for human consumption, there are probably four stages in developing a new treatment. Stage 1 involves a study of the efficiency of the decontamination in terms of the reduction in bacterial counts. Stage 2 involves the use of a trained sensory panel to investigate appearance, odour and flavour of the meat for possible 'taint' or other sensory attribute effects. Stage 3 investigates consumer acceptability of the meat. Stage 4 involves consumer attitudes to the introduction of new treatments and whether or not the image of 'wholesomeness' is affected. Following these stages should result in meat that retains sensory attributes and eating enjoyment whilst benefiting from improved safety and shelf life properties.

References

BSI (1982) *Sensory Analysis of Food. Part 2. Paired comparison test. BS5929.* British Standards Institution, Milton Keynes, UK.

BSI (1984) *Sensory Analysis of Food. Part 3. Triangular test. BS5929.* British Standards Institution, Milton Keynes, UK.

BSI (1992) *Sensory Analysis of Food. Part 8. Duo–Trio test. BS5929.* British Standards Institution, Milton Keynes, UK.

BSI (1993) *Assessors for Sensory Analysis. Part 1. BS7667. Guide to the Selection, Training and Monitoring of Selected Assessors.* British Standards Institution, Milton Keynes, UK.

Capita, R., Alonso-Calleja, C., Sierra, M., Moreno, B. and Camino Garcia-Fernandez, M. (2000) Effect of trisodium phosphate solutions washing on sensory evaluation of poultry meat. *Meat Science* 55, 471–474.

Dickens, J.A., Lyon, B.G., Whittemore, A.D. and Lyon, C.E. (1994) The effect of acetic acid dip on carcass appearance, microbiological quality and cooked breast meat texture and flavour. *Poultry Science* 73, 576–581.

Farnsworth, D. (1957) The Farnsworth–Munsell 100-Hue Test. Munsell Colour Company Inc., Baltimore, Maryland.

Griffiths, N.M., Hobson-Frohock, A., Land, D.G., Levett, J.M., Cooper, D.M. and Rowell, J.G. (1978) Fumigation of poultry food with methyl bromide; effects on flavour and acceptability of broiler meat. *British Poultry Science* 19, 529–535.

Hathcox, A.K., Hwang, C.A., Resurreccion, A.V.A. and Beuchat, L.R. (1995) Consumer evaluation of raw and fried chicken after washing in trisodium phosphate or lactic acid/sodium benzoate solutions. *Journal of Food Science* 60, 604–605.

Ishihara, I. (1967) *Tests for Colour Blindness.* Kanehara Shuppan Co. Ltd, Tokyo.

Janky, D.M. and Salman, H.K. (1986) Influence of chill packaging and brine chilling on physical and sensory characteristics of broiler meat. *Poultry Science* 65, 1934–1938.

Ngapo, T.M., Dransfield, E., Martin, J.F., Magnusson, M., Bredahl, L. and Nute, G.R. (2003) Consumer perceptions: Pork and pig production. Insights, from France, England, Sweden and Denmark. *Meat Science* 66, 125–134.

Van der Marel, G.M., De Vries, A.W., Van Logtestijn, J.G. and Mossel, D.A.A. (1989) Effect of lactic acid treatment during processing on the sensory quality and lactic acid content of fresh broiler chickens. *International Journal of Food Science and Technology* 24, 11–16.

6.7 Certification and Marking of Foods of Animal Origin

ALISON SMALL

Certification

Foods of animal origin travel freely within the country of origin, and between states united by common trade agreements, such as within the EU. In such trade, the foods are accompanied merely by a Commercial Document, which is used as evidence in tracing of foods. The commercial document is generated by the premises of origin of the food, and contains information such as the name and address of consignor and consignee, the approval number of the premises from which the food is to be transported, and the quantity and description of the product transported, including date of freezing in the case of frozen foods. Where foods of animal origin are to be transported to countries not included within the common trade agreement, known as 'third countries', veterinary certification of the food is required.

The veterinarian carrying out certification of foods of animal origin must be authorized by the competent authority of the country in which he/she is working, and will have undergone appropriate training in export procedures. The certificate to be completed is supplied by the competent authority, and contains particular declarations required by the importing country. Most certificates have been agreed with the importing country, but on occasion, full agreement has not been reached, and the certificate contains declarations of information judged to be appropriate by the competent authority of the exporting country.

Certification, of any sort, is an activity that can hold the greatest hazard to a veterinarian's professional reputation and career. False certification can be considered to be negligence, or could constitute a criminal offence. In the UK, the Royal College of Veterinary Surgeons Guide to Professional Conduct gives 12 Principles of Certification, which have been adopted internationally, and all parties involved in certification are advised to adhere to these principles.

It is important to read the certificate carefully before signing, and ensure that all declarations can be made truthfully and factually. Declarations can only be made on subjects that the certifying veterinarian knows to be true, or that are supported by documentary evidence, such as a certificate from the competent authority in the case of freedom from notifiable disease, or a certificate from the veterinarian involved in official controls at a premises earlier in the food chain. No blank spaces should remain on completion of the certificate, and all parts should be signed and dated, with the personal stamp of the certifying veterinarian applied. It is important to keep copies of the certificate and any supplementary evidence or documentation in the event of any challenge.

Marking of Foods of Animal Origin

Identification labelling of foods of animal origin is important. Proper identification allows tracing of the food back to the premises of production and – ideally – to the farm or even the animal of origin. Full traceability is vital in the event of a disease outbreak, or in the event of contaminants being found within a food product. Traceability allows recall of potentially unsafe foods, and also assists in the identification of the point in the food chain where contamination may have arisen. Correct identification of the source of illegal contaminants is vital to good enforcement of legislation. Individual countries and states have local rules on labelling of foods of animal origin; however, in general, foods will be marked with an identification mark showing the country of origin, and an approval number of the production plant where that food was produced. This therefore means that the component parts of a food sold at retail level may at some point in the chain have carried different approval numbers, as it progressed through the manufacturing process. For example, a pork sausage started as a pig, which carried the identification mark of the farm of origin. Then, the pig was processed and the carcass carried the approval number of the slaughterhouse. It may then have been sold to a cutting premise. From here the cut meat, bearing the approval number of this factory, is transferred to the sausage factory, and ultimately bears the identification mark of this final premises when displayed in the retail store. Each premises in the chain must keep records to allow that sausage to be traced back to the farm of origin.

In the EU, carcasses leaving a slaughter facility would bear a Health Mark, giving the required information of country and premises of origin. This Health Mark could be one of several different shapes, indicating the class of meat identified. For example, meat produced in export-approved premises would carry an oval mark, meat produced from animals that had been slaughtered on-farm as special emergency slaughter would carry a square mark, and wild game meat would carry a pentagonal mark. These Health Marks are under the control of the veterinary inspection service, and are an indication that the meat has been produced in accordance with the requirements of the current legislation, and has passed both ante-mortem and post-mortem meat inspection procedures. The Health Mark could also carry a code number indicating the individual official carrying out the health inspection of the meat. The dimensions of the mark and its lettering are laid down in the legislation (Fig. 6.4), and the colourant used in marking meat must be an approved food-grade dye. It is very important that the Health Mark is legible. Offals may be branded with the Health Mark, using a hot iron.

The Health Mark may be modified in certain circumstances. For example, carcasses from boars that demonstrate a sexual odour that is not pronounced, and may be used for manufacturing purposes only, may carry the Health Mark overlaid by two parallel horizontal lines, or carcasses from animals under movement restrictions due to notifiable disease control may carry the Health Mark overlaid by a cross.

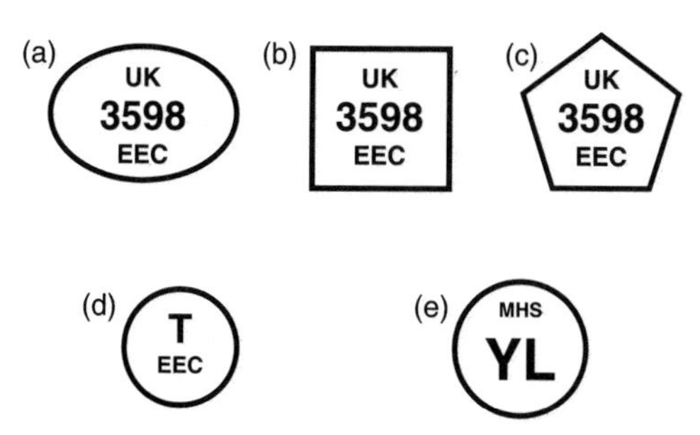

Fig. 6.4. Examples of marks applied to meats. (a) Oval mark; (b) Square mark for SES carcasses; (c) Pentagonal mark for wild game; (d) *Trichinella* mark; (e) Young lamb mark, for sheep under 12 months of age.

Carcasses may also carry other marks indicating that certain conditions have been met. For example, pig and horse carcasses are tested for the presence of *Trichinella spiralis*, and those that test negative are marked with a round 'T' stamp, or lambs may carry a round 'YL' stamp, indicating that the animal was under the age of 12 months, and therefore the spinal cord need not be removed under TSE control rules. Beef carcasses and carcasses of sheep over the age of 12 months may carry an inspector's personal stamp, indicating that TSE controls have been carried out.

Packaged products must also be identified with country and premises of origin, usually in the form of a Health Mark – as for carcasses in the case of wholesale supply, or as a smaller facsimile of the Health Mark on retail packages. Ideally, this label should be destroyed when the package is opened, so that it cannot be re-used by unscrupulous persons involved in illegal food production.

Other marks than the Health Mark may be seen on carcasses and foods, such as retailer brand labels or indications of compliance with Farm Assurance Schemes or Organic Standards. These are marketing strategies, and may not concern the certifying enforcement officer. However, the presence of the Health Mark, place of origin, dates of slaughter and processing and date of freezing are all important facets of the tracing and certification of foods of animal origin.

7 Meat Preservation and Processing

7.1 Conversion of Muscle to Meat

Paul Warriss

Introduction

Normally we do not eat carcass meat immediately after slaughter but, depending on the species concerned, wait for a period of between 1 and perhaps 21 days to elapse before doing so. During this time chemical changes in the musculature convert it into meat, generally improving its palatability. There are three main processes that are important: the muscles acidify, they go into rigor mortis and 'conditioning' takes place. In conditioning, also referred to as ageing, the meat becomes more tender and its flavour improves. These processes take place against a background of the carcass cooling, so that its surface becomes drier and the contained fat becomes harder. The hardening of the fat contributes to the general stiffening or firming of the carcass, facilitating the cutting of it into primal joints, and subsequent butchery. Traditionally, red meat carcasses are cooled by holding them overnight in refrigerated rooms operating at about 2°C. The muscle temperature therefore eventually falls from about 37°C to nearer 5°C in the first 24 hours post-mortem.

Muscle Structure

The overall structure of muscle is determined by a connective tissue skeleton. Within this is a hierarchical arrangement consisting of bundles of muscle fibres, the fibres themselves (equivalent to muscle cells), the contractile elements within the fibres, the myofibrils and the myofilaments within these. The myofilaments are of two sorts: thick filaments consisting mainly of the protein myosin, and thin filaments consisting mainly of the protein actin. The thick and thin myofilaments interdigitate and form the basis of the contractile mechanism.

So-called red, white and intermediate muscle fibres have different sorts of metabolism and contribute to the different characteristics of redder or paler muscles. The red colour is mostly due to myoglobin, which is related to the haemoglobin of blood.

Muscle Function

Muscle contraction is caused by myosin and actin molecules reacting together such that the thick and thin filaments slide over one another, shortening the muscle's length. The contraction is stimulated by calcium ions released from the sarcoplasmic reticulum membrane system within the muscle fibres, and requires adenosine triphosphate (ATP) as the energy source. ATP is also needed to maintain the working of the membrane systems. In the living animal ATP is produced from fatty acids or glucose delivered in the blood, or from glycogen stored in the muscle. Blood glucose and muscle glycogen are metabolized in very similar ways. First they are broken down to pyruvic acid (a process known as glycolysis), which produces a small amount of ATP, and then the pyruvic acid is oxidized completely to carbon dioxide and water (by oxidative decarboxylation and phosphorylation), which produces a lot more (a net yield of about 34 ATP molecules for every glucose molecule broken down). The oxygen for oxidation comes from the lungs via the blood. If it is not used immediately the ATP is stored in the muscle as creatine phosphate (CP). Muscles contain only relatively small amounts of ATP but much larger amounts of CP. However, immediately the available ATP is used, for example in supplying the energy for muscle contraction during exercise, it is replaced by the breakdown of CP. The reaction is reversible so that, in the period of recovery after exercise, ATP can be synthesized and used to replenish CP stores.

Post Mortem Changes in the Muscles

When an animal is killed, glucose and oxygen are no longer available via the blood stream. However, there is a continuing need for ATP to maintain membrane ion pumps and cell integrity. To continue to make ATP the muscle breaks down stored glycogen to pyruvic acid. Because there is no oxygen to complete the breakdown to carbon dioxide and water, and under the conditions found in the muscle at this time, the pyruvic acid is reduced to lactic acid. There is no blood circulation to remove the lactic acid, which therefore accumulates, and the muscle tissue acidifies. The pH drops from about 7.2 to 5.5 in a typical muscle. Acidification proceeds, and the generation of ATP continues, until the enzyme systems will no longer work in the acid conditions, or all the glycogen is used up. In beef an initial concentration of muscle glycogen of about 10 mg/g or more leads to normal acidification. The rate of acidification varies between species. It is most rapid in pork, followed by lamb then beef. The pH in beef may continue falling for

36 to 48 hours, while in pigs ultimate pH values are usually reached within 4 to 8 hours. The acidification leads to denaturation of some of the muscle proteins, and changes the characteristics and appearance of the muscle. It becomes paler and more opaque, and its ability to bind water decreases. If the muscle is cut the surface will exude moisture. This produces the drip (known in North America as purge) seen in retail packs of meat.

Meat quality problems associated with abnormal patterns of acidification

The pattern of acidification can have a large effect on meat quality. In extreme cases a very rapid acidification, caused by stress immediately before and at slaughter in pigs, can result in PSE (pale, soft, exudative) pork; a limited extent of acidification, caused by longer-term stress, that depletes muscle glycogen, can result in DFD (dark, firm, dry) meat in all species (often known as DCB – dark cutting beef – in cattle). Lesser variations in the pattern of acidification are the cause of much of the variation seen in the colour, particularly paleness or darkness, and in water-holding capacity in normal meat.

Development of rigor mortis

After slaughter, the muscles also gradually stiffen, signifying the onset of rigor mortis. The time of onset varies between species and between individual animals. ATP present in living muscle keeps it in a relaxed state, as well as being needed for contraction. When ATP can no longer be generated by glycolysis and is eventually exhausted, the muscles lose this relaxed state and pass into rigor. Their length becomes fixed because the actin and myosin molecules bind together irrevocably so the thick and thin myofilaments will no longer slide over one another. The onset of rigor is therefore controlled solely by the availability, or not, of ATP. It is not necessarily related to muscle pH, although normally the muscle will enter rigor as it acidifies. Factors that affect the level of muscle glycogen around the time of slaughter can also affect the rate of rigor development because lower than normal levels of glycogen provide only a limited supply of potential ATP. So, animals that have been very stressed, or exhaustively exercised, before slaughter may go into rigor more quickly than normal. If all the glycogen is depleted before slaughter the muscle will not acidify at all and rigor will occur very rapidly in this relatively alkaline state. This is therefore known as alkaline rigor.

The importance of rigor for meat quality

The thick myosin filaments and thin actin filaments are organized in the muscle in functional units called sarcomeres. Each myofibril within the muscle cell is composed of thousands of sarcomeres arranged end-to-end. The sarcomeres are shorter in contracted muscles and longer in relaxed muscles. Sarcomere length is a major factor influencing meat toughness. If contracted muscles are cooked they tend to be tough, while relaxed muscles tend to be tender. Rigor is important because it fixes the lengths of the sarcomeres, and therefore the muscle's length and the potential texture of the meat. Muscles entering rigor in a very contracted state will tend to produce tough meat; those entering rigor in a relaxed, or stretched, state will produce tender meat. This is taken advantage of in certain novel methods of hanging carcasses just after dressing has been completed. In these, by supporting the weight of the carcass from the pelvic girdle, rather than from the more usual hind leg, certain muscles are stretched before they go into rigor, so that the sarcomeres are extended. The longer sarcomere length is 'fixed' when rigor develops so that the resulting meat is more tender.

Before the onset of rigor, stimuli that cause muscle contraction may result in changes in meat texture. One stimulus that is especially significant is a cold temperature. If the carcass is cooled too quickly then some of the muscles may contract and, if as is likely, the contraction is not followed by relaxation, the resulting meat is tough, a phenomenon known as cold shortening. It tends to be mostly a problem in lamb carcasses because these are small and so cool quickly. Sometimes it occurs in beef but rarely in pork. Rapid chilling is desirable in limiting bacterial growth and in reducing carcass weight loss. To prevent cold shortening carcasses are sometimes stimulated electrically soon after death of the animal. This speeds up muscle metabolism so that the muscles can no longer contract when subjected to any cold stimulus.

The resolution of rigor mortis

Meat cooked immediately after the onset of rigor mortis is rather tough. With time the muscles soften and the meat becomes more tender when cooked. The rate of tenderization differs in the different species and increases with temperature. Chicken meat needs less than a day to achieve adequate tenderness but the texture of beef will improve with longer storage of up to 3 weeks or more. This variation leads to different recommended ageing times before meat is consumed: 4–10 days for pork, 7–14 days for lamb and 10–21 days for beef.

Conditioning

Tenderization occurs through the action of proteolytic enzymes called calpains, that break down structural proteins in particular parts of the muscle cell and so weaken its structure. However, there is no dissociation of the actin–myosin of the myofilaments. In the live animal calpains are involved in the normal breakdown of proteins associated with the body's protein turnover. Calpains are more active at higher pH values and are activated by calcium ions. These flood out of the muscle cell membrane systems when ATP is exhausted and energy for the membrane ion pumps is therefore no longer available, thus initiating proteolysis. For this reason, the infusion of meat with calcium salts (usually $CaCl_2$) can promote tenderization, and this has been suggested as a way of tenderizing meat commercially. In the absence of calcium, calpains are inhibited by calpastatin, to which they are bound. Eventually, however, the calpastatin itself is broken down by the calpains. Longer ageing also improves the juiciness and flavour of the meat, as well as tenderness, but it is not clear how this occurs.

Further Reading

Bendall, J.R. (1973) Post mortem changes in muscles. In: Bourne, G.H. (ed.) *The Structure and Function of Muscle*, 2nd edn, Volume II, Part 2. Academic Press, New York and London, pp. 243–309.

Bendall, J.R. and Swatland, H.J. (1988) A review of the relationships of pH with physical aspects of pork quality. *Meat Science* 24, 85–126.

Dransfield, E. (1994a) Optimisation of tenderisation, ageing and tenderness. *Meat Science* 36, 105–121.

Dransfield, E. (1994b) Tenderness of meat, poultry and fish. In: Pearson, A.M. and Dutson, T.R. (eds) *Quality Attributes and their Measurement in Meat, Poultry and Fish Products*. Blackie Academic and Professional (Chapman and Hall), London, pp. 289–315.

Fabiansson, S., Reutersward, A.L. and Libelius, R. (1985) Ultrastructural and biochemical changes in electrically stimulated dark cutting beef. *Meat Science* 12, 177–188.

Farmer, L.J. (1992) Meat flavour. In: Johnston, D.E., Knight, M.K. and Ledward, D.A. (eds) *The Chemistry of Meat-based Foods*. Royal Society of Chemistry, Cambridge, UK, pp. 169–182.

Warriss, P.D. and Brown, S.N. (1987) The relationship between initial pH, reflectance and exudation in pig muscle. *Meat Science* 20, 65–74.

7.2. Basic Methods Used in Food Preservation and Processing

Basic Characteristics of Meat

Fresh meat is a general term commonly used for chilled skeletal muscles with incorporated tissues (e.g. fatty tissue, connective tissue, lymph nodes, blood/lymph vessels, nerves), in which the main post-mortal changes have been completed but which have not been subjected to treatments such as freezing, salting/curing, drying and similar. Basic characteristics of meat include colour, water-holding capacity, aroma and texture.

Meat colour

Muscle pigment is myoglobin, a chromoprotein which – together with other coloured compounds such as haemoglobin – gives meat its normal red colour. Myoglobin comprises a porphyrin ring with an iron atom in the centre (haem) and an albumin-type protein globin. The iron in myoglobin is in the Fe^{++} form, but during oxidation changes to Fe^{+++}. The total myoglobin content, and hence intensity of red colour, in animal muscles varies with species (e.g. horse>cattle>pig), age (older>younger), sex (male>female) and diet. At slaughter, myoglobin is normally saturated with oxygen (oxy-Mb, Fe^{++}, having a pink–red colour), but after slaughter oxygen is spent and meat predominantly contains myoglobin (Mb, Fe^{++}, having a purple colour). Depending on conditions, e.g. partial oxygen pressure, pH and storage, met-myoglobin – in which iron is oxidized (met-Mb, Fe^{+++}, having a brown colour) – can be formed. Therefore, meat colour depends on relationships between, and proportions of, the three forms of the main meat pigment. Higher levels of oxygen (e.g. >20%) lead to formation of oxy-Mb, whilst met-Mb is formed at lower (e.g. <4%) levels of oxygen. Lower meat pH and higher storage temperature usually contribute to met-Mb formation.

Water-holding capacity (WHC) of meat

Meat has the ability to hold (bind) naturally contained or added water when exposed to some treatments such as heating, freezing or pressure. The proportion of water that is separated/released from meat after such treatments is called 'free water', whilst the proportion that remains within meat is called 'bound' water. The former comprises mainly water located extra-cellularly, and the latter comprises water firmly immobilized, i.e. chemically bound (electrostatically) to meat protein molecules. The amount of immobilized water in meat is variable. At higher pH, meat has a higher WHC than at lower pH, so the highest WHC is immediately after slaughter, whilst the lowest occurs during post-mortem rigor. During meat tenderization, the WHC increases.

Meat aroma

Meat aroma is a combination of sensations due to actions of hundreds of chemical compounds from meat on our taste and smell senses. The aroma-inducing meat compounds include sodium and potassium salts, lactic acid, ribose, nucleic acids, amines, glycogen and fatty acids. Meat aroma is affected by animal species, age, sex, diet and the extent of post-mortem meat ageing. A particular problem with meat aroma can be caused by the presence in meat of higher levels of compounds related to the male hormones androsterone, skatole and indole, which give meat (particularly fatty tissue) a sexual odour called 'boar taint'. It can become a problem in meat from uncastrated ('entire') male pigs slaughtered older than 6–8 months and >80 kg live weight. If too strong, boar taint can make meat unfit for human consumption, but individual tolerance can vary with culture, eating habits and sex; women appear to be more sensitive than men. Sensorially detectable concentrations of androsterone in meat are >0.2–0.5 mg/g.

Meat texture

The physical properties of meat that can be registered visually, by touch and hearing, as well as during mastication, are called meat texture. Meat structure comprising relationship and connection between different tissues can be sensed visually. Tenderness/toughness of meat can be sensed by touch and also during mastication. Sound produced during chewing of meat also can be sensed aurally. Meat texture is affected by animal species, age, sex, breed and condition; it is determined by muscle structure, characteristics of connective tissue, amount of intramuscular fatty tissue, and how all these are interconnected. In addition, texture is affected by the extent of post-mortem changes, i.e. ageing, intensity of rigor mortis and WHC. Immediately after slaughter, meat texture is soft and elastic, but loses elasticity and becomes much firmer after a few hours. Subsequently, meat becomes more tender only after sufficient ageing. Meat having a very high WHC (e.g. DFD meat) has a firm and dry texture, whilst meat with a low WHC (e.g. PSE meat) is soft and with loose structure.

Meat Refrigeration

Artificial meat refrigeration as a means to extend meat shelf life has been known for a long time; commercial use started in the late 19th century in the USA. Its effects are based on inhibition of multiplication and/or metabolic activity of contaminating microorganisms.

During refrigeration, the temperature of the meat decreases from normal animal body temperature (around 38°C) to 4–7°C, or even to 1–2°C in meat intended for longer storage. To achieve that, carcasses are hung in refrigeration rooms on rails around 3.2–3.5 m high (cattle) or 2.4–2.7 m high (pigs).

Carcass refrigeration technologies differ, but can be divided into dry (i.e. air) refrigeration used for red meat and poultry carcasses, and wet (i.e. water) refrigeration used for poultry. Air refrigeration of red meat carcasses includes three main types: slow, rapid and ultra-rapid (i.e. shock) refrigeration.

Slow air refrigeration is used rarely, in small abattoirs with traditional technologies, and comprises three steps: carcass 'draining' or 'drying' at ambient temperature lasting a few hours, pre-refrigeration (around 10°C; 75% relative air humidity – RH) and refrigeration (4–7°C, 85–90% RH). The resulting dry carcass surface is beneficial in terms of surface microflora supression, but the weight loss is relatively high (around 3%).

In the case of rapid air refrigeration, carcasses are exposed to air at −1 to +1°C, 90% RH and 1–3 m/sec circulation for 24–36 h (cattle) or 18–24 h (pigs, lambs); weight loss is around 1.5–2.0%.

Ultra-rapid air refrigeration is two-phased. Carcasses are first exposed to intensive circulation (2–4 m/sec) of very cold (−4 to −6°C) and humid (90–100%) air in special tunnels for around 1–3 hours. This is followed by refrigeration at −1 to 2°C for 18–22 h (cattle) or for 14–16 h (pigs) with circulation of only 0.1 – 0.3 m/s. Weight loss is around 1%. Whilst as rapid as possible refrigeration of carcasses is desirable from microbial safety and practical perspectives, too rapid cooling can lead to some meat quality problems. If muscle is cooled below 10°C before rigor is complete, i.e. before the pH drops below 6.0 and while glycogen and ATP are still present, meat becomes very tough (see also Chapter 7.1). This phenomenon is in practice called 'cold shortening'.

The following biochemical explanation for cold shortening has been offered. Contraction-stimulating calcium is stored in mitochondria and in the sarcoplasmic reticulum, and a 'pump' (ATP-powered) removes it from the cytoplasm. However, at cell temperatures below 10°C this pump is less efficient, which enables leakage of calcium from its stores. If ATP is still present at those low temperatures, i.e. if they are reached before rigor, the leaked calcium will stimulate shortening of the myofilaments, i.e. contraction. To prevent cold shortening, the refrigeration regime should be adjusted to ensure that meat temperature does not fall below 10°C in 10 h (for beef) or 7 h (for pork). Another way to prevent cold shortening is to 'electrostimulate' carcasses before refrigeration. The treatment is based on passing pulses of electrical current through muscles, which stimulates a large number muscle contractions in a short time so that glycogen and ATP are quickly used up. This accelerates rigor onset and enables rapid cooling without cold shortening. Electrical stimulation treatment can be either of the high-voltage type (e.g. peak 700–1000V; 14 Hz pulses frequency; 90 sec duration) or the low-voltage type (e.g. 90 V; 14 Hz; 60 sec). The former can be applied within 1 h post-slaughter, whilst the latter only immediately after slaughter. In addition, there are indications that electrical stimulation can improve meat tenderness, to a lesser extent, even in situations where cold shortening is unlikely, e.g. in slow-refrigerated meat. A potential third way of reducing meat toughness during chilling is by hip suspension of carcasses, which mechanically reduces shortening of the main muscles.

The storage shelf life of chilled red meat carcasses can be very variable, depending on both storage conditions and levels of initial microflora. Under good conditions (e.g. 2°C), carcasses can have a shelf life of 3–4 (cattle) or 1–2 (pigs, lambs) weeks. However, under the same conditions, offal has a much shorter storage shelf life (e.g. 3 days).

Wet refrigeration is used mainly for poultry and is based on either spraying poultry carcasses with cold water or on submerging them in basins (spin-chillers) with running cold water for around 1 h. The former system is hygienically beneficial from the perspective of preventing cross-contamination, but uses more water (up to 10–12 l/carcass) than the latter (up to 4 l/carcass).

Packaging of Chilled Meat and its Spoilage

In modern times and in developed countries, most chilled meats are sold packaged. The main intentions with packaging of meat are to protect the product from secondary contamination during the handling–retail display–consumer chain of events, or to suppress microflora, or both. Microbial spoilage of meat can be caused by various organisms (Table 7.1), but the most important group is bacteria. Under conditions suitable for growth of both bacteria and fungi (yeast and mould) on a given food, bacteria always out-compete and outgrow fungi, and thus are the cause of spoilage. Normally, fungi cause food spoilage only where bacteria are suppressed, e.g. in very acidic or very dry foods.

Table 7.1. The three main categories of microorganisms that can spoil meat.

Category and examples of microorganism	Approximate range of growth			
	Temperature	pH	Oxygen	A_w
Bacterium *Pseudomonas* *Lactobacillus* *Brochothrix*	> 0°C	>5	Can grow in presence and/or absence	High
Mould *Thamnidium* *Cladosporium* *Penicillium*	~–5°C	3.8–6	Require O_2	Low
Yeast *Debaromyces*	~–5°C	4–6	Require O_2	Medium–low

Aerobic packaging of raw meat and its spoilage

Packaging meat in oxygen-permeable materials has beneficial effects with respect to the stability of meat colour, as oxygen helps formation of red-coloured oxygenated forms of myoglobin. On the other hand, as oxygen is available on the product surface, after sufficiently long storage the meat will undergo an aerobic type of microbial spoilage.

Chemical aspects

During aerobic spoilage, various meat compounds are degraded by meat enzymes (minor contribution) and microbial enzymes (major contribution), which can result in numerous end products having unpleasant sensory characteristics. Proteinaceous elements of meat are first degraded to lower molecule compounds in the order: proteins–polypeptides–peptides–free amino acids. Such changes occur normally during meat maturation (ageing) and, up to this stage, no negative effects on sensory qualities are noticeable. However, when the changes include degradation of free amino acids resulting in accumulation of compounds such as ammonia, hydrogen sulphide and amines, this produces characteristic, putrid off-odours (so-called putrefactive type of spoilage). In addition, protein degradation includes changes of myoglobin into oxidized forms, which results in a change of the red meat colour to grey, brown or green. On the other hand, if the meat contains more carbohydrates – natural or added – their degradation will result in accumulation of acids, which characterizes the so-called souring type of spoilage. Chemical changes during meat spoilage also include oxidation of fats, along the following chain of events: fats–free fatty acids–aldehydes/ketones. This results in rancidity.

Microbial aspects

Aerobic spoilage of chilled meat can be caused by a range of psychrophilic or psychrotrophic microorganisms. Nevertheless, at $<5°C$, *Pseudomonas* is normally a dominant spoilage organism, particularly if the meat pH is lower (e.g. beef). At refrigeration temperatures $>5°C$, however, *Brochothrix thermosphacta* can become more dominant, particularly if the meat pH is higher (e.g. pork, lamb). Signs of spoilage become noticeable at microbial levels between 10^7/g (off-odour) and 10^8/g (slime). Nevertheless, the composition of microflora and the metabolic patterns of dominant microorganisms are more relevant for spoilage than are the microbial numbers. Also, it seems that microbial metabolites from amino acids appear in higher-pH meat sooner (i.e. at microbial level of 10^6/g) than in lower-pH meat (i.e. at level of 10^8/g).

Sensory aspects

The unpleasant sensory characteristic of aerobically spoiled meat is a consequence of the accumulation of a complex mixture of microbial metabolites. The first stage of spoilage is characterized by a sweet, fruity odour (ethyl esters). In the advanced stage, a putrid odour is noticeable due to accumulation of sulphur compounds, ammonia and amines – particularly if *Pseudomonas* is dominant – and of acetoin, diacetyl and 3-methylbutanol, particularly if *Brochothrix* is dominant. Ultimately, signs of spoilage include meat greening (with or without fluorescence) and slime layer.

Comminuted meats

The general course of spoilage in comminuted, aerobically stored meat is similar to that of meat cuts, but is faster. The reasons for this includes poorer microbial status due to usually higher initial microbial levels, distribution of surface meat contamination throughout the product during mincing, and to the higher growth rate of bacteria due to damaged tissue membranes, finer structure and larger surface area in minced meat. Dominant spoilage organisms include *Pseudomonas* and psychrotrophic Enterobacteriaceae, but if the former is suppressed (e.g. by certain added preservatives) spoilage can be caused by *Brochothrix thermosphacta*.

Bone taint

Surface spoilage of aerobically stored joints is similar to spoilage of other raw meats, but spoilage can also develop in deep meat where anaerobic conditions exist even if the joint is stored aerobically. Deep meat spoilage (commonly called 'bone taint') is associated particularly with joints including cured – such as shoulder, gammon – and is characterized by off-odours in deep meat close to bones and/or in bone marrow. It occurs more frequently during summer and in higher-pH meat. The causes are not yet fully understood, but possible explanations include internal contamination (invasion) by bacteria during the agonal phase of pig slaughter and poor distribution of curing agents. Bone taint can take the course of either a souring- or a putrefaction-type of spoilage, and a range of bacteria – including particular types of psychrotrophic *Clostridia* – have been isolated from such meat.

Poultry

Generally, poultry meat is packaged only aerobically as its colour is more sensitive than that of red meats. Bacteria on poultry carcasses occur in feather holes and on cut surfaces, but their distribution on carcasses can vary considerably depending on the abattoir technology. Aerobic spoilage of chilled (<5°C) eviscerated poultry is very similar to that of red meat, but is usually faster.

Vacuum-packaging of raw meat and its spoilage

Lack of oxygen within a vacuum package (in oxygen-non-permeable materials) has a profound effect on the course of microbial spoilage of meat.

Aerobic microorganisms often present on meat (e.g. *Pseudomonas*, *Shewanella*, etc.) – that would have been dominant were the meat stored aerobically – are now suppressed and unable to grow. However, the anaerobic conditions allow proliferation of micro-aerophilic members of the initial microflora, including lactic acid bacteria (e.g. *Lactobacillus*, *Leuconostoc*, *Carnobacterium*), particularly in the case of low-pH meat. The main end product of metabolism of these organisms is lactic acid, which has a 'dairy' or 'cheesy' odour/flavour that is much more acceptable to consumers than the putrefactive microbial end products present in aerobically spoiled meat. Therefore, the shelf life of vacuum-packaged chilled meat is much longer. However, this is not because all microbial development is suppressed, but rather because vacuum packaging selects for more tolerable type of microorganisms, producing sensorially more acceptable end metabolites (i.e. lactic acid bacteria). Nevertheless, the initially mild 'cheesy' odour increases with storage time and ultimately, after a long enough time, becomes unacceptably intensive, and spoils vacuum-packaged meat. Sometimes, particularly if (and contrary to good practice) high-pH meat is vacuum packaged, its spoilage can be caused primarily by *Brochothrix* producing sharp off-odours.

Packaging of raw meat in saturated (100%) carbon dioxide atmosphere and its spoilage

With this technology, gas-impermeable packaging materials – such as an aluminium-foil layer – are used. After removal of the air from the packaging by vacuum, the bag is filled with a sufficient volume of 100% CO_2 gas and sealed. A proportion of carbon dioxide dissolves in water on the meat surface ('meat saturation') and produces carbonic acid, which lowers the surface pH of the meat. This, in combination with CO_2-induced damage of bacterial cells' membranes' permeability and inhibition of bacterial enzymes, causes extension of the bacterial lag phase and generation times. Because of the lack of oxygen, the dominant microflora on saturated carbon dioxide-packaged meat include *Lactobacillus*, *Leuconostoc* and *Carnobacterium* (similar to vacuum packaging), producing lactic acid and having a more acceptable 'cheesy' odour. The net result is prevention of growth of aerobic spoilage flora, selection for lactic acid bacteria and extension of the meat shelf life. In addition, CO_2 eliminates oxidative rancidity of fats. Therefore, meat packaged in saturated carbon dioxide can be cold-stored incomparably longer (several months) than aerobically packaged meat (1–2 weeks), and significantly longer than vacuum-packaged meat (several weeks).

However, packaging of raw meat in saturated CO_2 poses one meat quality-related problem: 100% CO_2 causes a brown colour of the meat, which is unacceptable for consumers. However, when the meat is removed from such packaging and exposed to oxygen, its normal red colour recovers. Therefore, packaging in a saturated carbon dioxide atmosphere is used primarily for long-term bulk storage of raw meat, such as in the case of lengthy transport to remote markets, where it is subsequently removed and packed in oxygen-containing packaging for retail sale. On the other hand, cured meat products having a stable red colour (nitrites) can be, and often are, packaged and retailed in a CO_2 atmosphere.

Packaging of raw meat in a modified atmosphere (MAP) and its spoilage

Modified atmosphere meat packaging technology is aimed at simultaneously using the advantages, and avoiding the disadvantages, of oxygen and carbon dioxide. Modified atmospheres in the packages comprise a gaseous mixture of lower concentrations of oxygen (to maintain red colour) and higher concentrations of carbon dioxide (to inhibit microflora), but also can contain certain proportion of inert gas(es) to maintain targeted concentrations of the former two. Meat companies usually find the atmosphere composition that suits their own products best through trial and error. Nevertheless, generally, MAPs for raw meat comprise 60–75% CO_2, 10–25% oxygen and 15–30% nitrogen. The type of dominant flora in MAP-packaged meat depends on the gas composition. If high levels of oxygen are used, meat spoilage will be similar to aerobically stored meat – putrefactive (*Pseudomonas*). If lower levels of oxygen, but higher levels of CO_2, are used, the meat spoilage will be caused by lactic acid bacteria – similar to vacuum-packaged meat.

'Intelligent' packaging of food

This type of packaging is aimed at incorporation of certain indicators either of meat spoilage or of health hazards, or of both, that would easily and visibly warn when the meat is no longer acceptable. A number of various indicators have been researched:

- storage time–temperature indicators;
- leak indicators (e.g. for oxygen);
- freshness indicators that detect microbial metabolites, e.g. diacetyl, amines, ammonia, ethanol, hydrogen sulphide;
- indicators for activity of microbial enzymes;
- indicators of consumption of certain nutrients by microflora;
- food safety indicators based on detection of microbes as such or their toxins.

Although 'intelligent' packaging of foods probably has a great potential, the technology is still largely in the research/development stage.

'Active' packaging of food

With this technology, certain antimicrobial compounds – such as chemical preservatives or bacteriocins – are incorporated into, and subsequently are slowly released from, packaging material onto the food to suppress the microflora. Alternatively, such antimicrobials can be introduced (e.g. sprayed, injected) and contained within the package, i.e. between the packaging material and the food.

Freezing of meat

Freezing of meat in industrial abattoirs is normally carried out in so-called 'freezing tunnels' with air at temperatures of between −20 and −40°C, a relative humidity of 95–100% and a circulation of 2–4 m/s. These rooms must have effective insulation from the outside environment, and walls/doors made of appropriate materials to withstand freezing. Due to associated occupational health and safety risks, appropriate security measures are necessary in these rooms, including an appropriate locking system and door heaters which preventing their freeze-blockage in the shut position.

Meat freezes (cryoscopy points) at temperatures of between −1.5 and −1.8°C (muscle tissue) or −2.2°C (fatty tissue). Only the water in meat is actually frozen, and initially only a proportion of it. The concentration of various compounds dissolved in the water increases in the remaining unfrozen water which, in turn, decreases its freezing point. Consequently, approximately only 75% of water in meat is frozen at −5°C, around 90% at −30°C and 100% at −60°C.

Various freezing regimes are used in the meat industry, with freezing rates determined by factors such as air temperature and circulation, as well as by size, shape and fat content of the meat. The meat freezing rate can be expressed by at what depth, measured from the surface, meat becomes frozen within a given time unit. For example, air-mediated (convection-based) freezing regimes can be slow (freezing rate <1 cm/h), rapid (1–5 cm/h) or very rapid (>5 cm/h). In the case of contact freezing where the meat is in direct contact with cold plates (conduction-based), even higher freezing rates are achieved.

Freezing and defrostation have some profound effects on meat quality. Normal post-mortal biochemical processes are very inhibited. If the meat is frozen before the onset of rigor mortis, rigor will be delayed but will resume on defrostation – sometimes called 'defrostation rigor'. The volume of meat increases with freezing due to ice formation. Ice crystals cause physical damage to muscle cell membranes; this is more so during slow freezing, where larger crystals are formed, than during rapid freezing. Partial, freezing-induced denaturation of meat proteins also occurs which, in combination with damage to membranes, reduces the water-holding ability of the meat after defrostion. Consequently, a certain amount of meat juice (drip) is released from defrosted meat, usually causing weight loss of around 1–1.5%. The amount of defrostation drip depends on various factors, including the defrosting method. If frozen meat is defrosted slowly by placing it at refrigertion temperatures (e.g.

4–7°C), the drip will be less than if quickly defrosted at higher temperatures. As a simplified, practical guidance for frozen storage, it could be said that the rapid freezing–slow thawing system best preserves the quality of raw meat.

Microbial spoilage of meat during frozen storage is very inhibited or totally prevented. As indicated in Chapter 7.3, this inhibition is temperature-dependant. It can be assumed that bacterial activity ceases at temperatures of −7°C, whilst that of yeasts and moulds ceases at −12°C. Therefore, to prevent microbial spoilage, meat should be stored at −12°C (frozen meat) or preferably at −18°C or less (deep-frozen meat).

However, that will not prevent physical and chemical changes in the frozen meat resulting in slow, undesirable changes in the sensory qualities of the meat that will make it ultimately unacceptable, i.e. unfit for human consumption. If the frozen meat is stored non-packaged, the ice on the meat surface can evaporate (sublimation) and the exposed meat can oxidize producing dry, discoloured patches – popularly called 'freezing burns'.

The main cause of chemical spoilage of frozen meat is oxidation of the fat, i.e. free fatty acids resulting in compounds (e.g. aldehydes, ketones) characteristic of rancidity. Fatty tissues with a higher content of unsaturated and polyunsaturated fatty acids ('soft fat') become rancid sooner, so they have a shorter frozen shelf life than fatty tissues containing mainly saturated fatty acids ('hard fats'). As the saturation degree of fatty acids in meat of different animal species is in decreasing order: beef–lamb–pork–poultry–fish, their frozen shelf lives are in correlated decreasing order as well. They depend on pre-freezing freshness and composition of meat, storage temperature and the packaging material but, as a general idea, it could be presumed that frozen beef can be stored for up to 12 months, lamb 9 months, pork 6–7 months, poultry 4–5 months and oily fish 2–3 months.

Salting and curing of meat

The terms 'salting' and 'curing' of meat are often erroneously used as synonyms, not only among consumers. In fact, meat salting means treatment of meat with salt (sodium chloride) only, whilst in meat curing, the product is treated with cure (also called brine) – a mixture containing salt, nitrites and/or nitrates and possibly some other compounds (e.g. phosphates, reducing agents, sugars).

Methods for salting or curing

Salting and curing of meat are carried out in a similar manner, and the practical applications can be grouped into: (i) dry methods (mainly for dry meat products); (ii) wet methods (mainly for cooked products); and (iii) combined methods.

DRY METHODS. With dry methods, meat is first surface treated with dry salt or dry brine, and then held at 0–7°C for extended periods (2–4 weeks) depending on the meat cut's size, composition and pH. During that time, the salt or brine ingredients diffuse into the meat, whilst a proportion of non-bound water is released from the meat. For some dry meat products (e.g. country-style hams), release of water is desirable, so this can be enhanced by putting the meat under presure (e.g. weights) during the process.

WET METHODS. With wet methods, salting or curing can be conducted by submerging the meat in a solution of salt/brine in water for certain periods of time (with refrigeration), allowing the salt/brine ingredients to diffuse from the solution into the meat. The process can be speeded up by using machines with multiple, hollow needles to inject a more concentrated solution deeply into the meat, followed by mechanical treatments of the meat (in 'massaging' or 'tumbling' machines). This further enhances the diffusion and uniform distribution of the salt/brine.

COMBINED METHODS. With combined methods, meat is first dry-salted/cured and then additionally treated by salt/cure solution.

Salting or curing preparations and roles of the ingredients

DRY SALT. Dry salt normally contains >95% sodium chloride. Its main role is to lower the water activity (a_w) of meat so as to inhibit spoilage and pathogenic microorganisms, as well as to achieve desirable taste. Optimal concentrations of salt targeted in the meat depend on the type of the intended meat product, and range from 1.5–2.2% in different types of cooked sausages or 2.5–7% in dry meat products.

DRY BRINE. Dry brine can comprise: (i) salt with 0.5–0.6% sodium nitrite; (ii) salt with 1–3% potassium nitrate; (iii) salt with 0.5–0.6% sodium nitrite and 1% potassium nitrate; or (iv) salt with 0.9–1.2% potassium nitrate. Dry brines are normally pre-mixed and are commercial products, rather than composed on the plant's production line. Using commercial mixes avoids public health risks associated with either handling of concentrated toxic compounds (nitrites), their overdosing, or both, by the plant's staff.

SODIUM NITRITE. Sodium nitrite ($NaNO_2$) is a reactive, unstable, toxic compund, so is added to meat in concentrations of less than 100–200 mg/kg (i.e. <0.01–0.02%). For potential public health concerns related to use of nitrites in meat see Chapter 1.3. The roles of nitrites in meat processing are multiple: (i) meat safety-orientated: inhibition of spoilage and pathogenic bacteria (particularly of *Clostridia*, including *Cl. botulinum*); and (ii) commercial/meat quality-orientated: stabilization of meat colour, inhibition of fatty acid oxidation and improvement of aroma.

The effect of nitrites on meat colour is based on slow and complex chemical reactions, but the main aspects include reduction of nitrites ($NaNO_2$) to nitrogen monoxide (NO), which reacts with myoglobin (muscle pigment), producing red-coloured nitrosyl-myoglobin (NOMb). During further processing of meat (e.g. cooking, fermentation, drying) associated with lowering of pH and denaturation of globin, NOMb is converted into nitrosyl-myochromogen which has a desirable, stable pink-red colour that is maintained even after cooking of the product.

POTASSIUM NITRATE. Potassium nitrate (KNO_3) is much less toxic than nitrites and is a very weak inhibitor of microorganisms. It contributes to the desirable flavour of meat products, but in higher concentrations is bitter, so is not added to meat at levels greater than 0.5–0.6%. The main role of nitrates is to serve, through reduction of NO_3 to NO_2, as a source (precursor) for the formation of nitrites.

PHOSPHATES. Phosphates are chain molecules comprising two (diphosphates) or three (triphosphates) or several tens (polyphosphates) of phosphorus atoms linked with oxygen. Their role is to enhance both the water-holding capacity of meat proteins and the mixing of fat and water (emulsion). Therefore, phosphates are normally used for commercial/meat quality reasons in meat products that contain added water (e.g. hot dogs, cooked hams, etc.). There are numerous commercially available phosphate preparations that can be of a neutral, basic or acidic nature. Phosphates are added in concentrations of up to 0.3% (calculated as P_2O_3) in the finished product.

REDUCING AGENTS. Reducing agents include primarily sodium salts of ascorbic acid or isoascorbic acid. They are added to meat in concentrations of up to 500 mg/kg (i.e. 0.05%), normally towards the end of the production process. Their role is to reduce meat redox potential so to enhance both reduction of nitrites to nitrogen monoxide and the formation of nitrosyl-myoglobin (i.e. the red colour) in cured meat.

SUGARS. Sugars, usually a mixture of dextrose, saccharose and starch, are added to some meat products with the aim of improving the taste/aroma, including masking saltiness or bitterness (from nitrates), to contribute to red colour formation, as a reducing agent, and to enhance the growth of useful microorganisms in some products such as fermented meats (e.g. salami).

Smoking of meat

Smoke is a result of aerobic or anaerobic pyrolysis of woods, their polysaccharides: cellulose, hemi-cellulose and lignin. It starts at around 170°C, and at temperatures up to 270°C is endothermic, and above that has an intensive exothermic nature. Anaerobically, pyrolysis results in smoke containing a large number of chemical compounds such as organic acids, aldehydes, alcohols, furans and phenols, that are useful for meat production. At higher temperatures (>300–400°C), undesirable toxic polycyclic aromatic hydrocarbons (see Chapter 1.3) are formed, in increasing concentrations as the temperature increases. Aerobically, wood burns intensively, with smoke containing largely water vapour and carbon dioxide.

Therefore, for food-smoking purposes, smoke is produced mainly endothermically, from 'damp' wood chippings and by limiting the air supply.

Meat smoking can be based on traditional or modern technologies. In the former case (small plants), wood is pyrolysed in open containers placed inside or outside smoking rooms where products are hung; the conditions (and the smoke) are very difficult to control. In the latter case, smoke is produced in industrial generators, with wood either being spread on heated metal plates or being pressed against a fast-rotating plate (friction). With both type of generators, the conditions, and hence the smoke temperature (around 200°C) and composition, are controllable. The smoke generated can be treated in various ways to achieve desirable characteristics, e.g. be cooled or heated within a pipe system, or dissolved/condensed in water or other liquids to produce 'liquid smoke', and/or specially filtered to remove particles or unwanted compounds, before its application to the product. Applications include cold-smoking in the air (e.g. fermented sausage, dried meats), hot-smoking in the air (e.g. cooked sausage), electrostatically-aided smoking in the air, incorporation of liquid smoke into brine or product mixture and submerging/spraying of the product with liquid smoke.

The two main reasons for smoking meats are: (i) commercial/meat quality-orientated, to achieve popular sensory qualities of the product; and (ii) meat safety-orientated, to inhibit spoilage and pathogenic microorganisms. Product quality effects of meat smoking include typical colour due both to attachment–polymerization of smoke compounds on the product surface and to reactions between smoke carbonyls and meat amines (Maillard reaction); typical aroma; and better texture, i.e. physical structure of the product due to coagulation of meat proteins (e.g. collagen). Product safety effects of smoking include inhibition of microorganisms on product surface by a number of chemical compounds present in smoke (see above). However, the antimicrobial effects of smoke are relatively limited and, alone, are insufficient to control bacterial pathogens or toxigenic moulds. Nevertheless, smoking can contribute to the antimicrobial effects of other preservative factors acting in/on the product.

Drying of meat

Drying of meat is based on removal of the water, through two simultaneous processes: internal and external diffusion of moisture. Through the former, moisture migrates from the inner layers of the product towards the product surface, whilst through the latter it evaporates from the surface.

Drying can occur only if the partial water vapour pressure on the product surface is greater than the relative air humidity at a given temperature. During meat drying, loosely bound moisture diffuses first – initially only water located between myofibrils, but later also from within the muscle cells. A proportion of water firmly bound to the meat proteins can be removed under special conditions, e.g. under vacuum, but a proportion of water very firmly bound (hydrated water) cannot be removed even under vacuum. The net result of drying is lowering of water activity (a_w) in the product to values inhibitory for spoilage and pathogenic microorganisms (see Chapter 7.3). However, excessive drying to very low a_w values can result in a product with unacceptable sensory qualities.

Meat drying is most often carried out by keeping the product suspended in air. Initially, whilst the product's a_w is relatively high and non-inhibitory for pathogens, drying is carried at lower temperatures, e.g. 10–15°C. As drying progresses and the product's a_w decreases, air temperature can be increased. At higher temperatures relative air humidity is lower, which speeds up drying. Nevertheless, the drying process should be gradual because, if it is too rapid, a hard, very dry layer of coagulated proteins could be formed on the product's surface, which would prevent further drying of deeper layers. Generally, to achieve balanced meat drying, the relative air humidity should be 2–3 units lower than the a_w value of the product.

Another, less common drying method is lyophilization, in which the meat is first frozen and then exposed to a very low pressure of around 5–6 mbar ('in vacuum') at 20–40°C. In this way, even firmly bound water is removed (90% of the total) from meat, resulting in a very dry product – retaining the same volume but having only around 70% of the original weight. Lean meat is selected for lyophilization, to avoid the rapid rancidity to which it is prone, and later the product is used either for further processing into various industrially prepared dishes (e.g. soups) or for strategic reserves.

Based on their final a_w values, foods can be divided into three global groups:

1. High-moisture products having an a_w value of 0.9–1.0 (e.g. cooked sausage, cooked ham); those with $a_w \geq 0.95$ and pH ≥ 5.2 have to be refrigerated at ≤ 5°C, those with a_w 0.91–0.95 and pH ≤ 5.2 have to be refrigerated ≤ 10°C, and those with a_w 0.9–0.95 and pH ≤ 5.0 can be stored without refrigeration.
2. Intermediate-moisture products having an a_w value of 0.6–0.9 (e.g. dried ham, salami), that can be stored without refrigeration.
3. Low-moisture products having an a_w value of <0.6 (e.g. lyophilized meat) that are self-stable.

As indicated in previous chapters, generally it is considered that the lowest a_w value for growth of pathogenic bacteria is 0.88–0.9, but moulds can grow at an even lower a_w.

Heat treatment of meat

Meat can be heat treated either for product quality- or for product safety-orientated purposes, but in most cases the two are combined.

Heating has multiple and complex effects on meat. Heat induces change in meat pigments typical for raw meat (myoglobin and oxymyoglobin, with Fe^{++}, to metmyoglobin, with Fe^{+++}), resulting in a change of meat colour from red (raw) to brown–grey (cooked), e.g. in well-cooked steak. Only if the meat was cured (nitrites) before cooking, will the product still have a red colour post-cooking, due to the presence of nitrosyl-myoglobin, e.g. in cooked ham.

On the other hand, heating denatures proteins and decreases their water-holding capacity. As a result, during cooking of untreated meat a significant proportion of water is released, with weight loss – depending on species, composition and pH of meat – of up to 40%. However, when meat has been treated with water-retaining additives (e.g. phosphates), the cooking weight loss is much reduced or prevented. Heat-induced changes in proteins also cause reduction of both length and diameter of myofibrils, resulting in a firmer texture of the cooked meat.

Heating meat also contributes to the formation of a large number of compounds and changes in both protein and lipids, resulting in taste, smell and aroma typical of cooked meat that is also meat species-specific. Compounds that particularly contribute to these sensory characteristics include products of the Maillard reaction (occurring between reduced sugars and amino-compounds), aliphatic (aldehydes, ketones, amines, carboxyl acids, etc.) and aromatic (lactones, furans, thiazoles, pyridines, pyroles, etc.) carbohydrates. At pasteurization temperatures (e.g. cooking in water at 60–95°C) mainly aliphatic, whilst at high temperatures (e.g. frying, roasting, barbecuing at 150–190°C) mainly aromatic compounds are formed. Heat treatments generally reduce the nutritional (biological) value of meat, but the reduction degree depends on the cooking temperature. This is primarily due to heat inactivation of vitamins (e.g. riboflavin by 80%, niacin by 75%) and of some amino acids such as methionine, cysteine, etc.

With respect to practical application of heat treatments of meat, they can be divided into:

1. Pasteurization in water or steam at temperatures <100°C as applied, for example, to various sausages (e.g. 70–80°C), canned hams (e.g. 62–68°C) and hot-smoked meats; this normally destroys all vegetative cells of psychrophilic and mesophilic microorganisms, but some vegetative cells of thermophilic bacteria – as well as all spores – can survive. Pasteurized products are stored with refrigeration.
2. Boiling in water at 100°C, with the temperature at the product's centre reaching 80–90°C, e.g. with liver paté, black pudding, sausage, etc.; this kills all vegetative forms of microorganisms, but not spores. The products need refrigeration.
3. Commercial 'sterilization' at >100°C, usually in pressurized steam autoclaves, e.g. with canned meats sealed in a metal container with a non-

corrosive surface and treated at 105–130°C; this kills all vegetative forms; spores are either destroyed or injured to such an extent that they are rendered unable to germinate in the product. Sterilized cans, such as so-called botulinum-treated (e.g. 121°C for 20 min in the centre), can be stored for years with no refrigeration.

Food safety aspects of heat treatment relate to efficacy in killing of pathogenic microorganisms and inactivation of meat enzymes, e.g lipolytic enzymes contributing to fat rancidity. For details of the nature, dynamics and quantitive parameters of the effects of heat on microorganisms see Chapter 7.3. It should be kept in mind that antimicrobial effects of heating meat depend on a number of variable factors and their inter-relations, including: (i) temperature and duration of heating; (ii) product substrate characteristcs such as lean–fat ratio, pH, a_w and nitrites; and (iii) microflora characteristics such as species, type, growth phase and initial counts. In practice, substrate pH is a very relevant factor and, as a general guidance, it could be presumed that efficient killing (elimination) of pathogenic bacteria can be achieved in low-acid foods (pH >4.5, e.g. in meats) only by sterilization, in acid foods (pH 4–4.5) by boiling, and in very acid foods (pH <4.5) by pasteurization.

Fermentation of meat

Fermentation of meat is used only in the production of raw (uncooked) meat products, primarily fermented sausage. Fermentation can be defined as a phase of intensive growth and metabolism of lactic acid bacteria accompanied by production of lactic acid, causing a rapid fall in pH, which acts as a preservative.

Natural fermentation occurs when indigenous lactic acid bacteria in the raw materials proliferate and anaerobically metabolize sugars, producing acid. The fermentation takes place normally over 2–5 days, during which Gram-positive facultative anaerobes and micro-aerophiles (*Micrococcus*, *Staphylococus*, *Lactobacillus* – the lactic acid bacterium) rapidly increase in numbers and lower the pH, until it is typically 4.6–5 at the end of fermentation. The microorganisms which initially dominate chilled meat (the Gram-negative aerobes, e.g. *Pseudomonas*) become reduced in numbers and pathogens are suppressed.

To speed up fermentation and suppress undesirable bacteria/pathogens as soon as possible, selected lactic acid bacteria (called 'starter cultures') can be artificially added. In addition to contributing to suppression of pathogens via low pH, some starter cultures also produce antimicrobial metabolites such as bacteriocins – sometimes called 'protective cultures'. Bacteriocins are low-molecular weight proteins with antibacterial activity similar to, while not being, antibiotics. They are effective primarily against Gram-positive bacteria (e.g. *Listeria monocytogenes*, *Staphylococcus aureus*). Some purified bacteriocins are commercially available (e.g. nisin) and are used in dairy and bakery products. Starter/protective cultures have antimicrobial potential only when the product contains low numbers of indigenous bacteria, i.e. is produced under good hygienic practice. The effectiveness of protective cultures, when acting alone, is insufficient to guarantee food safety; rather, their use provides an additional safety factor working in parallel with other factors (e.g. low pH, low a_w, nitrites) within the hurdle concept.

Numerous factors affect the competitiveness of starter cultures during meat fermentation, since fermentation is a sophisticated and complex food preservation process. In practice, the suitability of starter or protective cultures can be assessed according to critical criteria and desirable criteria, described below.

Critical criteria:

1. Effectively compete against indigenous bacteria.
2. Produce adequate quantities of lactic acid.
3. Tolerate at least 6% NaCl and 100 mg/kg $NaNO_2$.
4. Grow in the temperature range 15–40°C.
5. Homofermentative – do not produce gas or undesirable metabolites.
6. Non-proteolytic, thus avoiding production of free amino acids, resulting in the lowest possible biogenic amine levels.
7. Do not produce biogenic amines (moulds or yeasts must not produce mycotoxins or aflatoxins).
8. Do not produce large quantities of peroxides (H_2O_2). Peroxides oxidize fats and produce undesirable rancid flavours and odours; peroxides also produce free radicals, which are undesirable in modern diets. In addition, products ultimately resulting from rancidity may cause liver damage in consumers.

Desirable criteria:

1. Catalase positive, to ensure that any peroxide produced is largely destroyed.
2. Nitrate reducing.
3. Flavour enhancing.
4. Do not produce slime.
5. Antagonistic to pathogenic and undesirable organisms.
6. Synergistic with other components in the raw materials and starter.
7. Produce MAO or DAO.

Finally, although starter organisms have the potential to be genetically modified to reduce undesirable and enhance desirable characteristics, at the present time, this approach would not be supported by consumers.

Further Reading

Bauer, F. and Burt, S.A. (1995) *Shelf Life of Meat and Meat Products: Quality Aspects, Chemistry, Microbiology, Technology*. ECCEAMST Foundation, Utrecht, The Netherlands.

Davies, A. and Board, R. (1998) *The Microbiology of Meat and Poultry*. Blackie Academic, London.

Varnam, A.H. and Sutherland, J.P. (1995) *Meat and Meat Products*. Chapman and Hall, London.

7.3 Basics of Food Microbiology

SHERYL AVERY

Introduction

Bacteria, moulds, yeasts, parasites and viruses can all be detected in foods. Parasites and viruses do not proliferate in foods, but may survive. In contrast, bacteria, moulds or yeasts can grow in foods under permissive conditions. Limiting microbial growth in food can:

- extend food shelf life;
- reduce the risk of food-borne bacterial pathogens proliferating to infectious dose levels; and
- reduce the risk of toxin production at toxic levels.

Techniques and methods used in food harvesting, processing and packaging can limit or control microbial contamination of food. Control of contamination, both pre- and post-harvest, is a pre-requisite for food safety and hygiene, but is not discussed further in this chapter.

Microorganisms in Food Production

A wide variety of foods that are a direct result of microbial growth are produced throughout the world. Safe production of such foods is dependent in part or wholly on correct microbial proliferation and on production of suitable metabolic products during processing. Foods produced and traded in large volumes which are traditionally produced as a direct result of microbial growth include fermented meat (sausage), fermented fish, fermented dairy products (hard cheese, yoghurt, sour cream, kefir, koumiss, cultured butter), pickled vegetables (gherkins, olives, sauerkraut), sourdough breads, soy sauce, shrimp paste, fish sauce, vinegar and alcoholic drinks (wine, spirits). Although these foods are all traditionally produced by the growth of microorganisms in the product, some of them can be produced using chemical and/or enzymatic methods.

Bacterial Growth

Four phases of bacterial growth are recognized during *in vitro* growth that are relevant to bacterial growth in foods (Fig. 7.1). The lag phase is the time taken for the population to adjust to the new environment, produce enzymes to exploit it, and to repair any damage resulting from previous injury (e.g. freezing, desiccation, heating), and bacterial numbers remain

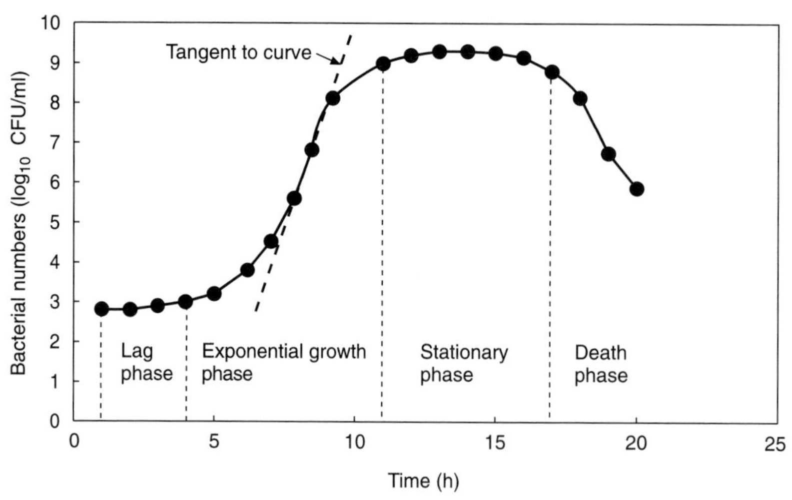

Fig. 7.1. Bacterial growth curve.

constant. Bacteria reproduce after chromosome replication, doubling in cell size, with subsequent division of the cell in two; the time taken for this to occur is the generation time. During the exponential growth phase (logarithmic phase), bacterial numbers increase exponentially. The generation time (doubling time) is the time taken for the cell number to double. The maximum specific growth rate (μ_{max}) occurs during the exponential phase, and is equal to the slope of the tangent of the exponential part of the bacterial growth curve (Fig. 7.1). During the stationary phase, the number of cells dividing becomes equal to the number dying, as key nutrients become depleted or toxic metabolites accumulate. Finally, bacterial cultures enter the death phase. *In vitro*, bacterial numbers decrease as cells die from factors including starvation, toxin accumulation and inability to maintain homeostasis.

Bacterial Death

Bacterial death can be logarithmic *in vitro* and in foods, if death is not instantaneous. The *D*-value, also called the decimal reduction time, is the time required to destroy 90% of the population (i.e. one log cycle). For killing by heat, plotting a range of *D*-values logarithmically against the temperatures used to generate them produces the thermal death time curve (Fig. 7.2). The *z*-value is the number of degrees required for the thermal death time curve to decrease by one log cycle, and allows calculation of equivalent thermal processes at different temperatures (Fig. 7.3). For example, if 9 min at 60°C produces a safe product and the *z*-value is 4.5, then 0.9 min at 64.5°C would also be safe, as would 90 min at 55.5°C. Similar calculations can be made for irradiation processing of foods.

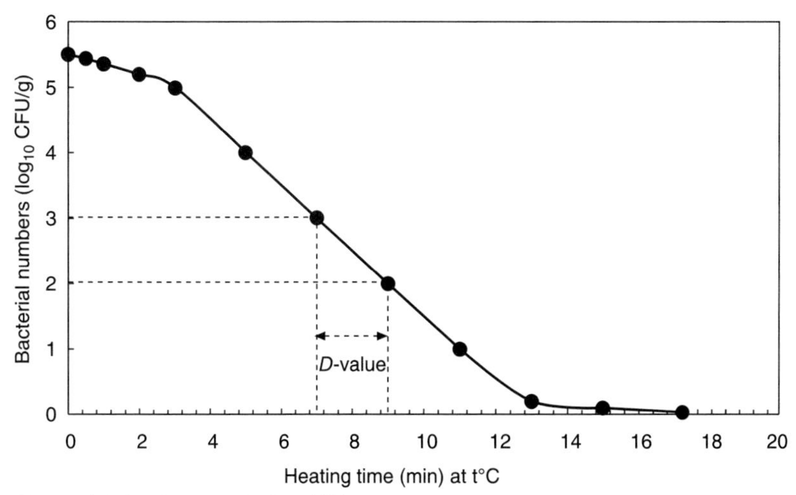

Fig. 7.2. Bacterial death curve in food (1).

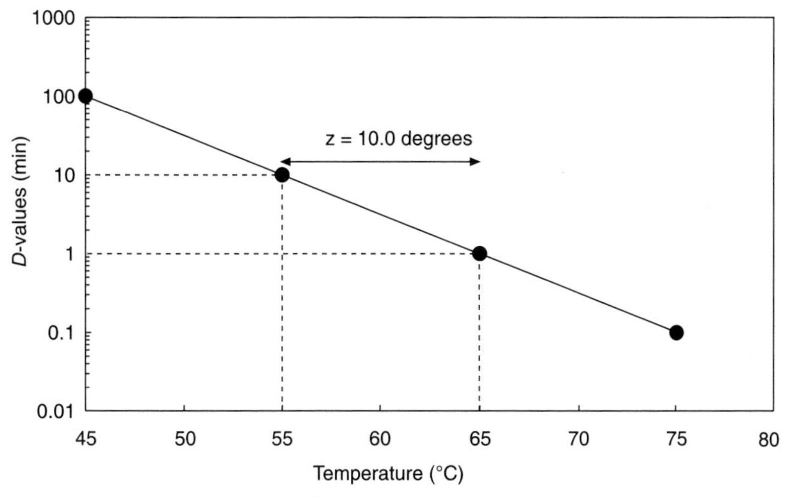

Fig. 7.3. Thermal death time curve (2).

Microorganisms in foods are killed mostly by heat or irradiation. In practice, the rate of bacterial death in foods depends on a variety of factors, including the population density, time of exposure, intensity of exposure, the nature of the heat applied, the physiological status of the cells and the food matrix.

Factors in Foods Used to Control Microbial Growth

Microbial behaviour in food is determined by extrinsic, intrinsic and microorganism-related factors. Some of these factors can be manipulated to alter growth and/or survival of microorganisms. As a result, production of toxins may also be affected.

Extrinsic factors include temperature and gas atmosphere (and related redox potential [*Eh*]). Intrinsic factors are properties of the food substrate itself, including pH, water activity (a_w), and the presence of added antimicrobials. In addition, microorganism-related factors in foods which are relevant to microbial behaviour include growth rate, physiological status, strain diversity and adaptation.

Factors acting against microorganisms in foods cannot always be clearly divided into those which enable microbial survival or growth, or cause injury or death. Some food environments may be microbicidal (lethal) to some organisms at some levels (e.g. high osmolarity, high CO_2 concentration, low pH), others may be microbiostatic (prevent growth), or merely reduce growth. Extrinsic and intrinsic factors may act synergistically, antagonistically or have little effect on each other.

Extrinsic food environment factors that affect microbial growth in foods

Temperature

Low temperature (freezing and chilling) is the most important factor used in slowing the spoilage of perishable foods, and in limiting growth of bacterial pathogens. Storage at low temperatures does not usually kill microorganisms: they mostly survive in a dormant state, recover and then proliferate when the temperature increases. In fact, bacterial survival in a variety of matrices including foods is enhanced at chill temperatures (<7°C) compared with that at higher temperatures (>20°C). Both freezing and chilling lower the temperature to below the activation level required by intracellular enzymes; lag time and generation time increase, and growth rate decreases until microbial growth is retarded or ceases. Low temperatures also induce alterations in fatty acid contents of lipids in cell membranes; these molecular changes can inactivate proteins in cell membranes, thus inactivating cross-membrane transport and causing cell death. Freezing also immobilizes liquid water, thus lowering the water available for growth, concentrating solutes and resulting in diffusion of water from microorganisms. Ice crystals may physically damage microorganisms. Air chilling lowers the water available for growth by desiccating surfaces.

Microorganisms can be classified into groups according to their growth behaviour at different temperatures (Table 7.2). Pychrophiles and psychrotrophs are defined by their growth at low temperatures and thermophiles by their growth at high temperatures.

Freezing (≤−18°C) can preserve foods for several months, by preventing bacterial growth and slowing oxidative rancidity. Most foods start to freeze between −1 and −3°C. Some moulds (*Thamnidium*, *Cladosporium*) and yeasts can grow on frozen foods stored >−10°C. Freezing is used to inactivate the nematodes *Trichinella spiralis* in pork and *Anisakidae* in fish, as well as cysticercus in beef/pork.

Table 7.2. Classification of microorganisms according to thermal groups and food environment relevance.

Description	Cardinal temperatures for growth[a]	Examples of microorganisms (but vary with strain)	Relevant food or food environment
Psychrophile	$t_{min} \leq 0°C$ t_{opt} <15°C t_{max} ~20°C	*Thamnidium elegans*	Frozen foods Chiller or freezer units
Psychrotroph	t_{min} 0–7°C t_{opt} >15°C t_{max} >25°C	*Listeria monocytogenes* *Yersinia enterocolitica* Lactic acid bacteria	Chilled foods
Mesophile	t_{min} ~0–7°C t_{opt} 35–37°C t_{max} ~44–46°C	*Staphylococcus aureus* *Escherichia coli* *Salmonella* *Shigella*	Foods stored at ambient temperatures
Thermotolerant		Spores of bacteria and fungi	Pasteurized foods
Thermophile	t_{opt} >37°C t_{max} ~44°C	*Clostridium botulinum*	Canned foods

[a] Accepted ranges.

Chilling (−1.5°C to 5°C) can stop some bacteria from growing (e.g. most strains of *Salmonella* and *E. coli*), or can slow but not prevent growth of other bacteria. Psychrotrophs, including some pathogens (e.g. *Listeria, Aeromonas, Yersinia*) and many spoilage organisms (e.g. lactic acid bacteria, *Pseudomonas*), can grow on foods ≤4°C. Additionally, some strains of some food-borne pathogens (*Salmonella, E. coli* O157) can proliferate slowly on permissive foods stored at or above correct chill temperatures (5 to around 10°C).

Holding cooked foods at high temperature (>60°C) is recommended for short periods just prior to serving, and prevents bacterial growth and associated toxin production. Generally, high temperatures are used to kill bacteria in foods, not prevent their growth, and so are discussed below.

Gas atmosphere

Gas atmospheres are manipulated primarily to control (slow or stop) the growth of microorganisms in food, and to promote the growth of specific microorganisms in particular foods. Microorganisms are classified as:

- aerobic (grow in the presence of O_2);
- facultatively anaerobic (grow in the presence and absence of O_2);
- strictly anaerobic (grow only in the absence of O_2); or
- micro-aerophilic (grow preferentially in atmospheres with reduced O_2 tension).

Fungi relevant to food hygiene and spoilage grow aerobically, while yeasts grow either aerobically and/or by anaerobic fermentation, and bacteria can be found in all groups. Therefore, composition of the gas atmosphere affects the fate and growth of microorganisms on food.

Alterations to gas atmospheres are achieved by vacuum- or modified atmosphere-packaging (MAP). The main gas used in food preservation is CO_2, commonly used to restrict microbial growth. The inhibitory effects of CO_2 increase with decreasing temperature.

Aerobic microorganisms generate ATP using O_2 as the terminal electron acceptor in their respiratory chain. Therefore, aerobes grow on food stored in air, in O_2-permeable wrap or in modified atmospheres containing O_2. Many common food spoilage organisms are aerobes, including *Pseudomonas*, *Micrococcus*, *Acinetobacter* and *Moraxella*.

Facultative anaerobes can use O_2 as their terminal electron acceptor, but, in the absence of O_2, they can use a variety of electron acceptors (e.g. NO_3^-, SO_4^{2-}), so they can grow in all permissive atmospheres. Yeasts and some bacterial facultative anaerobes generate ATP from fermentation (an anaerobic process) and not via respiratory chains. The lactic acid bacteria (facultative anaerobes) ferment glucose to produce lactic and other acids, and dominate in vacuum and MAP meat and fish stored at chill temperatures. *E. coli* and *Salmonella* occur naturally in the anaerobic GIT of man and animals, but can survive and/or grow in a variety of foods.

Strict anaerobes use terminal electron acceptors other than O_2, and grow only when O_2 is absent. *Clostridium* (anaerobic spore-former) is more likely to proliferate in improperly processed canned meat where the storage temperature (~15 to 20°C) allows its growth. Some anaerobes can tolerate O_2, whereas others will be killed in the presence of even small amounts.

Eh (redox potential) is a measure of the ease with which material loses or gains electrons. Generally, aerobes grow at *Eh* +500 to +300 mV; facultative anaerobes grow at +300 to −100 mV; and anaerobes grow at +100 to less than −250 mV. The *Eh* of foods can change with time as the growth of microorganisms and changes in the gas atmosphere and/or alterations in pH all occur. In addition, active enzymes can lower the *Eh* of respiring foods (fresh fruit and vegetables, fresh meats and fish).

Properties of the food itself can create environments that select for bacteria that can grow in differing oxygen tensions. During ageing of mould-ripened cheese, moulds grow on the surface of cheese, but do not grow in anaerobic cheese centres. Large volumes of cooked meat in gravy can be anaerobic in the centre, permitting growth of *Clostridium perfringens*.

Intrinsic food environment factors that affect microbial growth in foods

pH

The measure of acidity, pH, is defined as $-\log_{10} [H^+]$.

Foods are frequently acidic environments with low pH; high-pH foods are less common. The pH of preserved foods is normally lowered by the addition of either organic (weak) acids, strong acids or by fermentation.

Adverse pH affects microorganisms in two ways: the functioning of cellular enzymes and the transport of nutrients into the cell. Generally, microorganisms maintain pH homeostasis of cell interiors near neutrality by complex proton pump mechanisms, even in acidic environments. Microorganisms are affected by the concentration of free H^+ ions (i.e. the pH itself), and also by the concentration of undissociated weak acid in the food, which itself is affected by pH. Therefore, the pH tolerance of microorganisms is affected by the nature of acid in the environment. At any given acidic pH, weak organic acids have greater inhibitory effects than strong inorganic acids, as they can pass through cell membranes, dissociate and acidify cell interiors. Undissociated acid in the cell cytoplasm may have as yet undetermined, but negative, effects on cells.

Generally, the antimicrobial effectiveness of organic acids is in the order: lactate > benzoate > sorbate > propoinate > acetate.

The optimum pH for growth of many food-associated bacteria is in the range 6.5 to 7.5, but many species can proliferate in food with more acidic pH values. Yeasts and moulds grow at lower pH values than bacteria. However, the prehistory of bacteria, including previous exposure to low pH, can increase their acid resistance when they are moved to new environments.

Water activity (a_w)

Water activity (a_w) is defined as the ratio of the water vapour pressure of a food (p) to that of pure water (p_0) at the same temperature: $a_w = p / p_0$.

Most fresh foods, such as fresh meat, vegetables, and fruit, have a_w values that are close to the optimum growth level of most microorganisms (0.97–0.99). Bacteria usually grow optimally in the range 0.980–0.995, but they can also grow at a lower a_w. *Staphylococcus* is very tolerant to low a_w, and can grow at 0.86. Yeasts and moulds grow optimally on drier substrates (a_w 0.610–0.900) than can most bacteria. Bacterial heat resistance increases as a_w is lowered.

Drying is a classic method of food preservation – if the product is dry enough (a_w <0.900) and stored in an environment with low relative humidity (RH) so that it stays dry, bacteria will not grow. Drying can be achieved in four ways.

1. Air drying. Milk powder, dried fruits, vegetables, cheeses, meats and fish can be air dried. Dried products frequently have solutes added to increase the antimicrobial effect of physically removing water. Carcasses hanging in chillers are air dried, as circulating chilled air around the carcass effectively lowers the a_w of carcass surfaces.
2. Addition of solutes (NaCl, sugars) to food (meat products, jams, jellies, vegetables, pickles) lowers the a_w.
3. Freezing (see above) is also a method of reducing a_w, as it converts free water into ice, making it unavailable for microbial growth.

4. Altering the microstructure of a food. Butter is a water-in-fat emulsion prepared from cream, a fat-in-water emulsion. The process of manufacturing butter inverts the emulsion, and the small water droplets produced do not support bacterial growth.

The a_w of a food may be affected by the RH of the atmosphere surrounding it. If food preservation or safety rely on strict control of a_w, then the RH of the atmosphere must be controlled.

Presence of antimicrobials

Antimicrobial compounds can occur intrinsically in some foods (e.g. lysozyme in egg white, allicin in garlic or onion), can be added during processing (e.g. nitrite pre-formed bacteriocins, weak organic acids) or can result from microbial growth (bacteriocins, weak organic acids, alcohols). Many antimicrobial food additives are microbiostatic rather than microbiocidal, as they must be present in foods at levels that are not detrimental to humans.

1. Bacteriocins. Nisin, produced by *Lactococcus lactis*, prevents growth of germinating Gram-positive spores, including *Clostridium* and *Bacillus*, and is also effective against other Gram-positive organisms. Used in processed cheeses and canned meat. Bacteriocins generally deplete the proton motive force across bacterial membranes, by forming leaky pores in the membranes.
2. Nitrite. Commonly added to cured meat products to stabilize red colour and inhibit *C. botulinum*. Does not prevent spore germination but inhibits subsequent growth of *C. botulinum* and other clostridia. High levels may be required to prevent growth of vegetative cells. More effective at lower pH values. Nitrite inhibits growth by reducing intracellular ATP levels.
3. Sodium, potassium and calcium sulphite salts are common food additives which have multiple functions: as antioxidants, colour retainers, reducing agents and inhibitors of microbial growth. They inhibit both yeasts and moulds in low-pH and low-a_w foods, and also Gram-negative bacteria in higher-pH and higher-a_w foods. They affect many cellular processes, including production, protein synthesis and DNA replication.
4. Sorbate. Organic acid, added to foods as sodium, calcium or potassium salts, primarily to inhibit mould growth. Sorbate is also active against bacteria, and works synergistically with both nitrite and nisin. Most effective at pH < 6.0.
5. Woodsmoke compounds. Antimicrobial compounds including phenols, tars and formaldehyde deposit on meat during smoking. However, for most modern (lightly smoked) meat products, woodsmoke compounds impart desired flavour and colour but have little impact on microbial growth.

Microorganism-related factors that affect growth in foods

Some factors impacting on the behaviour or fate of microorganisms in food occur inherently. Gene alteration, or gene regulation, changes may account for some of these factors.

Microbial population and strain diversity

Even microbial populations in axenic (pure) cultures exhibit diversity with respect to tolerance of food-related factors, including pH and antibiotics. This naturally-occurring, probably gene-based diversity, probably contributes *in vitro* to adaptation of microorganisms to specific conditions over time, and can result in permanent changes in resistance. Additionally, significant within-species diversity with respect to lag phase duration, growth rate, virulence, bacteriocin resistance, heat tolerance and drying has been observed among bacterial isolates, even those belonging to one genus.

Microbial injury

Injury can be caused by exposure to the above parameters, if sub-lethal (insufficient to cause death). Injury also results from food processing and/or treatments including freeze-drying, aerosolization, and exposure to dyes, sodium azide, heavy metals, antibiotics, essential oils, EDTA and sanitizers. Injured bacteria have a lengthened lag phase duration, prolonging the time needed until they start proliferating.

Viable but non-culturable bacteria

Bacteria are viable but non-culturable (VBNC) when they cannot be grown on laboratory media even when a repair step is used to allow recovery of injured cells. *Vibrio*, *Campylobacter*, *Salmonella*, *Shigella* and enteropathogenic *E. coli* can enter the VBNC state. VBNC cells can have altered morphology and metabolism, including synthesis of novel proteins. The VBNC state can be induced *in vitro* by temperature downshifts, although whether this occurs in foods is not known.

The bacterial stress response

Bacteria can produce a stress response when exposed to some parameters used to control their behaviour (e.g. sub-lethal heat). Whether the stress response is related to bacterial injury and the VBNC state is unknown. The stress response is evidenced by the production of novel proteins, including heat-shock proteins. The stress response can alter bacterial behaviour in opposite ways to that normally expected, for example, making bacteria more:

- fast-growing; μ_{max} can be increased even if the lag phase is lengthened;
- toxigenic, and therefore more likely to cause food-borne disease;
- resistant to the factor that initially caused injury; and
- able to adapt to other adverse factors subsequently imposed along the food chain.

Cross-protection occurs when the recovery of a bacterium from injury caused by a sub-lethal stress results in that microorganism becoming more resistant to other, unrelated, stresses.

Therefore, the bacterial stress response may significantly impact on the efficacy of modern food processing techniques where multiple parameters are used to control microbial behaviour. This may be particularly significant in the style of food processing and distribution in developed nations, where the public are demanding 'less intervention' and 'more natural' methods of controlling food-borne pathogens.

Factors Used to Kill Microorganisms in Foods

Thermal treatments

Heat (cooking, pasteurization, canning) is used to destroy microorganisms in food. This reduction in microbial load can increase shelf life, destroy heat-labile toxins, and alter microbial composition. The efficacy of heat treatment depends on the type and intensity of the heating process used, the microbial load, the composition of the food and the type of microorganism. Spores are more heat resistant that vegetative cells.

Cooking

Cooking is the general term for heating where kills of specific organisms are not determined. Cooking is achieved by boiling in water, baking, broiling, grilling or frying.

Pasteurization

Pasteurization kills most vegetative bacteria, but spores are inherently more heat-resistant, and may survive later to grow in the product. Thermoduric organisms, including *Enterococcus*, may also survive and afterwards grow at abusive chilling temperatures. Used primarily for foods that are destroyed by excessive heating (e.g. milk, beer, honey).

Hot-filling

Hot-filling is a process used for high-acid foods (e.g. tomato juice), which are heated and immediately transferred into containers.

Aseptic packaging

Aseptic packaging is used for low-acid foods (e.g. puddings, sauces, soups), which are sterilized, usually by heat, and then transferred into sterile containers.

Canning

Canning produces foods that are 'commercially sterile', a process known also as appertization. This term refers to heat processing where the only organisms that survive are non-pathogenic and incapable of proliferating in the product under normal storage conditions. For canned meat stored at room temperature, this means that even if spores of thermophilic (heat-loving) bacteria survive the heating regime, they will not proliferate in the product under temperate storage conditions. Canned meat is exposed to a 'botulinum cook' – a heat process that will reduce numbers of *C. botulinum* to 10^{-12} of their original number. This is also called the 12*D* process, because the numbers of *C. botulinum* are reduced by 12 log cycles.

Survivor curves of log numbers plotted against time are not always linear, but can have shoulders and tails. These may be caused by clumping of cells, mixed microbial populations, spore germination before death, variation in heat resistance of individual cells in the population or by experimental design. Death rate is a function of a_w and RH; survivor curves of microorganisms exposed to moist heat are more commonly linear than those exposed to dry heat.

Irradiation

By 1989, irradiation of some types of foods using ionizing radiation was legalized in over 36 countries. However, consumer resistance has limited the practical application of irradiation. Irradiation causes chromosomal damage (single- or double-strand breaks in DNA, or hydroxylation of purine/pyrimidine bases) in microorganisms. Irradiation ultimately causes microbial death as microorganisms cannot divide (DNA replication is halted), or metabolic enzymes cannot be synthesized (DNA transcription cannot occur). Resistance to irradiation depends on the ability of microorganisms to repair the damage caused, and generally follows the sequence Gram-negative < Gram-positive < moulds < spores < yeasts < viruses.

Inactivation kinetics are generally logarithmic, so survivor curves similar to those that occur with thermal treatments can be constructed. *D*-values (the dose required to inactivate 90% of the population) can be derived from the linear portions of the survivor curves. *C. botulinum* spores are among the most radiation-resistant of the bacteria found on food.

The Hurdle Concept

In reality, in any particular food, multiple parameters ('hurdles') are used to control microbial behaviour in foods. Many hurdles used to control microbial growth in foods act either additively or synergistically on microorganisms. Therefore, each additional parameter provides an increased level of control over microbial behaviour (growth, toxin production, death, etc.). A large number of factors are known that can be applied to food systems as hurdles, and more and more producers of shelf-stable foods of the future are likely to employ this concept. Even though each novel/altered food or process creates new environments for microorganisms, using the hurdle concept should result in safer food for consumers.

7.4 Meat Products and Descriptive Assessment of Risk

General Considerations

When considering hygiene of meat processing and safety of meat products, it is not enough to focus only on the processing step, but also the events that take place both before and after meat processing should be taken into account. Consideration should be given to:

- contamination events during primary production;
- contamination events during meat processing;
- whether processing includes a microbicidal step and if any survivors exist;
- whether post-microbiocidal step contamination can occur;
- identification of antimicrobial factors acting in the final product, and their interaction;
- whether conditions during storage and retail stages may enable growth of, or toxin production by, pathogens;
- usual pre-consumption practices by consumers relevant to behaviour of pathogens; and
- infective dose for given pathogen(s).

It is difficult to determine the total number of different types of meat products produced and consumed in different countries, but it probably reaches hundreds, if not thousands. Therefore, it is impossible to address them individually here; rather, they will be considered in main, global groups.

Approaches to meat products' safety risk assessment can be qualitative (descriptive), semi-quantitative and quantitative. In this chapter, descriptive risk assessments of main groups of meat products will be illustrated, based both on descriptive evaluation of main environmental factors acting in a particular substrate (i.e. product type) and on the corresponding assessment of behaviour of relevant microorganisms when exposed to such factors (summarized in Table 7.3). In the following chapter, an example of semi-quantitative risk assessment is presented; whilst it is considered that details of quantitative risk assessment would be beyond the scope of this book.

Uncooked (Raw), Dried Meat Products

Fermented (dry, raw) sausages

Some typical examples from this group include salamis and tea sausages. With fermented sausages, meat and fat are chopped, brine and lactic acid bacteria starter cultures (alternatively, acidulants) are added, and the batter is stuffed into casings. The surfaces of some types of fermented sausage are also inoculated with selected strains of mould/yeast inoculum (optional).

Table 7.3. Summary of bacterial behaviour when exposed to some common environmental factors acting in processed meats.

Organism	Temperature (°C)	Heat resistance	pH	Oxygen tolerance	NaCl tolerance	A_w
C. botulinum	min. ~ 10; max. 45–50	–	min. 4.7; max. 8.5–8.9	Anaerobe	Growth in 5–10% NaCl	min. 0.940 max. 0.975
C. botulinum spore germination	min. 5.0	++++ (spores)				
S. aureus	min. ~ 7; max. 48; t_{opt} 37	++	min. 4.0; max. 9.8–10.0	Facultative anaerobe	Growth in 10% NaCl; some strains tolerate 20%	min. 0.830
S. aureus toxin production	min. 10 max. 46; t_{opt} 35–40	++++ (toxin)	min. 4.8; max. 8.0	Inhibited by anaerobic growth	Enterotoxin A can be produced in 10% NaCl; enterotoxin B production inhibited in 10% NaCl	min. 0.860
B. cereus	min. 4–5; max. 45–55; t_{opt} 28–35	++++ (spores)	min. 4.35–4.90; max. 9.3	Facultative anaerobe		min. ~ 0.950
B. cereus toxin production			min. 6.0; max. 8.5			
C. perfringens	min. ~12; max. 50; t_{opt} 37–45; growth slow below 20	–	min. 5.0; max. 8.5; pH_{opt} 6.0–7.5	Anaerobe, but can rarely grow in presence of O_2	No growth in 5–6% NaCl	min. 0.930–0.970
Brochothrix	min. −0.8; t_{opt} 20–25	–	min. 5.5–6.5	Facultative anaerobe	Growth in 10% NaCl	
Lactic acid bacteria	min. < 0		min. < 5.5; pH_{opt} 6.0	Aerotolerant anaerobes		
Streptococcus faecalis	min. 8–10	++	min. 4.4–4.7			

Listeria monocytogenes	min. – 0.7 to >1.00; max. 42–45; t_{opt} 30–35	–	min. 4.1–5.6; pH_{opt} 6–8	Facultative anaerobe Micro-aerophilic	Growth in 10% NaCl; survives 1 yr in 16% NaCl	min. 0.900–0.930
Salmonella	min. 4.0–6.2 to ~10; max. 47; t_{opt} 37	+	min. 4.0–5.5; pH_{opt} 6.6–8.2	Facultative anaerobe	9% NaCl bactericidal	min. 0.937–0.945
Campylobacter	No growth < 28; survive poorly at 20, but 15 days at 12; t_{opt} 37–45	–	min. > 5.5–5.8; pH_{opt} 6.5–7.5	Micro-aerophile For good growth 5–10% O_2 and 3–5% CO_2	No growth 3.5% NaCl	Very sensitive to dehydration when chilled
Yersinia enterocolitica	min. −2 max. 40–45; t_{opt} 29	–	min. 4.1–5.1; pH_{opt} 7–8	Facultative anaerobe	Growth in 5% NaCl; no growth 7%	
E. coli O157:H7	min. 8–10; max. 42; no growth 44.5	–	min. 4.5; survive in low pH well	Facultative anaerobe	Growth in 6.5% NaCl; no growth > 8.5% NaCl	
E. coli	min. 7–10; max. 44.5; t_{opt} 37	+	min. 4.4	Facultative anaerobe		min. 0.950
Pseudomonas	min. < 0	–	min. < 5.5–5.6	Aerobe		
Acinetobacter			No growth 5.4–5.6	Aerobe		

Depending on type, sausages are subjected to fermentation (see Chapter 7.2) at 15–40°C for 2–5 days, and then smoked (optional). This is followed by drying for 1–4 weeks (semi-dry fermented sausages) or for 12–14 weeks (dry salamis), before their retailing either as whole or as sliced and pre-packed.

Antimicrobial factors associated with these products:

- low pH (dry sausages 5.3–6.0; semi-dry with acidulants 4.8–5.2);
- salt 3–5%;
- nitrites;
- starters/protective cultures (via competition, bacteriocins);
- low a_w (dry sausages 0.80–0.90; semi-dry 0.90–0.95); and
- smoke (on the surface).

Potential hazards in whole fermented sausages originate either from the raw meat and/or from contaminated equipment during batter preparation, and include: (i) pathogenic bacteria; (ii) microbial toxins or their toxic metabolites; and (iii) parasites. Among pathogenic bacteria, if the pH fall is too slow or insufficient during fermentation, Gram-positive, salt-tolerant pathogens may grow, such as *L. monocytogenes* and *S. aureus*. Gram-negative pathogenic bacteria (e.g. *E. coli* O157, *Salmonella*) do not usually multiply, but can survive the entire production process. Among toxic compounds, enterotoxin can be produced by *S. aureus*, biogenic amines (especially tyramine – see below) by indigenous or non-tested starter organisms (see Chapter 1.3), and aflatoxins can be produced on the surface by contaminating toxigenic fungi. Among parasites, *Trichinella* can survive the fermentation and drying processes to a significant extent, whilst *Cysticercus* is mostly inactivated due to low a_w. If fermented, dry sausages are sliced and packaged, the possibility of secondary contamination (cross-contamination) with microbial pathogens from the processing environment must be taken into account.

One potential hazard in fermented sausages might be formation of higher quantities of tyramine, a toxic biogenic amine. The main factor determining tyramine production in fermented sausages is the presence of tyramine-producing microorganisms (natural or starter). Numerous physical and chemical factors determine the amounts of tyramine produced, including numbers of tyramine producers in the product and the rate at which the producer strain generates tyramine. The relative activities of the enzymes tyrosine decarboxylase, MAO and DAO also play a role. Substrate pH has an important role, since it influences both growth of microorganisms and enzyme activity. The low pH of fermented sausages enhances production of tyramine and other biogenic amines.

However, the best and safest fermented sausages generally have low pH values because the acid suppresses growth and toxin production by pathogens, enables better drying, and the finished product has the typical sensory qualities (colour, aroma, firmness) expected of fermented sausage. Since reduced tyramine levels are best achieved in higher-pH sausage, while microbiological safety is best achieved in lower-pH sausage, production of safe and desirable fermented sausages requires consideration of all factors. To satisfy both considerations, it may be desirable to avoid pH extremes, use the hurdle concept and to use starter cultures producing MAO or DAO (enzymes degrading biogenic amimes).

Dry, raw meats

Some typical examples include Parma hams, other Italian prosciuttos and pastrami. These are high-quality products, for which raw material is very carefully selected. Curing of these products is a lengthy process, using dry-curing methods at 0–7°C. This is followed by 9–18 months maturation and drying – first at 10–15°C and then at 18–20°C with relative air humidity of 70–80% – so that the total weight loss is 30–45%.

The production process can be carried either under particular natural environmental conditions (particular locations specific for geographic regions) or under industrially controlled conditions. Proteolytic enzymes of the meat itself play an important role in the formation of specific aromas in these products.

Antimicrobial factors associated with these products:

- salt 5–11%;
- nitrites;
- low a_w (0.70–0.90); and
- smoke (on the surface).

Deep meat from healthy, well-managed animals is sterile, so properly produced, sufficiently dry raw meat products are self-stable and safe. Nevertheless, potential risks relate to growth and toxin production of *Cl. botulinum*, mainly in case of products that were subjected to insufficient curing at higher temperatures.

Cooked Meat Products

Cooked, uncured meats

Undercooked uncured meats

Some typical examples from this group include grilled/barbecued meats such as steaks and burgers. Commonly, grilled pork is heated sufficiently so that it is properly cooked in the centre, which is noticeable as the original pink colour of the meat turns to grey–brown. However, beef (typically 15 mm-thick steak) is often grilled only to a 'rare' or 'medium-rare' degree, where temperatures in the centre reach only 40–45°C. As there are no other antimicrobial factors in these products (apart from mildly low pH), this temperature range cannot destroy a biological hazard if present. Therefore, any biological hazard present in the meat originally would be viable when ingested and could cause infection.

Antimicrobial factors associated with these products:

- higher temperatures achieved only on the product's surface; and
- slightly low natural pH (beef: 5.2–5.5; higher in other species).

Among microbial pathogens, the greatest risks would be from *E. coli* O157:H7, *L. monocytogenes* and *Salmonella*, as these are relatively frequent surface contaminants on meat. These risks would be greater with burgers, where the pathogens are distributed throughout the product (mincing), so are more likely to survive in the centre, than is the case in beef steaks. With the latter, microbial pathogens are located primarily on the surface – which is exposed to high temperatures during heating even if the centre remains rare. However, in the case of other parasitic hazards located inside the meat (e.g. *T. saginata/T. solium* cysticerci), the risks would not differ between steak and burger heated equally.

Lightly cooked (pasteurized) uncured meats

Some typical examples from this group include beef and turkey roasts. The meat is oven-heated with air temperatures reaching 150–180°C, but in the meat centre the maximum temperatures reached are only ≤100°C.

Antimicrobial factors associated with these products:

- pasteurization heat treatment; and
- slightly-low natural pH (beef: 5.2–5.5; higher in other species).

Therefore, although vegetative bacteria are killed, bacterial spores survive. The most common risks with this group are associated with *Cl. perfringens* spores. If the product is temperature abused – either due to too slow cooling of the large piece of cooked meat or to subsequent keeping without refrigeration – the spores can germinate and the pathogen proliferates. Subsequently, the meat can be a vehicle for intoxication/toxicoinfection. Other risks relate to meat being held at abusive temperatures before cooking, enabling *S. aureus* multiplication and the associated production of heat-stable enterotoxins not destroyed by subsequent cooking. In addition, post-cooking cross-contamination (from raw foods, people or equipment) with pathogens can occur (e.g. during carving/portioning), with *L. monocytogenes* and *Salmonella* most commonly involved. A particular problem in the safety of this group of meat products is due to the elimination by cooking of spoilage microflora. Their lack of growth means lack of spoilage signs that would warn of potential growth of pathogens.

Canned, commercially sterilized uncured meats

Some typical examples from this group include canned fish and canned vegetables/fruit, which are heat treated by various regimes, but all under pressure at temperatures >100°C, including so-called commercially sterilized 'Botulinum-cooked' cans (≥120°C for 20 min).

Antimicrobial factors associated with these products:

- commercial sterilization heat treatment; and
- salt 1–2%.

Because these properly applied heating regimes are expected to destroy or irreversibly damage even spores, any associated microbial safety risks relate to process errors leading to growth and toxin production of *Cl. botulinum*. This can be caused by insufficient heat treatment due to lack, or erroneous monitoring, of the time–temperature parameters. Another problem can be caused by the seal between the body and lid, if it physically contains microscopic pores. This porosity can be due to overfilling of the can before sealing, or to disproportion between body and lid, or to disoperation of the sealing machine. In any case, during post-heating cooling of these faulty cans, cooling water can be sucked (through seal pores) inside the cans aided by negative pressure generated as the content cools. In this way, microorganisms or their spores can enter the content, and multiply/produce toxin during subsequent storage. Because uncured content does not contain nitrites, and particularly if it is low-acid, the conditions could support *Cl. botulinum*.

Cooked, cured meats

Lightly cooked (pasteurized), cured meat joints

Some typical examples from this group include cooked ham/shoulder/gammon. Usually, production processes include: (i) curing of selected meat (commonly by the injection method); (ii) massaging–tumbling to distribute brine ingredients evenly within the meat; (iii) sometimes other treatments, such as with enzymes to aid restructuring and 'gluing' the meat pieces together; and (iv) placing in appropriate containers (cans) or casings, followed by heat treatment at pasteurization temperatures – often between 62 and 68°C. Too high temperatures cause separation of excessive amounts of gelatin from this product, which decreases product quality. Therefore, producers tend to choose lower temperature–longer duration heating regimes. The cooked product is chilled and then, commonly, taken out from the container/casing to be sliced and vacuum-packaged.

Antimicrobial factors associated with these products:

- pasteurization heat treatment;
- salt 2–4%; and
- nitrites.

Potential microbial safety risks associated with this product relate to two main scenarios. One is that if the product is undercooked due to process errors, some vegetative bacteria can survive. Another is that, even if all vegetative bacteria are killed by cooking, pathogens can recontaminate the product during the slicing and packaging phases. Among such survivors or contaminants, salt-tolerant *S. aureus* and *L. monocytogenes* provoke the greatest concern. Typical concentrations of salt and nitrites in these products are insufficient to control their growth. Growth of cold-tolerant *L. monocytogenes* would not be prevented even by refrigeration. For growth and enterotoxin production of *S. aureus* higher temperature and the presence of oxygen, respectively, would be necessary.

Lightly cooked (or hot-smoked) cured sausages

Some typical examples from this group include emulsion-type sausages (e.g. hot dogs, bologna) and the emulsion-coarse meat-type of sausages (e.g. Tyrolean sausage, Polish sausage). 'Emulsion' in meat processing terminology means preparation of sausage batter with a very fine, uniform texture and appearance, and it is prepared in the following way. Lean meat is very finely ground in a special, high-speed 'cutter' machine until meat pieces are no longer visible, then around 30% water is added in the form of ice (to prevent overheating of the mixture), as well as around 30% fatty tissue, whilst the machine keeps working. Finally, curing salt containing nitrites and phosphates is added and homogenized with the mixture. The very fine, sticky mixture obtained contains uniformly dispersed water and fat within the protein matrix, hence it is called 'emulsion'. The only components of the batter of emulsion-type of sausages are spices and the emulsion itself, which are mixed together and stuffed into casings. Emulsion-coarse meat-type sausages are produced by mixing pre-prepared emulsion with coarsely chopped meat/fatty tissue and spices, and then stuffing the sausage batter into casings. Although details of heat treatment regimes can vary significantly between different kinds of sausages from these groups, for all of them pasteurization temperatures well below 100°C (e.g. 70–80°C) are used. Heat treatments can be conducted simultaneously with smoking in special climatized chambers; such sausages are called 'hot-smoked'.

Antimicrobial factors associated with these products:

- pasteurization heat treatment;
- salt 2–4%;
- nitrites; and
- smoke (on the surface).

Most vegetative forms of microorganisms, including the main food-borne pathogens, are normally killed during the process. However, microbial safety risks, similar to those described above for pasteurized cured joints and for similar reasons, can arise. These particularly relate to re-contamination of emulsion-type sausages (e.g. hot dogs) during subsequent skinning and vacuum-packaging (for retail), or to recontamination of emulsion-coarse meat-type of sausages of larger diameter that are subsequently sliced and vacuum-packaged before sale. In both cases, *L. monocytogenes* is the greatest concern.

Canned, commercially sterilized cured meats

Some typical examples from this group include canned corn beef.
Antimicrobial factors associated with these products:

- commercial sterilization heat treatment;
- salt 2–4%; and
- nitrites.

Potential safety problems are very similar to those described for canned, commercially sterilized uncured meats. The main difference relates to the fact that in this type of product, being cured, the risks from *Cl. botulinum* are comparably much lower due to the presence and inhibitory role of nitrites.

Further Reading

Davies, A. and Board, R. (1998) *The Microbiology of Meat and Poultry*. Blackie Academic, London.

Lücke, F.-K. (1995) Microbiological changes during storage and spoilage of meat and meat products. In: Bauer, F. and Burt, S.A. (eds) *Shelf Life of Meat and Meat Products: Quality Aspects, Chemistry, Microbiology, Technology*. ECCEAMST Foundation, Utrecht, The Netherlands, pp. 57–74.

Varnam, A.H. and Sutherland, J.P. (1995) *Meat and Meat Products*. Chapman and Hall, London.

7.5 Risk Profiling of Meat Products

PHIL VOYSEY

Microbiological Risk Assessment (MRA), as defined by the Codex Alimentarius Commission, is a process made up of the following steps: Hazard Identification; Exposure Assessment; Hazard Characterization and Risk Characterization (Codex Alimentarius Commission, 1999). For clarification and ease of use, Campden & Chorleywood Food Research Association (CCFRA) advocates that three further steps are added to these as guidance for industry: Step 0 – Outline MRA; Step 1 – Statement of Purpose; and at the end of the MRA, Step 6 – Production of a Formal Report (CCFRA, 2000).

CCFRA suggests that, before carrying out a formal MRA, an Outline MRA (Step 0) should be performed. In the Outline MRA, the steps of the MRA as a whole are analysed, so that any gaps in the knowledge, information or data required to perform the MRA can be identified. One way of carrying out an Outline MRA is to perform a Risk Profile. This technique was developed by Unilever Research (CCFRA, 2000).

The Risk Profile is a simple paper-based approach to Risk Assessment. The technique contains all the elements of a risk assessment, but utilizes information which can be chosen from tables of values representing the likely ranges for the key determinants of risk. The Risk Profile allows the user to recognize the features of the process and the product exerting the biggest influence on the level of risk. However, it does not give the detail that would be obtained through carrying out a formal MRA.

The Risk Profile consists of a series of questions, which cover the four steps of the MRA described by the Codex Alimentarius Commission (1999). These questions need to be adapted to the product being considered and to the process used to manufacture it. After answering the questions, the uncertainty associated with the answers given has to be assessed. Both the questions and the uncertainty are rated on a scale from low (1) to high (5).

An example of a Risk Profile for *Listeria monocytogenes* in cooked ham is given in Box 7.1. The questions can be modified to describe the risk for any pathogen in any processed food. In this example, specific answers are taken from a range of five answers. For a complete range of possible answers, the reader is referred to CCFRA (2000), pp. 91 and 92.

Discussion

The main advantage of following the Risk Profile process is that it makes those doing the exercise think about and challenge their food and the way it is manufactured and handled.

Box 7.1. Risk Profile Example – *Listeria monocytogenes* in Cooked Ham.

Hazard identification	
1. What is the name and type of product?	Cooked ham
2. What are the pathogens realistically associated with the product?	*Listeria monocytogenes*, *Staphylococcus aureus*, *Salmonella typhimurium*
2.1 What is the microorganism covered by this risk assessment?	*Listeria monocytogenes*
2.2 Is it toxigenic or not?	No
Hazard characterization	
3.1 Who are the consumers of concern?	Families
3.2 How many distinctive sub-groups are there in the population of consumers?	Pregnant women, immuno-compromised
3.3 What is the severity of the hazard (the sensitivity of each group should be considered, or that of the most sensitive consumers should be used for a single assessment)?	**4** Severe symptoms, hospitalization, some deaths
3.4 What is the hazardous level of the microorganism covered by this risk assessment?	**4** Low minimum dose (100–1000 cells)
3.5 What is the uncertainty of this estimate?	**1** Accurate, precise data on relevant microbe and food
Exposure assessment (occurrence of the hazardous microorganism)	
4.1 What is the frequency of contamination of the raw materials making up the product?	**5** Always
4.2 What is the range of levels of contamination found in the raw materials?	**4** 0–10,000 cells/g
4.3 How uncertain is this estimate?	**4** Qualitative general information on similar microorganisms and food
Exposure assessment – effect of processing/decontamination	
5.1 What is the effect of storage before processing on the level of the hazard?	**5** More than 10,000 cells/g
5.2 What is the intended effect of all processing and any decontamination stages on the level of the microorganism?	**1** Inactivation: at least 6-log decrease in numbers
5.3 What is the uncertainty of this estimate?	**1** Accurate, precise data on similar micro-organisms and food

Continued

Box 7.1. *Continued*

Exposure assessment – occurrence of toxin (if the hazardous microorganism is toxigenic)	
6.1 What is the likelihood of toxin presence if the micro-organism can produce toxin and contaminates the raw materials or product?	Not Applicable
6.2 What is the uncertainty of this estimate?	Not Applicable
Exposure assessment – re-contamination after processing or decontamination	
7.1 What is the frequency of re-contamination of the product in the factory after processing or decontamination, so that the hazard is present in the final product?	**2** Very low frequency: 1/1000
7.2 What is the likely level of re-contamination after processing or decontamination?	**1** 0–10 cells/g
7.3 What is the uncertainty of this estimate?	**1** Accurate, precise data on similar micro-organisms and food
Exposure assessment – packaging	
8.1 Is the product put in its primary packaging before (yes) or after (no) decontamination step?	No (after)
8.2 If the answer to 8.1 is yes (before), what is the effectiveness of packaging in preventing recontamination before consumption?	Not applicable
8.3 What is the frequency of recontamination after packaging	**1** Never
8.4 What is the level of recontamination after packaging?	**1** 0–10 cells/g
8.5 What is the uncertainty of the estimate?	**1** Accurate, precise data on similar micro-organisms and food
Exposure assessment – effect of product storage	
9.1 How does the level of the microorganism change during product storage?	**4** Slow growth: less than 3-log increase in numbers
9.2 What is the uncertainty of the estimate?	**3** Quantitative general information on similar microorganisms and food
9.3 What is the effect of storage of the final product (according to the usage instructions) on the level of toxin?	Not applicable
9.4 What is the effect of storage conditions on toxigenesis (if the level of the microorganism changes and it is toxigenic)	Not applicable
9.5 What is the likelihood of toxigenesis in the product?	Not applicable
9.6 What is the uncertainty of this estimate?	Not applicable

Exposure assessment – consumer use	
10.1 Is the product intended as single use (yes) or multi-use (no), where will it be stored after opening?	No
10.2 If the answer to 10.1 is no, this means that the product is multi-use either in a domestic or food service application and 11 and 12 must be completed	
Exposure assessment – the effect of open shelf life on the microbial hazard	
11.1 What is the effect of open shelf life storage on the level of microorganisms?	**4** Slow growth: less than 3-log increase in numbers
11.2 What is the uncertainty of this estimate?	**1** Accurate precise data on similar micro-organisms and food
Exposure assessment – the effect of open shelf life on toxigenesis	
12.1 What is the likelihood of growth and toxin production during open shelf life?	Not applicable
12.2 What is the uncertainty of this estimate?	Not applicable
Exposure assessment – the effect of usage and preparation on hazards	
13.1 What is the effect of customer or food service preparation and usage on the level of the microorgansim?	**4** Slow growth: less than 3-log increase in numbers
13.2 What is the uncertainty of this estimate?	**5** Opinion/default, no hard data
13.3 What is the effect of usage and preparation on toxin level and production?	Not applicable
13.4 What is the probability of toxin presence at the point of consumption?	Not applicable
13.5 What is the uncertainty of this estimate?	Not applicable
Exposure assessment – food intake by a consumer	
14.1 What is the likely quantity of the food consumed by a customer on a specified occasion or over a period of time?	**3** Medium intake: 50–100 g
14.2 What is the uncertainty of this estimate?	**3** Quantitative general information on similar microorganisms and food

The values used in this table are for example purposes only. The figures in bold in the second column refer to the level of uncertainly (low (0) to high (5)). Once the appropriate list of questions and their answers have been decided upon, the answers can be plotted onto a profile chart, as in Fig. 7.4.

The exercise also highlights the areas where there is:

- a high level of risk associated with the process;
- a lack of information or knowledge about the answer; or
- a high level of uncertainty.

In Fig. 7.4 for example, high scores are associated with:

- the Hazard Characterization, indicating that *L. monocytogenes* is an important and dangerous pathogen;
- the occurrence of the bacterium in the ham prior to processing; and
- the storage and use of the ham.

From carrying out this exercise, the manufacturer can make better decisions on whether there is a need for a more detailed MRA. Alternatively they can make a decision on whether more information or data are needed on the 'hot spots' of their current process. In each case, the aim is to make the product more safely.

Acknowledgements

Professor Martyn Brown and Christelle Billon at Unilever Research are acknowledged as the developers of the basis of the Risk Profile. Keith Jewell at CCFRA is acknowledged for his further development of the concept.

References

CCFRA (2000) *An Introduction to the Practice of Microbiological Risk Assessment for Food Industry Applications*. CCFRA Guideline No. 28. CCFRA, Gloucestershire, UK.

Codex Alimentarius Commission (1999) *Principles and Guidelines for the Conduct of Microbiological Risk Assessment*. Codex Alimentarius Commission, Rome.

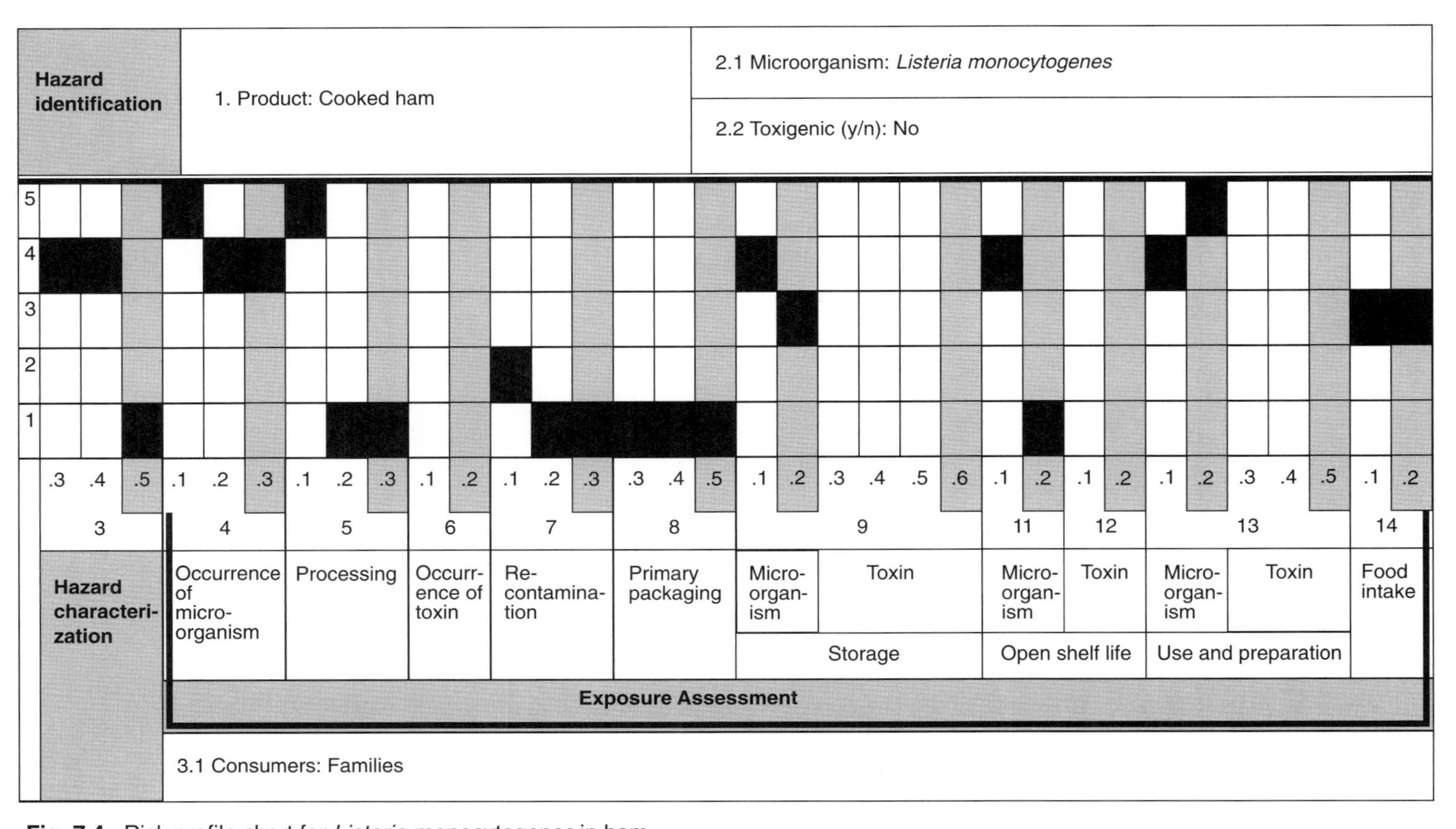

Fig. 7.4. Risk profile chart for *Listeria monocytogenes* in ham.
(NB blacked-out boxes indicate 'risk score')

8 Meat Safety Management at the Abattoir

8.1 GHP and HACCP Principles

Introduction

As indicated in previous chapters, the major causes of food-borne disease (*E. coli* O157, *Salmonella*, *Campylobacter*) are undetectable by traditional post-mortem meat inspection. The recommended systematic approach to managing process hygiene and controlling undetectable hazards in foods is based on Good Manufacturing Practice (GMP), Good Hygiene Practice (GHP) and Hazard Analysis and Critical Control Points (HACCP) principles. The HACCP-based approach uses risk analysis as one of its main tools, so this chapter is closely linked to Chapter 1.7.

The government is responsible for formulating a food safety policy and deriving Food Safety Objectives (FSOs) from that policy (see Chapter 10.2). FSOs are used in the design of food control systems, and they may incorporate end product criteria. Some examples are the levels of pathogens allowed in a meat product, or the level of indicator organisms allowed on carcasses.

The global targets for controlling food-related hazards (FSOs) set by government should be translated by the food industry into their own performance objectives (POs); these must be achievable. The role of industry is to implement risk management systems to achieve the FSOs, and these current systems can be illustrated by the following formula:

FSO to be achieved: Food producers + PO = GMP/GHP + HACCP (1)

GMP/GHP

GMP refers primarily to technical aspects of the whole production process; GHP concentrates on the hygiene aspects of production. However, these terms are frequently used interchangeably; indeed, with food operations, it would be very difficult to consider hygiene as stand-alone and without actual technical context.

GMP/GHP programmes are a prerequisite that must be in place before a HACCP plan can be developed and implemented. GHP describes the best hygienic practice for food production that is universally applicable, and is based on science. GHP alone is sufficient as a control mechanism for lower-risk food products (e.g. cereals, grains, nuts) and for many foods produced by traditional methods. However, GHP alone is insufficient for high-risk foods (e.g. foods of animal origin) and many newer types of foods produced using more complex, and novel, methods.

Within abattoirs, GMP/GHP programmes relate to a range of individual stages of the operation, including transport and lairaging, stunning and sticking, skinning or scalding/dehiding, evisceration, carcass splitting, washing and refrigeration. In simple terms, GMP/GHP provides general, basic principles for hygienic production of food, including:

- hygienic design, construction and operation of plants;
- hygienic use of machinery, equipment and tools;
- plan for maintenance, cleaning and sanitation;
- staff aspects, including training, health and personal hygiene;
- Standard Operating Procedures (SOPs); and
- identification and traceability.

HACCP

HACCP is a management system for food safety assurance and is based on Risk Analysis. The management of risks through HACCP is more systematic, more organized and more documented than through GHP. HACCP plans are process- and product-specific, targeting specific hazards. They include specified and quantified controls to manage risks, and they specify methods to measure whether controls are successful. In many cases, the same control measures are used in both GHP and HACCP; the difference is in the much higher specificity and measurability of their application within HACCP.

There are seven principles of HACCP:

1. Identify health hazards.
2. Identify Critical Control Points (CCPs).
3. Establish critical limits for each CCP.
4. Establish a monitoring system for each CCP.
5. Establish corrective actions if CCP is out of control.
6. Verify that the HACCP plan is working effectively.
7. Establish documentation and records.

Principle 1: identify health hazards

All hazards associated with each process step must be identified and enlisted. The most practical approach is first to construct a process diagram, with clearly defined individual process steps. All inputs, including raw materials at each step, must then be identified. Next, the hazards (microbial, parasitic, chemical, physical) that could occur at each step are identified. The methods by which hazards are transferred to the product are identified. Finally, any redistribution of hazards within/on the product is analysed.

Subsequently, the hazards that could occur in the product at a given step need to be categorized and ranked according to the risk they present. This is done in order to apportion appropriate levels of resources to their control. A simple method to determine risk categories, as shown in Table 8.1, can be used. The judged severity of the consequences of occurrence of a given hazard is correlated with the judged associated probability of its occurrence, resulting in quantitative conversion of that relationship into the final risk category. Hazards belonging to a high-risk category – e.g. Category 4 in the described method – are critical for product safety and must be efficiently controlled through CCP (see below). Hazards belonging to lower-risk categories are not critical, so can be controlled by application of general principles, i.e. by measures within GHP.

Principle 2: identify CCPs

A Critical Control Point (CCP) is any point along the production process where hazards can be efficiently controlled. A decision tree is useful to clarify CCPs (Fig. 8.1).

CCPs are sometimes divided into two types: CCP1s and CCP2s, where CCP1s can control the hazard fully (e.g. cooking or chilling processes at given temperatures), whilst CCP2s can only minimize the hazard, but do not afford complete control (e.g. hygiene of dressing, evisceration, etc.). In conventional slaughter and dressing processes, CCP1 controls are rare: some people even consider them as non-existent. Usually the hazards cannot be totally eliminated at the slaughterline. Within the EU, where presently carcass decontamination is not allowed, most CCPs in abattoirs are actually CCP2s; however only the use of CCP is generally accepted for use in the terminology.

Table 8.1. Determining risk categories.

Severity of hazard	Probability of occurrence				
	Frequent	Likely	Occasional	Seldom	Unlikely
Catastrophic	Very high (Cat. 4)	Very high (Cat. 4)	High (Cat. 3)	High (Cat. 3)	Medium (Cat. 2)
Critical	Very high (Cat. 4)	High (Cat. 3)	High (Cat. 3)	Medium (Cat. 2)	Low (Cat. 1)
Moderate	High (Cat. 3)	Medium (Cat. 2)	Medium (Cat. 2)	Low (Cat. 1)	Low (Cat. 1)
Negligible	Medium (Cat. 2)	Low (Cat. 1)	Low (Cat. 1)	Low (Cat. 1)	Low (Cat. 1)

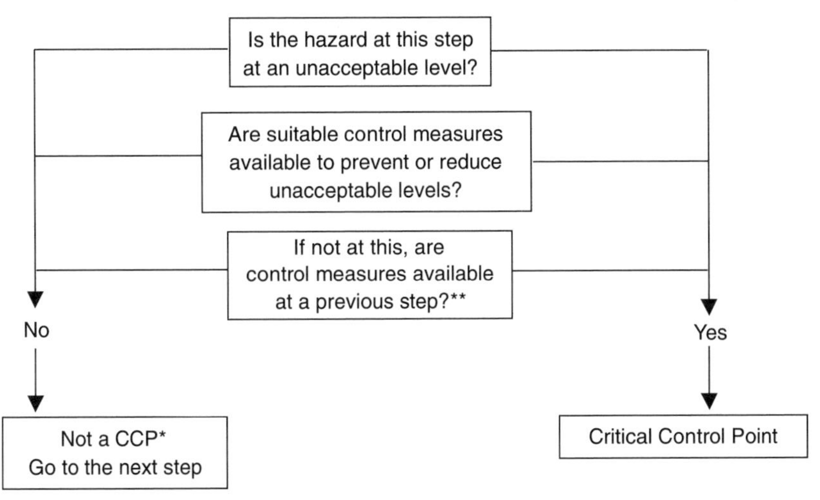

Fig. 8.1. CCP decision tree. *If the step is not a CCP, then consider control by GHP, or at a subsequent step; redesign the process if possible. **Assign retroactive CCP if control measures are available at a previous step.

Principle 3: establish critical limits for each CCP

For each CCP, defined and measurable critical limits must be determined, below which the hazard is controlled and the product is acceptable, and above which the hazard is not controlled and the product is unacceptable. The critical limits must be easily visualized or measured. Within abattoir operations, a common and useful critical limit states that no visible faecal contamination is allowed at a particular step (e.g. after dehiding or after evisceration). Other examples of critical limits on the slaughterline are that carcass refrigeration temperature is ≤7°C, and that the temperature of the hot water in the knife sterilizers is ≥82°C.

Principle 4: establish a monitoring system for each CCP

For each CCP, monitoring parameters must be established. Monitoring is often not continuous, but must be regular and of known frequency (e.g. checking temperature in sterilizers every hour). Sometimes monitoring is based on a sampling plan, but this has to be meaningful. Clearly defined methods (e.g. visual, for absence of faecal carcass contamination) must be used to monitor the CCP by trained staff. The monitoring system must state clearly who is responsible if the CCP is found to be out of control.

Principle 5: establish corrective actions

For each CCP, specific actions are taken when critical limits are exceeded. For example, in the case of carcass contamination, trimming, or altering its disposition, may be conducted. These actions are designed to regain rapid control of the CCP (e.g. retaining carcass on the slaughter line) and to prevent reoccurrence of the problem (e.g. replace or retrain the staff).

Principle 6: verify the HACCP plan

Each HACCP plan must be validated, i.e. analysed to determine that all the controllable hazards have been identified and included in the plan. The plan is then analysed thoroughly to ensure that it is complete and capable of achieving the company's performance objectives (POs), thus ultimately enabling achievement of the government's FSOs. Verification is conducted using measurable parameters and by comparing defined parameters with in-house and national performance; the aim is to verify that the plan is working and that all hazards are controlled. The outcomes of the HACCP system should be at least equivalent to, but would normally exceed, those of the GHP-based system. The HACCP plan must be subjected to periodic independent review. Revalidation of the HACCP plan is necessary after any changes in production or of other aspects affecting the plan. Often, product testing is used to verify that CCPs are under control and that the plan is working (see Chapter 8.2).

Principle 7: establish documentation and records

HACCP documentation must be thorough and include all details of the HACCP plan. All monitoring, corrective actions, verification procedures and results must be recorded. The HACCP plan must be adhered to by all staff involved. Some examples of summarized documentation are given in Boxes 8.1, 8.2 and 8.3.

Advantages and limitations of the HACCP-based system

HACCP is proactive and preventative, the aim being to anticipate problems and prevent their occurrence. It is owned by producers and staff, so compliance and participation is stimulated and motivation is usually high. HACCP is also specific, systematic and documented. These are all qualities that contribute to the effectiveness of HACCP-based systems in achieving hygienic production processes and, hence, a safe product (food).

On the other hand, HACCP is demanding on staff and time. Developing, implementing and monitoring HACCP requires a team of experts in the plant, covering a range of disciplines (e.g. slaughter personnel, engineers, veterinarians, microbiologists, chemists, management). This is achievable by large operators with a workforce having all the necessary skills, but is less achievable for small operators. Operators producing a large number of products may also experience difficulty developing/implementing a separate HACCP plan for each.

Box 8.1. Hazard analysis: an Example at a Selected Process Step

Process step	Hazard Identification, characterization	Risk evaluation			CCP?	Control measures
		Probability	Severity	Risk category		
1.						
2.						
etc.						

Box 8.2. Summary of CCPs

CCPs	Critical limits	Monitoring				Corrective actions		
		Procedure	Frequency	Responsibility	Records	Procedure	Responsibility	Records
CCP 1								
CCP 2								
etc.								

Box 8.3. HACCP Validation and Verification

Validation carried out by		Name:			Position:		Date:	Signature:	
Validation carried out BEFORE the plan is first implemented									
The scope is accurate?	Process flow chart complete?	All hazards are addressed?	Control measures in place?	CCPs are justified?	Critical limits are acceptable?	Monitoring procedures given?	Records are adequate?	Does the plan cover all hazards?	Does the plan control all hazards?
YES/NO	YES/NO	YES/NO	YES/NO	YES/NO	YES/NO	YES/NO	YES/NO	YES/NO	YES/NO
Verification carried out AFTER the plan is implemented									
Persons responsible for verification:			Part of the plan verified:		Part of the plan verified:		Part of the plan verified:		Whole plan verified:
			Part	Date	Part	Date	Part	Date	Time frame
Person 1:			*		*		*		
Person 2:									
etc.									

For each part, a separate signed verification record must be prepared comprising any corrective actions required, as well as whether and who carried them out.

However, external organizations can be contracted to assist small operators to design the HACCP plans necessary for their plant; support can also be obtained from producers' associations. Finally, HACCP systems are designed to assure product safety, whilst the normal Quality Assurance systems operating in abattoirs are designed to reassure commercial clients about varying aspects of the product. Both programmes are necessary, but in some aspects they may have opposing goals.

Further Reading

Anon. (2004) *Good Practices for Meat Industry*. FAO Animal Production and Health Manual. FAO, Rome.

Bolton, D.J., Sheridan, J.J. and Doherty, A.M. (2000) *HACCP for Irish Beef Slaughter*. Teagasc–The National Food Centre, Dublin.

Brown, M. (2000) *HACCP in the Meat Industry*. Woodhead Publishing Ltd, Cambridge, UK.

National Advisory Committee on Microbiological Criteria for Foods (NACMCF) (1993) Generic HACCP for raw beef. *Food Microbiology* 10, 449–488.

National Advisory Committee on Microbiological Criteria for Foods (NACMCF) (1998) Hazard analysis and critical control point principles and application guidelines. *Journal of Food Protection* 61, 762–775.

8.2 Microbiological Examination for HACCP Verification

Introduction

Verification of HACCP involves comparing the performance parameters of each operator – with their own parameters obtained in different periods – with the parameters of other operators, and with the parameters from national and international baselines (databases); they all should be compatible with related Food Safety Objectives (FSOs) provided by the government. The absence of microbiological hazards on carcasses cannot be guaranteed by any microbiological testing, since the entire surface of every carcass cannot be examined, and the hazards may be present infrequently and/or at levels below the limit of detection, or even be non-culturable. Therefore, the process hygiene parameters are usually monitored by testing for selected indicator organisms, rather than for hazards (i.e. pathogens) themselves.

Current national legislation on the microbiological examination of carcasses and surfaces in the context of HACCP verification, using indicator organisms, is based on EU Commission Decision 2001/471/EC. According to this Decision, meat operators must conduct regular microbiological checks, to establish whether general hygiene is being maintained; the checks must cover the hygiene of utensils, fittings and machinery and, if necessary, products, at all stages. This system for HACCP verification is currently mandatory in the EU, so will be briefly described here.

Checks on the hygiene of carcasses

Carcass sampling sites

After slaughter, carcasses must be sampled and tested for the presence of two groups of indicator organisms (described below). The samples are taken after post-mortem inspection but before the final wash/chill steps. This is because the carcass microflora at the end of the slaughter line (but before chilling) directly reflect the process hygiene of the operator; the microflora changes qualitatively and quantitatively during chilling so no longer directly reflect the level of slaughterline hygiene.

Samples from carcasses are taken from the following sites:

- cattle: neck, brisket, flank, rump;
- sheep/goat: flank, lateral thorax, brisket, breast;
- pig: back, jowl (or cheek), medial hind limb (ham), belly; and
- horse: flank, brisket, back, rump.

The chosen sites for each animal species are those most typically contaminated.

The frequency of microbiological sampling is specified in the legislation: a minimum of five carcasses must be examined on one day each week. The day of sampling must be rotated. In plants slaughtering multiple species, alternate species must be sampled each week. The samples are taken halfway through the slaughter day or production run, to produce a realistic average of the bacterial numbers on the carcasses. Samples should not be taken at the start or end of the day, since bacterial numbers may be abnormally low or high, respectively.

Carcass sampling methods

The reference microbiological sampling method is tissue excision, a destructive method which removes tissue from the carcass surface. A sample consists of a piece of tissue, 20 cm^2 and up to 5 mm thick, excised from the carcass surface either by square slicing or using a borer. Deeper cuts into the tissue must be avoided, since this could transfer bacteria into sterile deep tissue, where they may be protected from the effects of drying and chilling.

Other alternative sampling methods, including wet–dry swabbing, can be used to take samples, provided they have been fully validated. Wet–dry swabbing uses systematic stroking to remove bacteria from the carcass surface, within an area delineated by a disinfected metal template. The wet swab is used first, and is rubbed in ten horizontal, ten vertical and ten diagonal strokes. The swab must be rotated, and constant pressure evenly applied. The procedure is then repeated using a dry swab. Both swabs are collected together in one container to produce one sample. Any instruments used for sampling must be disinfected between samples, usually by alcohol (ethanol).

The most effective microbiological sampling method is excision sampling, since it is assumed that 100% of the microorganisms present are physically removed from the carcass surface. Wet–dry swabbing is less effective, since only a proportion of the bacteria actually present are removed from the carcass surface. The bacterial recoveries routinely achieved by this technique are highly variable, ranging from 1% to 90%. In spite of that, the non-destructive wet–dry swabbing is preferred by the meat industry, as the excision method damages the carcass surface, affecting its commercial value.

Microbiological methods for sample examination

After sampling, the samples from four carcass sites can be pooled together to produce a single sample from each carcass. Pooling of samples is not permitted when an unacceptable result is not resolved by corrective action. The excised tissue portions, or the wet–dry swabs, are held refrigerated at <4°C for 24 h (at most) until examination.

In these samples, two microbiological parameters are determined: Total Viable Count of bacteria (TVC – meant to be an indicator of general hygiene) and Enterobacteriaceae count (meant to be an indicator of contamination of faecal origin).

The laboratory conducting the microbiological testing must be either accredited, or must be supervised by an accredited laboratory. Suitable laboratory quality assurance programmes must be in place. The actual microbiological methods used are published by the International Standardization Organization (ISO; Geneva) and are the following:

- Method for sample preparation, homogenization and dilution (ISO 7218 and ISO 6887).
- Method for determination of Total Viable Count of bacteria (TVC; ISO 2293:1998).
- Method for determination of Enterobacteriaceae count (ISO 7402:1993).

Other, alternative methods that produce equivalent results may be authorized by the OVS on a case-by-case basis if they are validated; preferably, their validation should be previously recognized by ISO or a similar body.

Keeping records on microbiological testing

Microbial counts from the pooled carcass sample are initially calculated as average colony-forming units (CFU)/cm^2 of the carcass. These counts are then converted to logarithms, taken to the base 10. The mean logarithm is then calculated for all the carcasses sampled on each day. Subsequently, daily variations in the mean logarithms can be used to observe the longer-term trends. The most recent (at least 13) daily mean logarithm values must be provided to the OVS, in the form of process control charts, on his request. The records should include sample type and origin, identification, sampling date and time, testing laboratory, personnel names and details of the analysis; all records must be kept for 18 months.

Microbiological criteria for carcasses

A three-class system, classifying microbiological results from carcasses (for each animal species) into acceptable, marginal and unacceptable is used to determine the performance of the operator (Table 8.2). The criteria in Table 8.2 apply when the excision sampling method was used. If the wet–dry swabbing method is used, then all the values in Table 8.2 would have to be adjusted to take into account lower bacterial recoveries normally obtained by swabbing. However, this is a very difficult question; because of the very high variability of the swabbing method, it is unclear what exactly the adjustment factor would be. Therefore, from a scientific perspective, it would be much more advisable to use the excision sampling method universally.

Interpretation of the results of microbiological testing of carcasses

It is important to keep in mind that the results of microbiological carcass testing do not relate to safety or fitness of the carcasss: individual carcasses do not ‘pass’ or ‘fail’ based on these results. This is because there is no

Table 8.2. EU criteria for classifying microbial test results from carcasses.

	Microbial load on carcasses (Log10 CFU/cm^2)		
Microbial test	Value m[a] (Results <m are satisfactory)	Marginal range (Results >m but <M are marginal)	Value M[b] (Results >M are unacceptable)
Total Viable Count of bacteria (TVC)	3.5 (cattle, sheep, horse) 4.0 (pig)	3.5 to 5.0 (cattle, sheep, horse) 4.0 to 5.0 (pig)	5.0 (cattle, sheep, horse, pig)
Enterobacteriaceae count	1.5 (cattle, sheep, horse) 2.0 (pig)	1.5 to 2.5 (cattle, sheep, horse) 2.0 to 3.0 (pig)	2.5 (cattle, sheep, horse) 3.0 (pig)

[a] m = border value between 'satisfactory' and 'marginal'.
[b] M = border value between 'marginal' and 'unacceptable'.

proven correlation between indicator organisms and prevalence/levels of pathogens. Whilst higher levels of indicators can mean the process hygiene was inferior and, therefore, that potential meat safety risks could be higher, the indicators themselves are no proof that the meat actually contains pathogens. Instead, the microbiological data based on the indicators should be interpreted only to assess general trends in the process hygiene of the operator.

Checks on the hygiene of environmental surfaces

Environmental surfaces include meat contact surfaces such as utensils, machinery, conveyor belts or cutting boards, and other, non-meat contact surfaces. According to the EU Decision, environmental surfaces must be examined before work begins each day, but after cleaning and disinfection; a minimum of ten samples must be taken fortnightly. Approximately two-thirds of the total number should be taken from food contact surfaces.

Environmental surfaces must be examined for TVC, while testing surfaces for Enterobacteriaceae is voluntary unless demanded by the OVS. The EU criteria for surfaces are: TVC counts of <10 CFU/cm^2 or Enterobacteriaceae counts of <1 CFU/cm^2 are acceptable; values above these are unacceptable.

HACCP Verification

In the context of the related EU Decision, if the trends of the microbiological results from regular checks of carcasses and surfaces (outlined above) fall consistently over the long term into the acceptable range of the related criteria, the HACCP plan is verified. However, an unacceptable result should trigger a review of process controls that must ensure the cause is determined, and prevention of recurrence. Feedback of unacceptable results must be conveyed to the operator's staff. Generally, unacceptable results can be due to several factors, or their combination, including: changes in technology, false or inadequate working procedures, inadequate staff training or instructions, unsuitable cleaning and disinfection regimes, inadequate maintenance and inadequate supervision.

However, one could argue that HACCP verification based on microbiological results described above, used alone, may be insufficient. The results are obtained only at the end of the slaughterline, so whilst they may indicate that some problems exist in the production process, they do not provide any information on what and where the source of the problem is. For more substantial assessment of process hygiene and HACCP verification, more complex information would be beneficial; these aspects will be briefly commented on in the next chapter.

Further Reading

Anon. (1999) *The Evaluation of Microbiological Criteria for Food Products of an Animal Origin for Human Consumption*. European Union, Brussels.

Brown, M.H., Gill, C.O., Hollingsworth, J., Nickelson II, R., Seward, S., Sheridan, J. *et al.* (2000) The role of microbiological testing in systems for assuring the safety of beef. *International Journal of Food Microbiology* 62, 7–16.

Hutchison, M.L., Walters, L.D., Avery, S.M., Reid, C.-A., Wilson, D., Howell, M., Johnston, A.M. and Buncic, S. (2005) A comparison of wet-dry swabbing- and excision-sampling methods for microbiological testing of bovine, porcine and ovine carcasses at red meat slaughterhouses. *Journal of Food Protection* 68, 2155–2162.

McEvoy, J.M., Sheridan, J.J., Blair, I.S. and McDowell, D.A. (2004) Microbial contamination on beef in relation to hygiene assessment based on criteria used in EU Decision 2001/471/EC. *International Journal of Food Microbiology* 92, 217–225.

Pepperell, R., Reid, C.-A., Nicolau Solano, S., Hutchison, M.L., Walters, L.D., Johnston, A.M. and Buncic, S. (2005) Experimental comparison of excision and swabbing microbiological sampling methods for carcasses. *Journal of Food Protection* 68, 2165–2168.

8.3 Hygiene Performance and Auditing of Abattoirs

Meat safety systems in abattoirs, GHP- and HACCP-based, are owned by the operators but must be independently audited to ensure that they are designed and implemented properly, are verified, and work correctly.

Auditing GHP and related prerequisite programmes

The Hygiene Assessment System (HAS scoring) was developed by the UK Meat Hygiene Service to evaluate general hygiene practices in abattoirs. During HAS scoring, all stages of abattoir operation are observed systematically and individually with respect to their hygiene and to any associated public health risks; they are compared with scientifically accepted correlated 'best practices', and then a resultant quantitative score is allocated to each stage. Finally, the total sum of all scores gives a numerical final HAS score for that abattoir. However, the main drawback of HAS-based auditing is that it is reasonably subjective, so the final HAS score for the same abattoir may differ when given by different auditors. In addition, HAS scoring is not connected directly to methods for HACCP verification and auditing.

Auditing HACCP

Auditing HACCP is more complicated than that for HAS, since it is more complex and tailored to each individual abattoir. Presently, within the EU, clear regulatory or government guidance on auditing HACCP is lacking. Nevertheless, it can be assumed that the main elements of HACCP auditing would include the following: (i) the HACCP documentation must be studied, to determine whether all seven principles of HACCP are being addressed; (ii) on-site determination of whether the written HACCP plan and the actual practices correlate; (iii) determination of whether all actual hazards are covered; (iv) determination of whether all CCPs are verified and monitored; (v) assessing HACCP validation; and (vi) trend analysis of hygiene performance parameters, such as regular microbiological checks, used for HACCP verification – this aspect will be further considered below.

Interpretation of microbiological verification results from different HACCP types

The suitability of methods and parameters for determining the microbiological verification of HACCP is controversial, but naturally must involve sampling plans and performance criteria. Between-plant and between-country comparisons of performance parameters may be conducted, although it is necessary to compare only those plants and results which are directly similar.

For example, different HACCP approaches can be used in different meat industries, so hygiene performance parameters differ between those. One example of a significant difference in approaches includes those having a HACCP system with interventions and those with a HACCP system without interventions. Abattoirs having HACCP without interventions presently do not have a CCP based on meat decontamination treatment to eliminate hazards. Therefore, in these abattoirs, the CCPs can reduce, but not necessarily eliminate, the hazards on the finished carcasses (Table 8.3). This situation occurs in the EU, where HACCP-based control measures are the same as those which are GHP-based, although their application is more systematic. In contrast, abattoirs having HACCP with interventions have a CCP based on meat decontamination treatment which is capable of eliminating the hazards on the finished carcasses (Table 8.4). This situation occurs in the USA, where antimicrobial treatment of carcasses is incorporated in HACCP as a mandatory CCP. Understandably, the parameters used for hygiene performance assessment, and for HACCP verification, can significantly differ between these two types of abattoir.

Overall, the general approach to assessing HACCP verification could be illustrated by the following formula: HACCP verification = HACCP validation + auditing. Sources of validation data include, but are not restricted to, results of product testing, research results, regulatory requirements and computer modelling. Auditing involves inspection of HACCP plans, records and testing results, followed by evaluation of the results against databases and performance criteria.

Which process hygiene performance criteria to use when comparing abattoir operations?

Presently, comparison of abattoirs' hygiene performance commonly utilizes the results of end product microbiological testing. 'End product'-based assessment has microbiological criteria based on final carcasses, and some current examples are shown in Table 8.5. Such criteria do indicate the status of final carcasses, but they do not characterize the process itself in depth, since initial contamination is not taken into account.

'Process-based' microbiological criteria are based on criteria measured at various stages of the process, including final carcass values. These criteria indicate the microbiological status of final carcasses, but also characterize the process itself.

Two recent examples of process-based abattoir hygiene performance have been proposed.

First, the Irish approach (Bolton *et al.*, 2000) involves microbiological sampling at different stages of the slaughterline with two aims: (i) to grade the carcasses; and (ii) to determine the 'process dynamics' of any contamination. This approach enables much better understanding of the process, and the roots of any problems, than if only final carcasses were tested.

Table 8.3. Examples of typical CCPs in HACCP schemes in abattoirs where intervention is not allowed post-slaughter.

	Typical CCP				
CCP criteria and actions	Acceptance of animals	De-hiding	Evisceration	Splitting and spinal cord removal	Chilling
Critical limits	Cleanliness score, e.g. MHS 2 (or 3?)	(a) No visible contamination or (b) % contamination rate (c) Sterilizers at 82°C	Same as de-hiding	No residual tissue	≤ 7°C Air humidity, velocity, spacing are also quantifiably controlled
Monitoring	Visual, and conducted on every animal	(a) Visual and conducted on every carcass or (b) Computerized, push-button	Same as de-hiding	Visual, and conducted on every carcass	(a) Instrumental or (b) visual
Corrective actions	Rejection or cleaning	Trimming; retraining; repairing or replacing equipment	Same as de-hiding	Same as de-hiding	Reject; retraining; repairing or replacing equipment

Table 8.4. Examples of typical CCPs in HACCP schemes in US abattoirs where intervention post-slaughter is conducted.

	Potential CCP				
CCP criteria and actions	Pre-skinning hide decontamination?	Post-evisceration/ after trimming; hot water washing	USDA final inspection	USDA veterinarian	Chilling
Critical limits	?	75–85°C; 0–15 Pa; 5–12 seconds	Zero tolerance for contamination	Zero tolerance for contamination	≤ 7°C, RH, spacing
Monitoring	?	Water temperature, pressure and time continuously monitored	Continuous visual inspection on every carcass	Verification that previous CCP (continuous visual inspection) has been properly conducted	(a) Instrumental or (b) Visual
Corrective actions	?	Re-processing carcass	Re-trimming, re-inspection; if three failures: HACCP revision	HACCP revision?	Reject; retraining; repairing or replacing equipment

Table 8.5. Examples of end product-based abattoir performance criteria (for carcasses).

Criterion	Country and purpose		
	EU, UK – regular checks	USA – HACCP	USA – pathogen reduction
TVC (log CFU/cm^2)	m <3.5[a] M >5.0[b] (≥5/week)		
Enterobacteriaceae (log CFU/cm^2)	m <1.5[a] M >2.5[b] (≥5/week)		
E. coli (CFU/cm^2)		m < 5[a] M >100[b] (≥1/300)	
Salmonella (Positives: no more than)			Steer/heifer: 1/82 Cow/bull: 2/58

[a] m = border value between 'satisfactory' and 'marginal'.
[b] M = border value between 'marginal' and 'unacceptable'.

A second potential approach is based on evaluation of process hygiene by comparison of bacterial loads on final carcasses with bacterial loads on correlated incoming animals (i.e. hide). The derived BOIF factor (Bacterial Output–Input Factor) is a numerical parameter showing the relationship between hide and carcass microflora, i.e. the microbiological reduction achieved (Vivas Alegre and Buncic, 2004). The results of a study comparing the EU microbiological criteria for final carcasses, BOIF and HAS scores at two selected abattoirs, A and B, are shown in Table 8.6. End product testing according to EU criteria showed that the actual microbial counts achieved on carcasses produced by abattoir B were lower than those found on carcasses produced by abattoir A. In contrast, BOIF results showed that abattoir A succeeded in reducing the microbial levels on carcasses compared with the levels on hides – to a greater extent – than abattoir B. This was in agreement with HAS, in which abattoir A was judged to be more hygienic than abattoir B.

Table 8.6. Comparison of process hygiene assessment systems.

Process hygiene performance criteria	Comparison of abattoirs A and B	Resultant ranking
EU (microbiological criteria for final carcasses)		
TVC[a]	A > B	B is better
EC[b]	A > B	B is better
BOIF (microbial level on final carcasses as proportion of that on hides)		
TVC	A < B	A is better
EC	A < B	A is better
HAS scores	A > B	A is better

[a] TVC, total viable counts.
[b] EC, Enterobacteriaceae counts.

Evidence for the efficacy of HACCP

Very often, both in practice and in science, a simple but understandable question is asked: does HACCP in abattoirs work? To answer this question, one would need to have and compare the same data from the same operators, obtained both before and after implementation of the HACCP system; these data could show whether post-HACCP data are better than pre-HACCP data. Such evidence of the success of HACCP is scarce, but some is available for the meat industry in the USA (Table 8.7). The data shown indeed indicate that introduction of HACCP resulted in significant global reduction of pathogens on meat. However, similar data from within the EU are lacking.

Table 8.7. *Salmonella* prevalence data before and after the introduction of HACCP in the USA (Anon., 2004).

	Salmonella prevalence in animals (%)		
	Cattle	Pigs	Broilers
Pre-HACCP	1–2.7	8.7	20.0
Post-HACCP	0.4–2.2	5.4	10.7

Further Reading

Anon. (2004) *Progress Report on Salmonella Testing of Raw Meat and Poultry Products 1998–2003*. Food Safety and Inspection Service, US Department of Agriculture, Washington, DC, pp. 1–10.

Bolton, D.J., Sheridan, J.J., Doherty, A.M. (2000) *HACCP for Irish Beef Slaughter*. Teagasc – The National Food Centre, Dublin.

Brown, M.H., Gill, C.O., Hollingsworth, J., Nickelson II, R., Seward, S., Sheridan, J.J. *et al.* (2000) The role of microbiological testing in systems for assuring the safety of beef. *International Journal of Food Microbiology* 62, 7–16.

McEvoy, J.M., Sheridan, J.J., Blair, I.S. and McDowell, D.A. (2004) Microbial contamination on beef in relation to hygiene assessment based on criteria used in EU Decision 2001/471/EC. *International Journal of Food Microbiology* 92, 217–225.

Vivas Alegre, L. and Buncic, S. (2004) Potential for Use of Hide-Carcass Microbial Counts Relationship as an Indicator of Process Hygiene Performance of Cattle Abattoirs. *Food Protection Trends* 24, 814–821.

III Hygiene of Production – Processing of Other Foods and Retail–Consumer Food Safety

9 Hygiene of Production – Processing of Other Foods

9.1 Hygiene of Milk and Dairy Products

ALISON SMALL

This chapter aims to outline the dairy production chain, introducing the reader to the process steps involved and examining public health and hygiene issues throughout.

Milk

Milk is produced in the udder of all mammals, in order to feed and nourish the newborn of the species. It is composed primarily of water, containing proteins, carbohydrate, minerals and fat. The proportion of each of these nutrients present in milk from different species of animal varies, and has evolved in order to provide the correct balance required for the development of the newborn of that species. For example, the protein content of human milk is substantially lower than that of other species, and the lactose level quite high. These differences mean that the formulation of milk replacers, used extensively in the rearing of infants and other newborn animals, is an exceedingly complex task, and also mean that milk replacers formulated for one species are not appropriate nutrition for another. There are two groups of proteins present in raw milk, the caseins and the whey proteins. Caseins form over 80% of the total protein in milk, and do not possess an organized molecular structure, so cannot be denatured in the conventional sense. Within the casein molecule, there are areas that are highly hydrophobic, and other areas that are extremely hydrophilic. Cross links between these areas form readily, and these cross links form the basis of cheese formation. Whey proteins, which include various enzymes, are organized, globular proteins and are readily denatured, e.g. by the application of heat. The primary sugar in milk is lactose, comprising around 4.5% of the total milk solids. Lactose is a disaccharide of glucose and galactose, which itself is a reducing sugar, and reacts with the free amino acids present in milk producing a brown discolouration. The fat content of milk is very variable, from low fat in the horse (around 2% of milk solids) to high in sheep (7%) and buffalo (8%), and is comprised of globules of triglyceride surrounded by a phospholipid membrane.

Milk-borne Disease

In the early part of the 20th Century, milk and dairy products probably constituted the most dangerous parts of our diet, being the vector for thousands of cases of diseases such as brucellosis, paratyphoid fever, Bovine Tuberculosis (which at this time often led to the death of the affected individual), as well as food poisoning. Human illness and deaths as a result of milk-borne disease have fallen dramatically since the 1920s. Disease due to bovine tuberculosis and brucellosis has been controlled through milk pasteurization, and through the implementation of eradication programmes in livestock in the latter half of the 20th Century, but milk-borne infection with *Salmonella* and *Campylobacter* still occurs, causing substantial morbidity and subsequent cost to society. Most of these infections originate with raw or improperly pasteurized products, or through recontamination of a pasteurized product, for example wild birds pecking through the bottle tops on doorstep-delivered milk to reach the cream below can introduce organisms such as *Salmonella* or *Campylobacter* into the bottle contents, thus presenting a risk of infection to the householder consuming that product. Recontamination may also occur from a food handler carrying and excreting pathogens, and summer-long enteric disease outbreaks in popular seaside holiday resorts may commonly be traced back to a particular ice cream vendor who happens to be excreting, for example, *Salmonella paratyphi* B. Globally, dairy products are responsible for approximately 21% of outbreaks of infectious intestinal disease where a food vehicle has been identified; 8% is attributable to milk and milk products and 13% to cakes and ice cream (Fig. 9.1). For comparison, 23% of outbreaks are attributable to eggs and egg products, and 15% to meat and meat products.

The Dairy Production Chain

Milk is first produced on the farm, and in the majority of cases is removed in a raw state to a collection centre or processing plant. There do exist small producer–processors, where the milk is harvested from the lactating cattle, sheep, goats or buffalo, and processed on the farm of origin for direct sale to the final consumer. In countries with a highly industrialized dairy industry, these private operations are in the minority,

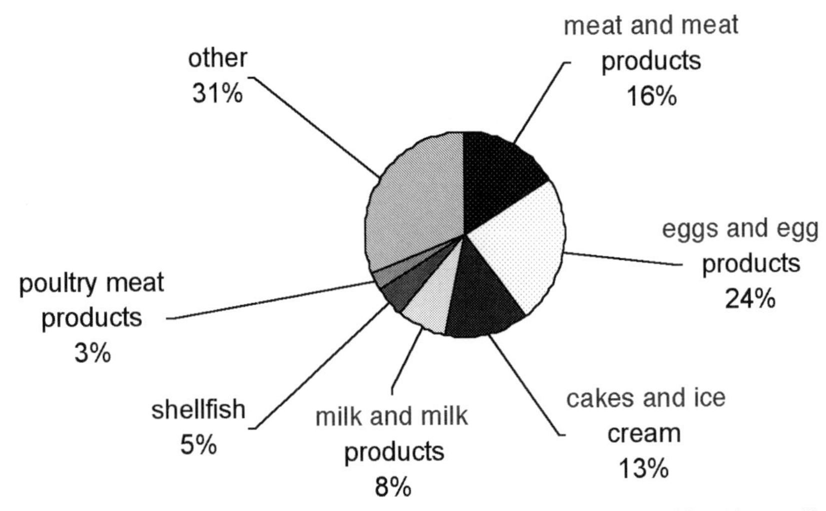

Fig. 9.1. Estimated contribution of different food groups to outbreaks of food-borne illness.

but in other countries they may form the greater proportion of the dairy supply. Equally, although this chapter considers milk produced by cattle and sheep, throughout the world the milk of many species is harvested and used for human consumption. The hygiene considerations however, are similar.

In an industrialized system, the milk is removed from the farm in bulk tanker vehicles to a collection point, where it is mixed with milk from many different farms, standardized and stored under refrigeration until processed. Most milk is pasteurized, before packaging or bottling and distribution, or further processing into dairy products (Table 9.1). Some products and some markets, however, demand raw, unpasteurized milk.

Table 9.1. Production of milk for human consumption.

Site	Stages in production
On-farm	Milking Cooling
Transportation	
Processing plant	Storage in silos Clarification Pasteurization – heating and holding Cooling to below 10°C Pre-filling holding tank, agitated Filling cartons or bottles Chilling
Distribution to cold store and retail outlets	

Primary production

Primary production occurs on the farm, and farm and livestock management can have a significant impact on the productivity of the herd. There is also a genetic effect on milk yield from individual cows, but, using the UK as an example, improvements in genetic quality, health and nutrition of dairy cows over the last 20 years of the 20th Century have resulted in an increase in average milk yield per dairy cow from 3900 l per annum to 6500 l per annum. To put this figure into perspective, 6500 l would be sufficient to supply 26 families with their liquid milk requirement for 1 year. On average, in the UK, each person drinks around 1.5 l of liquid milk each week.

On the dairy farm, cleanliness and the use of good farming practices are paramount. Cleanliness of the premises, personnel, animals and equipment will not only protect public health, by reducing the risk of milk contamination, but also protect the health of the animals, by reducing the risk of mastitis. A reduction in mastitis in the dairy herd also results in improvements in milk quality as measured by the somatic cell count (SCC) in the milk. Also, healthy animals are capable of maximum performance as regards milk yield, and thus the overall farm income is supported. One of the hidden costs of endemic and subclinical illness in dairy herds is a reduction in milk yield, and this reduction often remains unobserved until the disease problem is solved, and milk yields rise, because the reduction in yield is often insidious in onset rather than sudden.

Hygiene of premises

Milk is highly vulnerable to contamination by both pathogenic and spoilage organisms, so it is important that the premises are laid out in such a manner that there is complete separation between animal/'dirty' operations and food/'clean' operations. When the dairy is first constructed, regard should be given both to the topography of the land and to the services available. Flood plains and sewage outlets should be avoided, whilst a sufficient supply of potable water and power is essential. Sources of contamination, such as manure heaps and tanks, should be separated from the animal housing, and particularly from the milk-handling and storage areas, as should lavatories. The premises should be well drained and ventilated, to prevent excessive humidity and the build-up of moisture in animal bedding, and dung channels should be cleaned and droppings removed regularly.

Within the animal housing, the premises should be kept in such a manner that the animals themselves remain clean and healthy. There should be isolation facilities for sick animals, and species constituting a high risk of carrying food-borne pathogens, for example pigs and poultry with *Salmonella* or *Campylobacter*, should be housed separately from lactating dairy animals. Similarly, animals and substances that may pose a risk of tainting the milk should be separated from the lactating animals, and the dairy parlour itself. Breeding rams and billy goats have been known to impart an odour taint in sheep milk, whilst certain chemicals or combinations of chemicals may result in tainting: for example the use of phenolic detergents alongside hypochlorite results in the liberation of chlorophenols, which would taint milk. The choice of chemicals used on the dairy farm should be chosen with care to avoid problems with taints, and also to avoid residues of unauthorized substances in milk. In fact, any activity which may pose a risk to the hygiene and quality of the milk, for example feeding, mucking out or cleaning, should not be carried out in the same place or at the same time as milk harvesting is under way.

Feedstuffs should be kept separate from the milk production and storage areas. Animal feeds may contain components that carry a risk of tainting milk, and also feeds have been shown to be a source of contamination for the farm with food-borne pathogens such as *Salmonella*. Even feeds purchased from a reputable supplier and tested for certain pathogens are not likely to be sterile, and so present a risk of introduction of spoilage and other organisms if kept close to milk.

Equipment used on the farm should be kept clean and well-maintained, and store rooms and feed stores clean and pest-proof. Vermin should be actively discouraged throughout, and there should be hygienic arrangements for the disposal of waste materials and discarded milk. Personnel should be provided with clean protective clothing to be used only within the milking parlour, separate from clothing to be used in the animal housing, and facilities for washing and drying hands should be available. The milking parlour itself should be easy to clean, with good drainage and ventilation, and good lighting is important so that cleanliness of both equipment and animals can be adequately assessed. Chemicals used in cleaning, and medicines used on the farm, should be correctly stored in lockable facilities.

Traditionally, milk was harvested by hand, into open buckets, which would then be covered for transportation to the milk store, where the buckets would be tipped into milk churns for collection or processing. In a modern facility, the milk is collected automatically through a milking system comprising a cluster of teat cups that attach to the udder, drawing the milk off by a pulsing vacuum system into a primary receiver bottle. The bottle is then emptied via a milk transfer line into the bulk milk storage tank, where it is held under refrigeration (6°C or less) until collection by the milk tanker vehicle. The bulk tank should be housed in a separate room, considered to be a 'high-risk' area, which is used for no other purpose. In some areas, the 'milking bail' is commonly used for milk harvest while cows are at summer pasture. The 'milking bail' is a mobile milking parlour which is positioned at a site close to the cows, often in a corner of the pasture, close to the gate. When choosing the site for a bail, the farmer should take into account the same factors as when building a permanent dairy parlour, such as potential for flooding, position of manure heaps, sewage outflows and drainage and cleanliness of the land. Adequate protection for the milk is important, and the bail must be kept clean. The farmer will need to bring to the site a power supply, potable water and storage/transport containers for the milk produced, and the equipment must be cleaned as thoroughly as the equipment in the permanent facility. An outline of a milking system is given in Fig. 9.2.

Where a farm is a producer–processor, and the milk is to be further processed on the same site, the processing unit should be a separate building, accessed via dedicated hygiene facilities, and using separate equipment and protective clothing from the rest of the operation. Milk may be transferred from the dairy parlour to the processing unit using milk churns or via hygienic pipes. The latter arrangement is more suitable, as it involves an entirely closed system, so the milk will not be exposed to external sources of contamination.

The equipment used in the dairy plant must be smooth in nature, to prevent the build-up of milk residue, which would be an ideal medium for the growth of microbes. It must be corrosion resistant and easy to clean and disinfect, and also must be made of a substance which itself will not cause tainting of the milk. Metal piping is commonly used, usually a steel–nickel alloy, or stainless steel. Glass tubing may be used, but with this material there is the risk of breakage, resulting in foreign body contamination of the milk, and also safety issues with personnel. Rubber is often used to form corner-pieces, gaskets to provide good seals, and for teat cup liners. All these items are therefore prone to deteriorate with time as the rubber slowly perishes. Perished rubber is characterized by a myriad of tiny cracks, and these allow harbourage of microorganisms including spoilers, human pathogens, and mastitis-causing organisms.

Cleaning of a dairy facility usually involves a clean-in-place system, where hot water – or a solution of hot water and chemical – is flushed through the pipes, effecting cleaning through the turbulence of the liquid in the pipes. Where dead areas occur in the system, such as where the layout of the pipes has been modified, leaving a closed branch, the

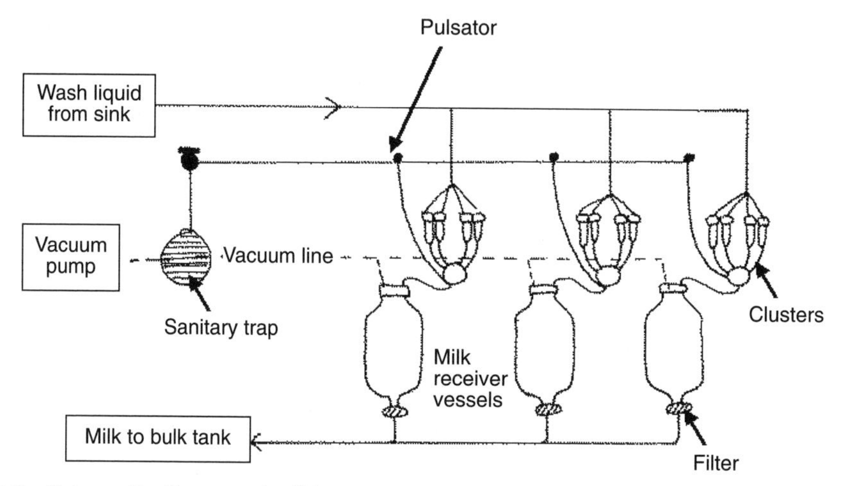

Fig. 9.2. Schematic diagram of milking system, showing clean-in-place wash line.

cleaning liquid often bypasses this area, allowing deposits of milk to build up, and thereby giving harbourage to microbes. Once cleaned, the system should be rinsed with potable water to prevent taint occurring. The outlet valve on the bulk tank should be left open to allow complete drainage and drying of the tank, as pools of residual liquid can present a reservoir of contamination to the subsequent batch of milk stored in the tank.

Health and hygiene of animals

Milk for human consumption should never be harvested from animals showing clinical signs of infectious diseases that may be transmitted to humans through ingestion of contaminated milk, for example tuberculosis or brucellosis, or from animals suffering from enteritis, mastitis or metritis. Sick animals may be treated with therapeutic medicines, and during and after treatment their milk should be discarded, until such time has passed that there is no risk of residues of those medicinal products being present in the milk.

When harvesting milk, it is important that the udder and teats are clean. They should be cleaned and dried each time the animal is milked, and the foremilk drawn off, prior to application of the teat cups, or drawing off of the milk. This action will not only aid in prevention of contamination of the milk, but will also assist in the prevention of mastitis, and the discarded foremilk can be examined as part of the herd mastitis screening programme. However, rather than focusing solely on the udder, the stockman should assess the cleanliness of the cows as a whole, as there is a correlation between cow cleanliness and milk hygiene. Clean cows also tend to have a lower incidence of mastitis, and hence lower somatic cell count, meaning that the milk is of a higher quality grade. Assessing the cleanliness of cows objectively can also assist the stockman in identifying possible management problems, and thereby to take appropriate action to correct these. The primary cause of coat soiling in dairy cattle is loose faeces, but other factors also play a part in the overall appearance of the cows on a farm.

Where cows have dirty legs, the passageway in the cow house is often insufficiently cleaned, and the cows may be walking through slurry. Modern dairy cows are substantially larger than their counterparts of 30 or 40 years ago, consume more food and water, and subsequently void more faeces and urine. A dairy cow can produce up to 30 l of each of these daily, and the practice of scraping passageways twice daily is no longer sufficient to adequately remove this waste. All too often, scraping produces a tidal wave of slurry that slops back over the scraper and into the beds.

Cows with dirty tails may be housed in cubicles that are too small. Again, the modern dairy cow, being larger than her predecessors, requires a larger bed, and where the bed is too small, her tail and udder may hang over into the dung passage and become contaminated. Tails may also be excessively dirty where the faeces are too loose. A healthy faecal consistency, where the dropping is moist but forms a distinct pat on the ground, indicates cows that are on a well-balanced diet. Cows which are fed diets with insufficient long fibre and a crude protein content greater than 18% often show sloppy faeces and dirty tails. A dirty tail not only indicates health and diet problems in the cows, it also poses a significant risk of contamination in the dairy parlour, the tail will flick faecal matter onto the equipment and personnel surrounding the cow and faecal contamination of the milk may result.

Where the flanks of the cows are identified as being dirty, this suggests that the beds are dirty and damp. Bed cleanliness is affected by the substrate used, drainage and the humidity of the cow house. Unused bedding should be stored under cover to keep it dry, and its moisture content should be maintained at less than 20%. Wet straw wads together, becomes mouldy and loses absorbency; wheat straw has a higher lignin content than barley straw, so is less absorbent; and all natural beddings such as straw, paper and wood shavings may support microbial growth and survival.

Processing of milk for human consumption

Approximately half of the milk produced by dairy cattle is ultimately sold as liquid drinking milk, the rest being processed into milk products such as butter, yoghurt or cheese. Milk is transported from the farm of origin in specially designed refrigerated tankers that are used solely for milk transportation, to prevent the risk of taint. The tank is often constructed of stainless steel, and designed in such a way as to allow thorough cleaning and complete drainage, as residual fluids can be a source of contamination for subsequent batches of milk. Tankers are often cleaned using a clean-in-place system, where superheated steam is circulated through the milk lines and the tank until sterilization temperatures are achieved. A tanker may collect milk from up to eight farms on a circuit before returning to the dairy processing plant to be emptied and cleaned.

When the milk arrives at the processing plant, a sample of the milk is taken and tested for odour, temperature and microbiological status. At this stage a rapid indicator test is used as a primary screen, and the sample removed to a laboratory for full microbiological analysis, which takes a matter of days. The milk is stored in a refrigerated silo prior to processing. On average, silos in use in modern dairy plants would hold the contents of three milk tankers, around 60,000 l. On arrival at the collection point, the milk should be at a temperature of no more than 10°C, and is cooled to below 6°C for storage prior to processing. Microbiological and quality standards to which the raw milk must comply have been set by the competent authority in most countries. For example, in the European Union (EU), raw cows' milk must have a somatic cell count (SCC) of no more than 400,000/ml, and some dairy processors pay a premium for milk of SCC $< 100,000$ cells/ml. Microbiologically, raw cows' milk is required to have an Aerobic Plate Count (APC) at 30°C of no more than 100,000 organisms/ml, whilst milk from sheep, goats or buffalo must have an APC of no more than 1,500,000 organisms/ml if the milk is going to be heat treated, and no more than 500,000 if it is to be sold without heat treatment.

Raw milk may undergo a number of treatments such as filtration, clarification and homogenization, as well as pasteurization, whilst at the processing plant. Usually the milk is passed from the silo through a coarse filter to remove large particles and foreign bodies. Further filtration may occur before the pasteurization process begins, whilst the milk is cold, during pasteurization, or immediately after pasteurization. Where filtration is carried out during pasteurization, this is effected by filters placed in the milk line, usually after pre-heating. A disadvantage of warm filtration is that some undesirable material, for example some dirt particles, becomes soluble when heated, and therefore will not be trapped in the filter. Cold milk filtration, however, reduces the butterfat content of the milk, and thereby affects its composition.

After pasteurization, ultrafiltration is often used to concentrate the proteins in skimmed milk, and the retentate from this process can be used as a concentrate in the process of milk standardization. The process of clarification involves the use of centrifuges to spin off foreign material. Centrifuges are also used to separate milk in modern processing plants, to remove the cream and for production of skimmed or semi-skimmed milk. The process of clarification is very important when the milk is homogenized, as it removes leucocytes and epithelial cells from the milk. These cells are naturally sloughed from the udder during lactation, are not removed by filtration and are present in raw milk. In milk that has not been homogenized, the cells remain in suspension and are not detected by eye, but in homogenized milk, they precipitate out and settle at the base of the container, leaving an unsightly, though harmless, grey sediment. Homogenization is carried out by forcing the milk through a tiny aperture under high pressure (around 210 kg/cm^2 or 3000 lb/in^2). This process breaks up the fat globules in the milk to give an even and stable dispersion of the butterfat, and breaks down any cross-links formed between caseins, reducing the curd tension of the milk. This makes the milk easier to digest and more palatable, but it can activate lipase in the milk, which will impart a rancid flavour. Lipase can be denatured by heat treatment, so homogenized milk is immediately pasteurized.

Milk may be heat treated by one of a number of ways – holding method pasteurization, High Temperature Short Time (HTST) pasteurization, Ultra High Temperature (UHT) treatment or sterilization. The aim of these treatments, of pasteurization, is the application of sufficient heat for sufficient time to destroy pathogenic microorganisms. This heat treatment, in a modern plant, is normally a batch process, with milk travelling through a long pipe in a heat exchanger. In the heat exchanger, the milk line is tightly coiled round a pipe containing superheated water or steam, so thermal energy is transferred from the steam to the milk without direct contact. The speed of flow of the milk and the length of the milk line is such that the milk remains in the heat exchanger for sufficient time to achieve the desired temperature and holding time. In a small dairy, the pasteurizer may be a small tank with a heated jacket and agitator, or a tank with rotating heated coils, stirring the milk continuously to ensure even heat distribution. When tank pasteurization is used, it is common practice to preheat the milk to reduce the energy load on the pasteurizer.

Holding method pasteurization, developed in the late 19th Century, requires milk to be heated to between 62.8°C and 65.6°C, and held for 30 min at this temperature. HTST pasteurization requires a temperature of 71.7°C, with 15 s holding. This method was developed from a technique called 'flash pasteurization', used in the early part of the 20th Century, where milk was heated to around 72°C with no holding period. The holding period of 15 s was added when it was realized that 'flash pasteurization' without holding often gave an inadequate kill of pathogenic microorganisms.

UHT milk has been held at 135°C for one second. This process is effected by indirect or direct heating. Indirect methods would use a heat exchanger as described above, while direct methods may involve passing steam directly through the milk, similar to the preparation of certain speciality coffees, e.g. caffe latte, or by passing an electric current through the milk. Sterilized milk has been heated to above 100°C. This tends to apply to canned products; milk in filled and seamed cans is placed in a retort and steamed at 115–120°C for 15 to 20 min, dependent on can size.

After pasteurization, it is important that the milk is protected from recontamination from any source. Pasteurization is the Critical Control Point in a HACCP for liquid milk. It should be cooled immediately to below 10°C, and packaged without delay. Processors should keep records of the pasteurization process, and plants are often fitted with automatic fail-safe devices, where milk that has not achieved proper pasteurization is diverted back to the raw milk silo for re-pasteurization, and there can be no cross-contamination of treated milk with untreated milk.

Pasteurization denatures milk enzymes, and this can be used as a test of correct pasteurization. Phosphatase is a natural milk enzyme, and it is used as the indicator enzyme. Properly pasteurized milk is phosphatase negative, and this is often used in legislation as a milk standard. To test for phosphatase activity, milk at 37°C is mixed with a phenylphosphoric ester, and a colour change indicator (2,6-di-bromoquinonechlorine) added. If phosphatase enzyme is present, phenol is liberated and the indicator develops a blue colour. This test is sensitive enough to detect 0.1% raw milk added to pasteurized milk, a 5-min reduction in holding time if using the holding method of pasteurization, or a 1°C loss in temperature during the pasteurization process. Heat treatment also reduces the Vitamin C content of milk by around 20%, and the Vitamin B_{12}/Thiamin content by around 10% (this has no significant effect on our dietary intake of these vitamins, as milk is not an important source in a balanced diet); this causes a slight disaggregation of the fat globules in the milk, giving a reduced cream line (this too has no nutritional significance). In UHT and sterilized milk these effects are increased due to the higher temperatures achieved, and also there is some caramelization of the sugars in the milk, giving it a sweeter flavour.

An outline of process control for milk production is given in Table 9.2.

Cream and Ice Cream

Cream is the portion of milk, rich in butterfat, that rises to the surface when milk is allowed to stand. Commercially it is separated from milk by centrifugation. Different types of cream are sold dependent on the butterfat content. For example, half cream has at least 12% butterfat, single cream at least 18% and double cream at least 48%. Cream sold as whipping cream has a butterfat content of 35% or more, and clotted cream 55%. Cream is pasteurized at a slightly higher temperature than milk; the holding method uses 63°C over a 30 min holding period, whilst the HTST method uses 73°C, held for 15 s. Once again, the phosphatase test is used as the indicator of correct pasteurization, and the cream must be immediately cooled and protected from recontamination. Cream is considered to be sterilized if it has been held at 108°C for 45 min, and UHT treatment of cream involves 140°C for 2 s.

Table 9.2. Process control in milk production.

Process step	Hazards	Controls
Arrival of raw milk	Raw milk may be contaminated with pathogens	Check bacterial quality of raw milk Keep raw milk separate from pasteurized milk
Pre-processing storage below 5°C	Growth of psychrotrophic bacteria	Limit length of holding time Thorough cleaning of equipment between batches
Pasteurization	Failure to destroy pathogens	Record time/temperature and flow rates Test milk – phosphatase test should be negative Clean and disinfect thoroughly between batches
Cooling to below 10°C	Bacterial growth Recontamination	Chill rapidly Prevent contact with raw product Thorough cleaning and disinfection between batches
Holding	Bacterial growth Recontamination	Temperature control Prevent contact with raw product Thorough cleaning and disinfection between batches
Filling	Recontamination from cartons	Store cartons hygienically
Cold Storage	Bacterial growth	Temperature control

Ice cream is a frozen product made from a combination of any of the following ingredients:

- eggs;
- sugar;
- cream;
- butter or butter oil;
- milk yoghurt;
- skimmed milk;
- evaporated milk;
- dried milk;
- dried skimmed milk;
- condensed milk;
- sweetened condensed milk;
- condensed skimmed milk; and
- sweetened condensed skimmed milk.

Flavourings and colourings are usually added to the ice cream base after pasteurization. The 'milk' in ice cream may begin in a number of forms, but once the base is prepared, it should be pasteurized at 65.6°C for 30 min, 71.1°C for 10 min or 79.4°C for 15 s. The ice cream base may also be sterilized using 148°C for 2 s.

Immediately after heat treatment, the ice cream base is homogenized and cooled. Flavourings and colourants are added in a storage vat, mixed with a mechanical paddle – either during the initial cooling phase or once the holding temperature of 7°C is reached. Ice cream must be cooled to below 7°C within 90 min of heat treatment, and held at this temperature until freezing begins. A temperature of below 4°C will improve the shelf life of the ice cream. Solid items such as fruits or cookies may be added to the base during cool storage, or at primary freezing. Primary freezing involves the cool ice cream mix being sprayed onto a cold surface and this soft-frozen mix is scraped off and placed into the final containers, which are transferred to the freezer store for final freezing to below −2.2°C. If the temperature of the product exceeds −2.2°C after this point, the ice cream must be re-pasteurized before sale.

Ice cream is a high-risk food product, as pathogenic organisms may be introduced to the base mix with ingredients such as fruit and cookies added after the pasteurization step, and some ice creams are made with pre-pasteurized milk, and no further pasteurization step after the eggs and gelatin have been added to make the base. The critical controls in ice cream production are pasteurization of the base (monitored using the phosphatase test) and strict temperature control thenceforth, combined with great care over the status of added ingredients (Table 9.3).

Further Processing of Milk

Milk used for further processing into milk products must achieve certain minimum standards prior to processing. In the EU, immediately before

Table 9.3. Outline of production process for ice cream.

Process stage	Notes
Mixing of base ingredients, e.g. milk, cream, sugar, eggs	Ingredients are potentially contaminated
Pasteurization or sterilization	Temperature control, negative phosphatase test
Homogenization	
Cooling to below 7.2°C within 1.5 h of heat treatment	Temperatures of below 4°C will improve keeping quality
Addition of flavourings and colourants	Added ingredients may carry contamination
Primary freezing to below 2.2°C	The temperature must remain below −2.2°C henceforth; if the temperature is allowed to rise, the product must be re-pasteurized
Addition of fruits, nuts, cookies	Added ingredients may carry contamination
Package	Ensure packaging is stored hygienically
Hardening	

processing, raw cows' milk must have an APC of less than 300,000 organisms/ml, whilst previously pasteurized or heat-treated cows' milk must have an APC of less than 100,000 organisms/ml. When milk arrives at the processing plant, it must be refrigerated and held at no more than 6°C until processed, unless processed within 4 h of arrival. If milk is to be stored for long periods (up to 48 h) it should be refrigerated to below 4°C. Milk for further processing may undergo a process called 'thermization', where it is warmed to 57–68°C and held for 15 s. This treatment improves the keeping quality of the milk pending processing, but is insufficient to destroy pathogens, and the phosphatase test will yield a positive result. This treatment cannot be used to 'improve' poor-quality milk – if the APC is greater than 300,000 organisms/ml, the milk must be discarded.

Cheese

Cheese is produced by coagulating the caseins in milk, using rennet or other suitable enzymes, or by the development of lactic acid produced during bacterial fermentation. Commonly, cheesemaking involves a combination of enzyme action and bacterial fermentation. The curd produced is then modified using heat, pressure, special moulds, ripening ferments and seasoning to produce cheeses of many flavours and textures. Cheese may be classified based on the raw material used in production: for example 'whole-milk cheese', 'skim-milk cheese', 'pasteurized cheese' or, more commonly, as hard or soft cheeses. Hard and soft cheeses can be further sub-classified based on the ripening process (Table 9.4).

Table 9.4. Examples of types of cheese.

Cheese type	Sub-type	Examples
Hard cheeses	Without gas holes	Cheddar Red Leicester
	With gas holes	Emmental Jarlsberg
Semi-hard cheeses	Ripened by moulds	Roquefort Stilton
	Ripened by bacteria	Edam Gouda
Soft cheeses	Ripened by moulds	Camembert Gorgonzola
	Ripened by bacteria	Limburger Brie
	Unripened	Cottage cheese Fromage frais

Very hard cheeses would traditionally be made using partially skimmed milk, but at least 32% fat must be present to impart flavour to the cheese, whilst soft cheeses would traditionally be made with full-fat milk. However, in recent years, the use of skim milk in the production of soft cheese has resulted in the availability of numerous low-fat varieties.

In cheese manufacture, a starter culture of selected microbes is added to the milk to assist the action of rennet, to expel whey due to acidification of the curd, to inhibit undesirable organisms, and to assist in curing of the cheese. In Cheddar cheese, the predominant organisms in the starter culture are *Streptococcus lactis* and *Lactobacillus casei*. In other cheeses, *S. thermophilus* and *L. bulgari* may be the organisms of choice, imparting a different flavour. Organisms that produce propionic acid as a by-product of fermentation are used to impart a particular flavour and for holes in certain cheeses. Rennin is added, and the caseins in the milk begin to form cross-links and coagulate. As the proteins coagulate, particles of curd are produced, and the acidification within these particles, caused by the starter culture organisms, pushes the whey out so that the curds shrink and become firm. Hard cheeses are traditionally made in large, open tanks, which contain up to 10,000 l of milk. As the curds develop the cheese is scalded, causing a marked contraction of the curd. During scalding, the curd is stirred or 'raked' to prevent it coalescing completely, and to allow the whey to be expelled.

Cheddar cheese is scalded to 40°C, whilst Emmental cheese is scalded to 53–60°C, which alters the microbial population in the cheese and thereby alters the flavour and textural characteristics of the cheese. The scalding process takes around 35 min, after which the whey is drained off through a strainer. The curds are then piled onto the sides of the tank, where they form a uniform mass. This mass of curd is then repeatedly cut and turned to encourage further shrinkage and whey expulsion, a process known as 'cheddaring'.

Once cheddaring is completed, the cheese is milled (cut into small pieces) and salt added at a ratio of 0.10–0.25% of the initial weight of milk used, and the cheese is then pressed into moulds and allowed to stand for 48 h while more whey is released. This 'green' cheese is then allowed to dry for several days before being coated in hot paraffin wax, which prevents any further moisture loss, and kills any surface moulds. The cheese is then cured in a humidity-controlled environment at around 8°C prior to sale. To make softer cheeses, the process involves less cutting and heating, as these steps increase firmness by allowing whey to be expelled, and there is a greater emphasis on acid curdling through the action of the starter culture than on rennet action.

In a hard, rennet cheese, ripening occurs uniformly throughout the curd, so large cheese wheels can be produced, and the cheese has good keeping quality. In soft cheese, where microbial growth and acid fermentation are important, the wheels must be small, as the microbial growth occurs on the surface, and the acid must diffuse into the centre of the cheese. If a soft cheese is over-ripened, abnormal flavours develop, and hence the shelf life of soft cheese is short. If blue-mould cheeses are made, the moulds (*Penicillium roquefortii* or *P. glaucum*) are added during preparation of the curd. It is vital to add *S. lactis* in the starter culture to produce sufficient lactic acid to control putrefactive spoilage organisms. The *P. roquefortii* breaks down the fats and proteins in the milk into simpler compounds, which gives the cheese its characteristic flavour. Salt is added to soft cheeses at 2.5–3.0% to restrict growth of spoilage organisms, and the cheeses are ripened at 95% relative humidity and 10°C for 60 days. Outlines of process controls for hard and soft cheeses are given in Tables 9.5 and 9.6.

Fromage frais is an unripened soft cheese, which may or may not be produced using pasteurized milk. There is a heating stage in the process, but it is insufficient to kill pathogenic organisms, and the ripening phase is insufficiently short to allow acidification of the product to a level where microorganisms will be inhibited. Fromage frais is a short shelf life, potentially high-risk product. An outline of process controls for fromage frais is given in Table 9.7.

Rennet

Rennet, used in cheese manufacture and also in the manufacture of powdered milk puddings and desserts, contains the enzyme rennin, which is the active ingredient, causing the coagulation of casein in milk which results in the formation of an insoluble calcium complex. Natural Rennet is harvested from the stomach lining of unweaned calves at slaughter, as rennin is the main digestive enzyme in the calf stomach. Calf stomachs are harvested at slaughter, dried and finely ground. The resultant material is added to a vat of water and acid, and slowly stirred for a period of 24 hours. The mucin is separated from the ground stomachs and rises to the surface, where it is skimmed off and dried before packaging. Each batch of rennet produced undergoes laboratory analysis for rennin activity, to allow a standardized

Table 9.5. Process control in hard cheese production.

Process step	Hazards	Controls
Standardization of cheese milk	Raw milk may be contaminated with pathogens	Check bacterial quality of raw milk; keep raw milk separate from pasteurized milk
Pasteurization	Failure to destroy pathogens	Record time/temperature and flow rates; test milk – phosphatase test should be negative; clean and disinfect thoroughly between batches
Addition of starter culture	Slow acid development may allow growth of bacteria including pathogens	Obtain starter cultures from a reliable source; check acid development
Addition of rennet	Rennet may be contaminated with pathogens	Obtain rennet from reliable source
Cutting	Contamination from equipment	Clean and disinfect thoroughly between batches
Scalding at 40°C	No incoming hazard, but note that this temperature is not sufficient to destroy pathogens	
Draining whey off; cheddaring at pH 5.2–5.3; milling and salting; pressing; wrapping	Recontamination Note that salt will assist in the suppression of bacterial growth	Check pH to ensure that fermentation is proceeding normally Clean and disinfect thoroughly between batches; monitor environment and product
Ripening	Outgrowth of contaminants	Clean and disinfect thoroughly between batches; monitor environment and product

product to be marketed. Rennet itself has a rather low proteolytic activity, so is commonly combined with, or replaced by, other combinations of enzymes such as papain (harvested from the papaya tree), ficin (from figs), pancreatin or pepsin (other digestive enzymes), and commonly by synthetic enzymes.

Microbiological hazards in cheese and dairy products

Listeria monocytogenes is the organism most commonly associated with food-borne disease from cheeses, particularly from unpasteurized soft and unripened cheeses. *L. monocytogenes* is a soil-borne organism that can multiply at temperatures between 0 and 3°C, and can persist in the environment in dairy plants, acting as a source of recontamination post-pasteurization. The competent authority may set limits on *Listeria* contamination in cheeses; for example, in the UK, each batch of cheese

Table 9.6. Process control in soft, mould-ripened cheese production.

Process step	Hazards	Controls
Standardization of cheese milk	Raw milk may be contaminated with pathogens	Check bacterial quality of raw milk; keep raw milk separate from pasteurized milk
Pasteurization	Failure to destroy pathogens	Record time/temperature and flow rates; test milk – phosphatase test should be negative; clean and disinfect thoroughly between batches
Addition of starter culture	Slow acid development may allow growth of bacteria, including pathogens	Obtain starter cultures from a reliable source; check acid development
Addition of rennet	Rennet may be contaminated with pathogens	Obtain rennet from reliable source
Drain whey off; shape or mould curds; salting or brining	Recontamination; note that salt will assist in the suppression of bacterial growth	Check pH to ensure that fermentation is proceeding normally; clean and disinfect thoroughly between batches; monitor environment and product
Ripening e.g. 10–14 days at 12–15°C, relative humidity 90–95%; storage at 4°C	Outgrowth of contaminants	Clean and disinfect thoroughly between batches; monitor environment and product

Table 9.7. Outline of production process for fromage frais, an unripened soft cheese.

Process stage	Notes
Thermization	Heat to 57–68°C for 15 s; improves keeping quality pending processing; does not destroy pathogens
Separation to obtain skimmed milk	Cream is a by-product
Pasteurization	This step may not occur in some processes
Addition of rennin and starter culture	
Ripening for 16–24 hours at 18–25°C	Produces pH of 4.5–4.6
Heat at 65°C for 4–5 min	Contracts the curd and gives a denser texture; insufficient to destroy pathogens
Centrifugal separation to remove whey	Product should attain 13–20% solids
Addition of sweet cream	Aim is to increase fat content to 40%
Cooling to 2–6°C	
Packaging	This product must be marketed within 2–4 days

other than hard cheese must be tested for *L. monocytogenes* five times, and each of these samples must be negative, whilst other milk-based products need be tested only once. Dairy products must also be tested and found negative for the presence of *Salmonella*, and there are maximum limits set for *Staphylococcus aureus* and *Escherichia coli*. For these two organisms, in the UK, a scale of acceptable, marginal and unacceptable has been set, and five samples are tested, of which at least three must comply with the acceptable standard, and all five must be below the unacceptable level.

Butter

Over a third of milk produced in the developed world is made into butter. The raw material for butter production is fresh cream, separated from milk using centrifugation. Cream may be pasteurized prior to butter-making, but even so, it must be used fresh. Holding cream for any length of time, even under refrigeration, can allow microbial growth of organisms present in raw cream, or re-contaminants in pasteurized cream. Also, heat-stable proteolytic or lipolytic enzymes that occur in cream and survive pasteurization can quickly give rise to off-flavours in the cream. The quality of the cream is very important in butter-making: poorly handled cream quickly develops lactic acid as a result of microbial fermentation, which, if not excessive, may be neutralized using calcium hydroxide. The cream will be assessed for acidity, flavour, odour and the presence of foreign particles. Cream and butter are very susceptible to taint, and strong odours in the milking parlour and bulk tank room on a farm can render cream and butter inedible, as can the presence of certain weeds in the forage consumed by cattle.

Salt is added to the cream at around 10–13% to improve keeping quality. This level of salt inhibits microbial growth, particularly of yeasts and moulds, and also inhibits proteolytic and lipolytic organisms and enzymes. A starter culture comprising *Streptococcus lactis* (to aid preservation), *S. citrovorus* and/or *S. paracitrovorus* (to promote flavour) may be added, in which case the cream must be allowed to ripen for 3–4 h at 3°C to allow the acidity to build up to a level of 0.3–0.4% lactic acid prior to churning. Churning inverts the emulsion of the cream from an oil-in-water emulsion to a water-in-oil emulsion, the butterfat particles coalesce to form butter grains and the buttermilk is drained off. The butter grains are washed in potable water, then further salt may be added before the grains are pressed into butter moulds. If spreadable butter is desired, vegetable oils are added to the butter grains, and this mixture whipped to the desired consistency for packaging and sale.

Butter, on average, comprises 82% fat, 14% water, 1% curd and 3% salt, and its low moisture content would be expected to inhibit microbial growth. However, its structure, being a water-in-oil emulsion, means that there is sufficient moisture and soluble nutrients distributed evenly throughout the product for microbial growth to occur between the fat globules. An outline of process control for butter is given in Table 9.8.

Table 9.8. Outline of production process for butter.

Process stage	Notes
Mixing of cream with salt and colourants	Cream quality is very important; addition of 10–13% salt improves the keeping quality; a starter culture may be used to promote certain flavours – if so, the cream must ripen for 3–4 h at 3°C to acidify
Churning	Fat droplets in the cream coalesce, and butter grains break away from the liquid
Washing of butter grains	Use potable water
Pressing and moulding to form hard butter, or addition of vegetable oils and whipping to produce spreadable butter	More salt may be added

Yoghurt

Yoghurt (also spelled yogurt or yoghourt) is fermented milk, and contains over 1,000,000 cells/ml of both *Streptococcus thermophilus* and *Lactobacillus delbrueckii* subsp. *bulgaris*. Both these organisms are natural inhabitants of milk and it is their interaction during growth that gives yoghurt its unique organoleptic properties. Other organisms may be added during the production of yoghurt, particularly those that may be probiotic in nature, for example *Bifidobacterium* spp. and other *Lactobacilli*.

The first step in the process of yoghurt making is to increase the solids non-fat content of the milk, by condensing or fortifying the raw milk. Traditionally this would have been achieved by heating the milk slowly on an open pan and allowing water to evaporate, but in modern yoghurt processing the milk is fortified by the addition of skim milk powder, whey or buttermilk powder, or condensed by evaporation of water under vacuum or removal of water by membrane filtration (ultrafiltration or reverse osmosis). In membrane filtration the membrane is a molecular sieve, through which milk is forced under pressure. Cells and large particles cannot pass through the membrane, so these are retained and water passes through the membrane and is drawn off. The condensed or fortified milk is next homogenized and heat treated at 90–95°C with a 2–5 min holding period. This treatment is greater than the treatment used for pasteurization of raw milk due to the increased solids content of the condensed or fortified milk. As well as effecting pasteurization, these temperatures promote the desired texture of yoghurt by linking β-lactoglobulin to caseins within the milk, break down the whey proteins into simpler compounds that will assist in fermentation later in the process, and also remove oxygen from the milk, which is desirable as the starter cultures used contain organisms that are micro-aerophilic. After heat treatment, the starter culture is added and fermentation begins.

When a set yoghurt product is being produced, the mix is packaged at this stage, and the fermentation occurs in the pot, but for stirred yoghurts, the fermentation of the 'base' occurs in a large vat. Fermentation is allowed to proceed until the pH reaches 4.2–4.3, at a concentration of 1.2–1.4 g/100 ml of lactic acid. This will take around 12–16 h, but fermentation in bio-yoghurts is stopped after 4–5 h by chilling, at around 1.0 g/100 ml lactic acid, and the product is marketed. Fermentation is allowed to continue in mesophilic yoghurts for a further 7 to 10 h, as acid production plateaus over time. The development of the acidity is carefully monitored, either manually by titration of samples, or more commonly by measuring the electrical conductivity of the base, which increases as pH falls (Fig. 9.3).

Once acidity exceeds 1.0 g/100 ml lactic acid, the caseins in the base coagulate, and the yoghurt sets. Over-acidification gives the yoghurt a sour taste, and the protein gel shrinks, expelling whey. This is often noticed in set yoghurts after purchase, as the fermentation will continue within the pot, and a domestic refrigerator often does not achieve temperatures required to inhibit fermentation, so whey is seen to develop on the surface of the yoghurt. In stirred yoghurt products, the base is agitated from pH 4.6 to break down the gel and give the desired texture. Slight over-

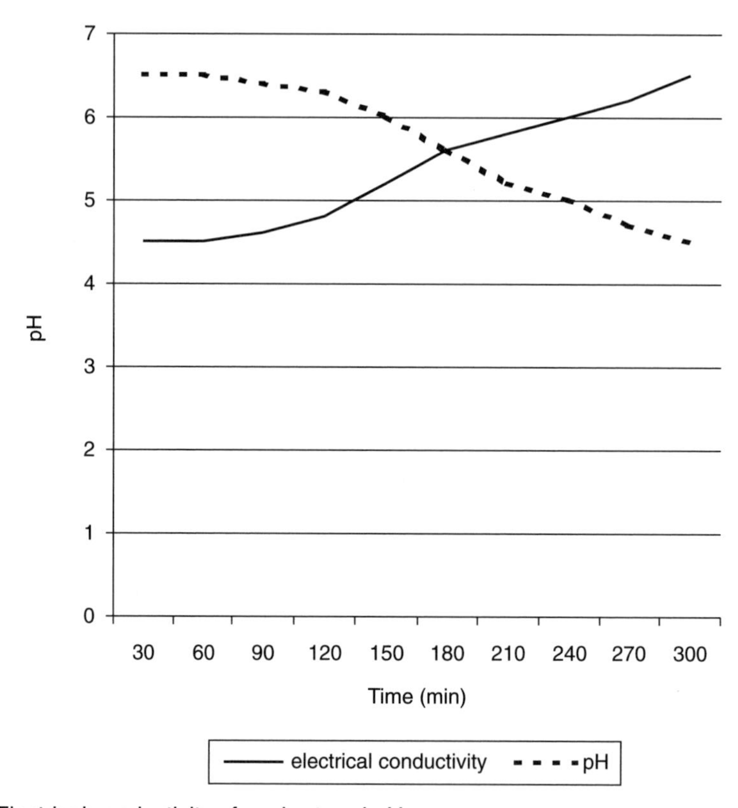

Fig. 9.3. Electrical conductivity of yoghurt and pH.

acidification of stirred yoghurts is not the major problem that it is in set yoghurt, as added flavourings and fruit will mask the sourness.

When fermentation is complete, the stirred base is cooled to 15–25°C (the temperature rises during fermentation) and fruits and flavourings added before the product is packaged. All ingredients added after pasteurization carry the risk of introducing pathogenic or spoilage organisms to the product, and yoghurts destined for consumption by infants and young children will be re-pasteurized as a final control on the microbiological status of the product, but there is a risk if caramelization of sugars in the yoghurt, and the development of off-flavours. Fruited yoghurts cannot be re-pasteurized for this reason and, therefore, yoghurts labelled as 'Children's' will not contain fruit pieces.

An outline of process control for yoghurt is given in Table 9.9.

Table 9.9. Process control in yoghurt production.

Process step	Hazards	Controls
Raw milk intake	Raw milk may be contaminated with pathogens or foreign material	Check bacterial quality of raw milk; pre-pasteurization filter (1 mm); keep raw milk separate from pasteurized milk
Pasteurization	Failure to destroy pathogens	Record time/temperature and flow rates; test milk – phosphatase test should be negative; clean and disinfect thoroughly between batches; many processing plants have automatic divert systems to return incompletely pasteurized milk to the silo
Addition of starter culture and fermentation	Slow acid development may allow growth of bacteria, including pathogens	Obtain starter cultures from a reliable source; check acid development
Filtration of base	Presence of foreign material in the white base	Filter (0.1 mm); check integrity of mesh filter
Addition of fruits	Presence of pathogens within the fruit; pathogens present on outer surface of fruit package	Obtain fruit from a reliable source; dip fruit packages in 336 ppm chlorine for 2 minutes prior to opening
Packaging	Recontamination from cartons	Store cartons hygienically
Storage	Outgrowth of contaminants	Cool to below 5°C

Further Reading

Roginski, H.J., Fuguay, J.W. and Fox, P.F. (2003) *Encyclopedia of Dairy Sciences*. Academic Press, Amsterdam

9.2 Hygiene of Eggs and Egg Products

Introduction

Poultry and eggs, together, are the most prevalent source of food-borne human infections in the UK, as well as in many other developed countries. *Salmonella* is one of the most important causes of gastrointestinal diseases in humans, and eggs are a major source of food-borne salmonellosis. The problem of *Salmonella* in poultry and eggs is largely associated with primary production (on-farm), so veterinarians are significantly involved in, and hold many of the responsibilities for, related control measures. A typical egg production chain is shown in Fig. 9.4. Different flock types are normally held in geographically separate locations.

Salmonella can contaminate the eggs internally, which is probably the most common route of egg contamination. However, external contamination of eggs with *Salmonella* also occurs, although more rarely. Egg structure is shown in Fig. 9.5.

Internal infection/contamination

Salmonella enteritidis, and to a lesser extent, *S. typhimurium*, are currently the most important serotypes causing food-borne human salmonellosis via eggs or poultry. *S. enteritidis* is the main *Salmonella* serotype infecting tissues and persisting in birds. *Salmonella* serotypes can have differing, serotype-specific characteristics, but *S. enteritidis* and *S. typhimurium* both have invasive potential since they carry genes necessary for the invasion of host cells and proliferation in host tissues. Infection of poultry and eggs is a consequence of this host cell invasion ability.

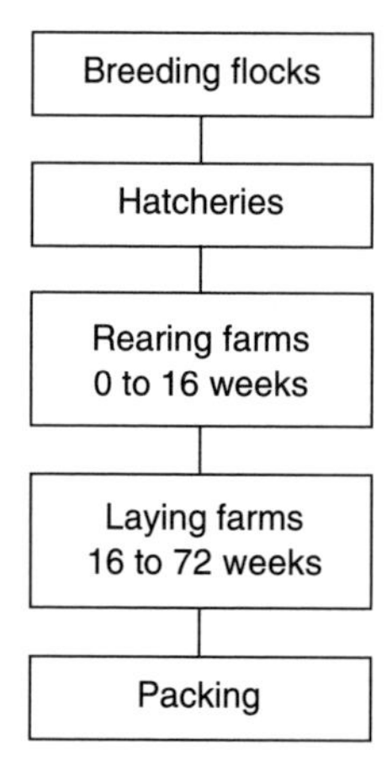

Fig. 9.4. Egg production chain.

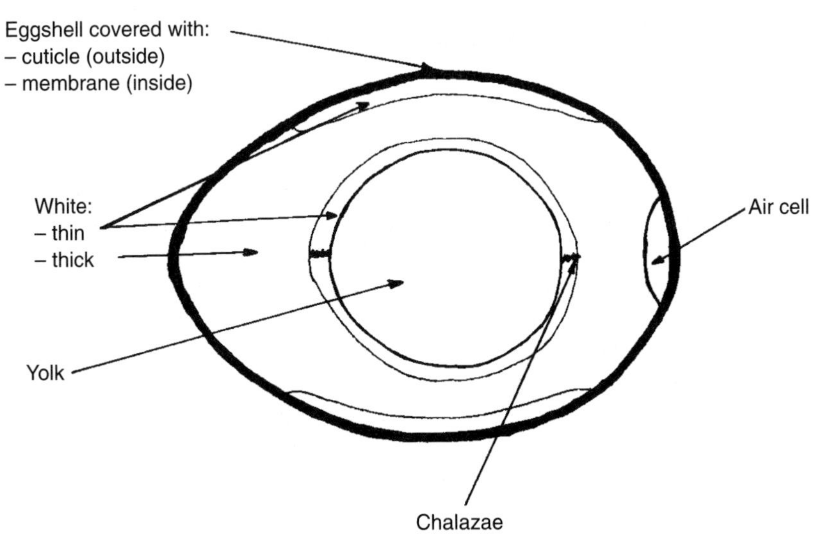

Fig. 9.5. Egg structure.

The *Salmonella* in an infected egg primarily originate from an infected layer bird. Birds become infected with *Salmonella* by two routes: orally or via the air. Most laboratory-based challenge studies on contamination routes have used the oral route of infection and inoculation doses in excess of 10^7 CFU/g. Even with such high inoculation levels, the oral route of infection results in a very low percentage of birds, and their eggs, being infected with *Salmonella*. On the other hand, *Salmonella* survive well in air; exposure to the airborne route of infection results in more *Salmonella*-positive birds and eggs, compared to the oral route (see Table 9.10). Therefore, *Salmonella* control in poultry feeds is unlikely to successfully control *Salmonella* infection of flocks, since airborne contamination is a more likely route of infection.

Salmonella can infect the developing egg while it is contained in the oviduct, and can later be found in the albumen or in the yolk. *Salmonella* in the developing egg originate from the bird's genital organs (Fig. 9.6). Surprisingly, no correlation between the presence of *Salmonella* in eggs produced by a bird and *Salmonella* in that bird's faeces has been reported. In the developing egg, the yolk is formed first, then albumen is deposited on the surface of the yolk, followed by the hard shell formation.

The cellular and molecular mechanisms leading to infection, and the serovar-specific differences between differing *Salmonella* isolates, are not fully understood. There are indications that infection of birds may be stress-related, since clustering of positive eggs occurs. Stress changes the chemistry and mucosal properties of the oviduct, and stress hormones act as iron-scavengers. Obtaining iron from the relatively iron-poor tissues of infected hosts is a challenge for all intracellular pathogens, including *Salmonella*.

Table 9.10. Infection routes with *Salmonella typhimurium* DT104.

Infection route and dose	Percentage of tissues		
	Egg contents	Muscle[a]	Blood[a]
Oral 10^8	1	0	0
Airborne 10^3	25	27	6
Airborne 10^2	14	27	0

[a] Birds examined 2 weeks post-infection.

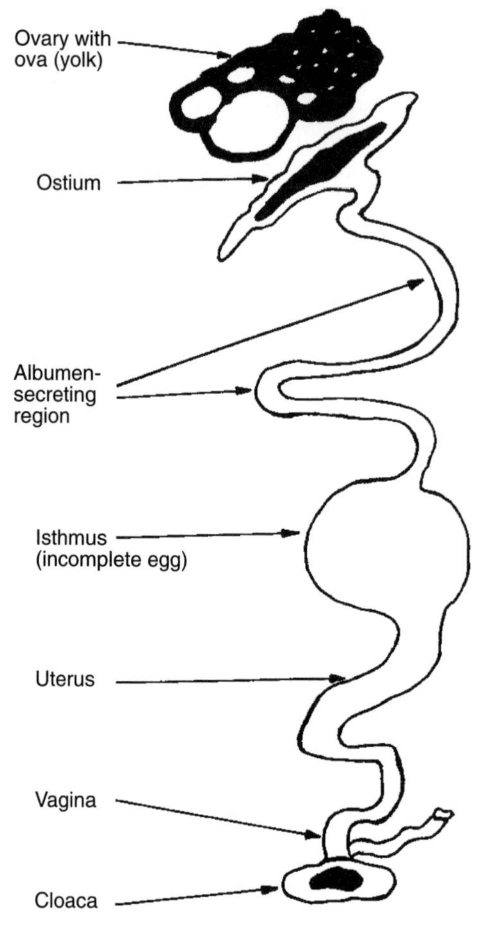

Fig. 9.6. Avian genital organs.

Salmonella located in egg albumen cannot proliferate, and should be killed over time by inherent antibacterial properties in the albumen; the resultant low numbers of the pathogen are unlikely to cause human disease. If the pathogen is deposited in albumen, its active movement towards the yolk becomes a critical factor. *Salmonella* attach to the yolk membrane using fimbriae. The yolk membrane starts to break down if the egg is subjected to long storage, particularly at high (>20°C) or fluctuating temperatures. This enables the pathogen to pass through the membrane more easily. Once it has passed through the membrane, *Salmonella* proliferates rapidly in the nutritious yolk, particularly if the egg is stored at higher temperatures. The egg contamination becomes visually detectable only when *Salmonella* reaches large numbers (>10^7 CFU/egg), but normally the numbers stay below this value, so *Salmonella* in eggs cannot usually be detected by consumers.

Surface infection/contamination

Eggs can also become contaminated with *Salmonella* externally on the shells, but this is less common than internal contamination of eggs. With external contamination, *Salmonella* in the faeces from the cloaca contaminate the surface of the egg while it is being laid. Eggshells can also become contaminated outside, from dirty, contaminated nests, and can also be cross-contaminated from other surface-contaminated eggs.

Egg content has high levels of available water, proteins and other nutrients, and so would be expected to support microbial growth. In spite of that, it is known that eggs can be stored for substantial times at ambient temperatures – without spoilage. This is due to innate protective antimicrobial systems existing in fresh eggs.

The external physical barrier of the eggshell provides the first level of protection. Eggshell is calcium carbonate with an organic matrix, containing around 12,000 gas exchange pores, and is covered by a proteinaceous cuticle. Egg contamination is most likely if the cuticle becomes wet or physically damaged, because bacteria adhere to the protein more readily when it is wet, but also because wetting or damage opens some pores – enabling microorganisms to penetrate. If eggs are stored dry, then microorganisms cannot penetrate the shell via the pores.

A second level of protection, comprising multiple factors, exists within eggs. First, two inner shell membranes impede microbial penetration of the eggs. Secondly, the albumen pH rises to ~ 9 during the first 24 h after laying (Fig. 9.7), which is relatively alkaline for microbial pathogens. Also, lysozyme present in the albumen has potent antibacterial activity. Iron-sequestering mechanisms ensure that the albumen is a low-iron environment, limiting pathogenic growth and survival. Finally, the viscous nature of albumen hinders bacterial movement.

Preservation/processing of eggs

Eggshell treatments

Egg washing can damage or destroy the protective protein cuticle. Although egg washing is practised in some countries, in the EU it is not

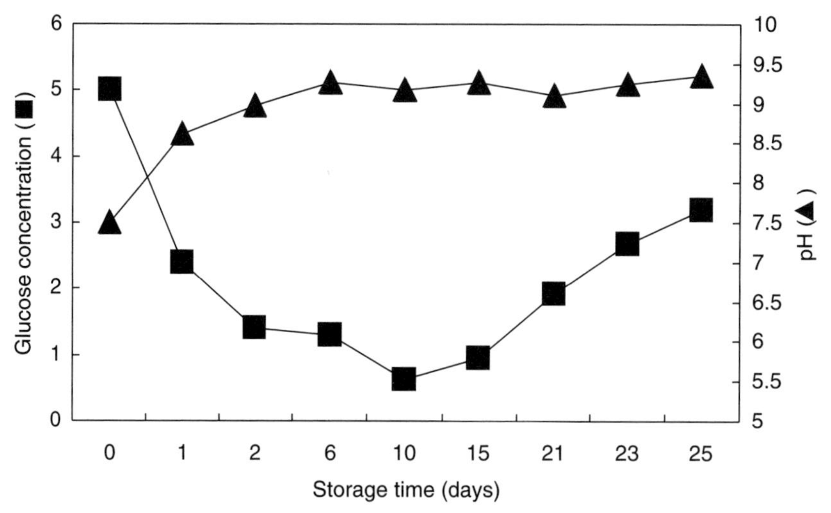

Fig. 9.7. Changes in egg chemistry during storage (Cogan, 2002).

allowed for Class A (retail; table) eggs. However, eggs intended for further processing, or for immediate use, may be subjected to washing. The temperature is critical during the washing procedure. The eggs and the wash water must be at similar temperatures (usually 10–14°C). If the eggs are warmer than the wash water, any surface contamination on the shell, together with bacteria, is effectively sucked through the pores and into the egg content. Post-washing, eggs must be dried quickly, since wet shells increase the spoilage rate. If the water contains iron, it can neutralize the antimicrobial effects of conalbumen (a proteinaceous compound with affinity to iron). Eggs for washing, as well as the wash water itself, must be of high microbiological quality. Shell coating has been proposed as a method of decreasing the movement of bacteria through the shells; this can be effective but is expensive and, therefore, is normally conducted only under exceptional circumstances.

Liquid egg

During processing of eggs into liquid form, they are washed (optional), broken, separated, and then homogenized. Every egg passes the same egg-breaking machine, so there is potential for cross-contamination, and the hygiene of this equipment is critical for production of safe, pasteurized liquid egg. The initial microflora of liquid eggs are derived from the shell, contaminated egg content (rare), processing equipment and handlers. In the UK, pasteurization of liquid egg was introduced in 1963; the current time/temperature regime for whole egg (mixture of albumen and yolk) is 64.4°C for 4 min. Pasteurization of liquid egg has reduced human food-borne disease significantly in the past. After pasteurization, the product is chilled, salted and can be frozen or irradiated to ensure microbiological risks remain low during storage.

Dried eggs

The first step during production of dried eggs is similar to that of dried milk production; glucose is removed to prevent discolouration due to the Maillard reaction. Drying technologies include spray-drying, heated surface-drying and freeze-drying. Post-drying, hot storage is used to inactivate any remaining bacteria. However, the process is not bactericidal. Nevertheless, bacteria are unable to grow in the low a_w of dried egg. Bacteria, including *Salmonella*, can remain viable, but dormant, until dry eggs are reconstituted. Typically, the presence of *Salmonella* in dried eggs is problematic in catering, where large volumes of dried eggs are reconstituted and can be stored at room temperature, allowing the pathogen to proliferate.

Further processed egg products

Many processed foods contain eggs as an ingredient. Some products are uncooked, whilst others contain uncooked egg, including some pies, egg-nog, dry diet mixes, etc. These products represent a higher risk category for *Salmonella*. Cooked products, including custard, cream cakes, etc. are a lower risk category, since proper cooking should eliminate the pathogen. Acid foods, including salad dressing and mayonnaise, can contain raw egg, and may be a public health risk if they are prepared with eggs containing *Salmonella*.

Spoilage of shell eggs

There are a large number of bacterial species present on the egg surface, although geographical- and bird-related variations occur. Nevertheless, relatively few bacterial species are involved in egg spoilage, including *Pseudomonas*, *Alcaligenes*, *Escherichia* and *Proteus*.

Main vehicles of egg-borne infection

Products containing raw egg, such as tiramisu, ice cream, egg-nog and mayonnaise, carry the highest risk for *Salmonella* infections. The presence of raw egg may be declared on labels, and usually these products mostly have additional innate control mechanisms (low storage temperature, acidity, etc.), which help prevent *Salmonella* growth. However, these types of product can cause human disease if they are prepared with eggs containing high numbers of *Salmonella*, or if these additional controls fail. Some processed foods can contain undercooked egg, including Scotch eggs, meringue, egg sandwiches and soft boiled or fried eggs; these are lower-risk foods, but have caused human infection when sufficient numbers of *Salmonella* have survived the sub-lethal heat treatments.

Global control measures for *Salmonella* in eggs

Controls of *Salmonella* infections in poultry are covered by legislation related to poultry feed, flock testing and registration. In some countries, including the UK, the first level of control is to slaughter flocks if they become *Salmonella*-positive. However, slaughter of positive flocks is not undertaken in all countries; instead, flocks may be treated with antibiotics or antimicrobials. *Salmonella* controls are prescribed by the EU zoonoses directive, requiring regular testing of breeding flocks. In the UK, eggs from the so-called 'Lion Code' are retail-labelled, fully traceable, and originate from registered *Salmonella*-free flocks where vaccination is used as a preventative measure. The code stipulates general hygiene measures, time/temperature requirements for storage, and the packages/eggs are stamped with a 'best before' date. Regular independent audits of the 'Lion Code' participants are conducted, with penalties for non-compliance.

In the UK, the government's advice to consumers on egg safety states:

- do not eat raw eggs;
- susceptible individuals should eat only well-cooked eggs;
- consume within 3 weeks of laying;
- refrigerate to ≤7°C after purchase to limit growth of any contaminating *Salmonella*; and
- wash hands after handling shell eggs to limit cross-contamination of *Salmonella* to other foods.

Further Reading

Cogan, T.A. (2002) Factors affecting the growth of *Salmonella* Enteritidis in eggs. PhD thesis, University of Exeter, Exeter, UK.

ICMSF (1980) *Microbial Ecology of Foods: Vol. II: Food Commodities*. Academic Press, New York.

Lund, B., Baird-Parker, J. and Gould, G. (2000) *The Microbiological Safety and Quality of Food*. Aspen Publishers, London.

9.3. Hygiene of Fish

Introduction

Seafood is a generic term, which includes all edible animals originating from seas, including invertebrates. The term 'fish' refers to free-swimming fin fish, members of the genera *Pisces* and *Elasmobranchii*. The Crustaceae include lobsters, crabs, shrimps and prawns; they have chitinous exoskeletons. Molluscs include clams, scallops and oysters, and are shellfish animals of a sessile nature. Cephalopods include octopus, squid and cuttlefish. Other invertebrates from the sea are eaten, including sea cucumber. Both fish and invertebrates that originate from fresh water are also eaten (e.g. trout, carp, lobsters, prawns).

Fish and seafood contain low levels of lipids, but are regarded as a good source of protein (Table 9.11). Fish lipids are highly unsaturated and contain high levels of phospholipids; together, these are regarded as beneficial in modern diets. Fish contain negligible quantities of carbohydrates, with the exception of molluscs, which contain 3% glycogen. The mineral content of fish is low, although normally comprises a comprehensive range; this can depend on the water in which the fish live. Fish muscle contains little connective tissue and high levels of water (Table 9.11). These conditions facilitate bacterial growth and movement within fish flesh, leading to rapid microbiological deterioration of the tissue and short shelf life compared with other muscle meats. The initial microflora of fish are largely derived from the microflora of the water in which it lived, so the shelf life is not usually very predictable.

The recommended storage temperature for fish and seafood is lower than for red meat, since fish spoils more readily. Consequently, fish are regularly stored on melting ice (~0°C), and four typical spoilage stages are recognized (Table 9.12). Trimethylamine (TMA) is a major component associated with the unacceptable odour of fish spoilage, and starts to increase in the tissues after 5–10 days. Degradation of proteins produces total volatile acids (TVA) and total volatile bases (TVB; ammonia), which are components used for the chemical detection of fish spoilage. Sensory organoleptic evaluation of fish flesh is the standard technique for assessment of fitness for human consumption. However, standard chemical analyses can also be used to determine levels of TVA and TVB in fish.

Table 9.11. General composition (%) of fish and seafood types.

Fish or seafood type	Water	Protein	Lipids
Fish[a]	69–82	16–20	0.5–10
Crustaceans	75	18	2
Molluscs	80	13	1.5

[a]Species-dependent variations.

Table 9.12. Spoilage of fresh fish stored on melting ice.

Spoilage stage	Days required to complete stage	Physicochemical and microbiological properties
1	0–5	Flesh undergoes rigor mortis; ATP is converted to inosine; the dominant bacterial types change
2	5–10	Inosine is converted to hypoxantine; level of NH_3 increases; Trimethylamineoxide (TMAO) is converted to trimethylamine (TMA); bacterial growth occurs
3	10–14	Hypoxantine is converted to xantine and uric acid; TMA, total volatile bases (TVB) and total volatile acids (TVA) increase; rapid bacterial growth occurs
4	>14	Proteolysis; TVA and TVB levels increase rapidly; H_2S is produced; physical deterioration of flesh occurs

Organoleptic assessment of raw fish freshness

Immediately after catching, fish eyes are convex, with a crystal-clear cornea. The gills are bright red or pink and covered with clear mucus. The skin has well-differentiated colours and is glossy with transparent slime. The odour is described as sharp, sea-like/iodine-like or metallic.

During the medium stage of spoilage (e.g. between stages 3 and 4 as indicated in Table 9.12), fish eyes become flat or slightly sunken, and there is some loss of corneal clarity. The gills undergo slight loss of red colour and brightness, while the skin fades slightly and the slime turns slightly milky. Odour becomes slightly ‘fishy’, shellfish-like, musty, garlicy, lactic acid-like or like cut grass.

With increasing spoilage, the eyes become sunken and cloudy with a discoloured cornea. Gills are bleached and/or discoloured, and coated with thick slime. The skin loses colour and becomes coated with yellow, knotted slime. The odour of spoilt fish is described as like stale cabbage-water, sour drains, wet matches or ammoniacal. The odour of TMA dominates.

It can be difficult to distinguish the different stages of fish spoilage, particularly between medium-spoiled fish and spoiled fish, as individual assessors have differing perceptions of spoilage at these stages.

Average storage life

The two main methods for storage of fish are melting ice and freezing. The recommended storage temperature for frozen fish is −18°C. This low temperature delays the oxidation of unsaturated fatty acids and the onset of rancidity. Storage life may relate to the longest storage time possible, but can also refer to the maximum storage time enabling production of high-quality food. Average storage times are shown for differing fish types in Table 9.13. Naturally, these average storage times are largely dependent on the water quality and microflora from the waters from which the fish were harvested.

Table 9.13. Maximum average storage times allowing production of packed fish of differing qualities.

	Days of storage if kept on melting ice		Months of storage if frozen at −18°C	
	High quality	Edible	High quality	Edible
White-fleshed fish (cod, etc.)	3	15	4	6
Dark-fleshed fish (tuna, etc.)	5	21	3	4
Shellfish	2	6	3	4

Public health hazards associated with fish

There are fewer public health issues and zoonotic diseases associated with fish than with farm animals. Fish are inherently more distant in evolutionary terms from humans than farm animals, so have comparably fewer organisms and parasites in common with humans. In addition, the indigenous microorganisms present in many fish originate from low-temperature salt waters, so are not adapted to infecting mammals at 37°C. However, pathogenic microorganisms, histamine (scombroid) intoxication, parasites, algal toxins and some natural toxins do cause public health problems for consumers.

The flesh and organs of freshly caught, healthy fish are sterile, although bacteria occur on the skin, gills and in the intestines. Fish from clean, cold ocean waters generally harbour fewer bacteria than do fish from warm, inshore waters, since the fish microflora reflect the water microflora. Fish caught in inshore waters, which may be subject to waste, agricultural and industrial pollutants, pose the highest public health risks. Molluscs pose particularly high public health risks, due to their filtration-feeding mechanism.

The main contributing factors to fish-borne infections are faecal contamination of the harvest water and consumption of raw or undercooked fish. Raw fish is commonly consumed and is a cultural delicacy in many countries, including Japan and other Pacific Rim countries, the Netherlands, Pacific island nations and certain northern latitude countries.

The most common aetiologic agents of fish-borne human disease in the USA are shown in Table 9.14. The two most common bacteria are *Vibrio* species, which are not a public health risk from farm animals. Those bacterial species which are a public health risk from farm animals (*Clostridium*, *Salmonella*) cause significantly less fish-borne disease than do *Vibrio*.

Processed fish

Processing can also add to the total bacterial load on fish. Fish processing is normally a lengthy process, and involves substantial handling of the product. Some critical points during production of smoked salmon include:

Table 9.14. Cases of fish-borne diseases in the USA annually (1994).

Aetiological agent	Percentage of fish-borne diseases in food-borne disease
Gram-negative bacteria	
Vibrio vulnificus	24
Other *Vibrio* spp. (e.g. *parahaemolyticus*)	43
Shigella	7
Salmonella	2
Campylobacter	2
Gram-positive bacteria	
Clostridium perfringens	7
Cl. botulinum	4
Other microbial agents	
Viruses	Not known

- transport (2–18 h) of slaughtered fish to processing factory;
- evisceration (machine);
- filleting (machine or hand);
- salting (by hand, injection, or brined);
- rinsing;
- pellicle removal (machine);
- trimming/slicing (hand); and
- vacuum packaging.

Cold-smoked salmon has been the vehicle of infection for outbreaks and cases of listeriosis. *Listeria monocytogenes* occur commonly in cold-smoked salmon, since the organism is ubiquitous, can be present in the harvest waters and can inhabit the processing plant. In addition, it survives the processing steps well, since it is relatively salt tolerant. Some types of *Clostridium botulinum* associated with waters and fish can potentially grow in vacuum-packaged products, even if stored at low temperature (~3°C). Although subsequent cooking will destroy the organism and the toxin, consumption of raw vacuum-packaged products can be a risk.

Histamine (scombroid) poisoning

Histamine is a biogenic amine with great heat-stability; it is not destroyed by even the high temperatures achieved in canning. Some fish (e.g. mackerel, tuna, sardines) contain high levels of the amino acid histidine. A number of non-pathogenic, spoilage bacteria convert histidine into histamine using the enzyme histidine decarboxylase. Healthy humans normally produce diamino oxidase (DAO), which degrades ingested histamine. However, people with a deficiency in the production of DAO, or who have been treated by DAO-inhibitors – including anti-tuberculosis drugs and anti-depressants, may develop histamine intoxication. The symptoms are allergy-like and include rash, oedema and hypotension. Several outbreaks have occurred in mental hospitals and nursing homes. The main control for histamine intoxication is to prevent its formation in fish flesh immediately after catching, by limiting microbial growth using low-temperature refrigeration or freezing.

Zoonotic parasites

Anisakis simplex

The natural hosts for *Anisakis simplex* (Fig. 9.8) are sea mammals (whales, dolphins, seals, etc.). *Anisakis* eggs are excreted into seawater, and are subsequently ingested by other sea animals, including fish. In fish, the larvae normally occur in the gastrointestinal tract. However, once fish are caught, the larvae migrate into fish muscle and remain viable in the tissue. Therefore, the main control is immediate freezing after catching. Proper cooking will also kill this parasite. The symptoms are relatively mild in humans.

Diphyllobothrium latum

This parasite (Fig. 9.9) is associated with freshwater fish, which are commonly eaten in Europe. The symptoms in humans are similar to those that occur from *Taenia* infestation. The main controls for this parasite are freezing or cooking.

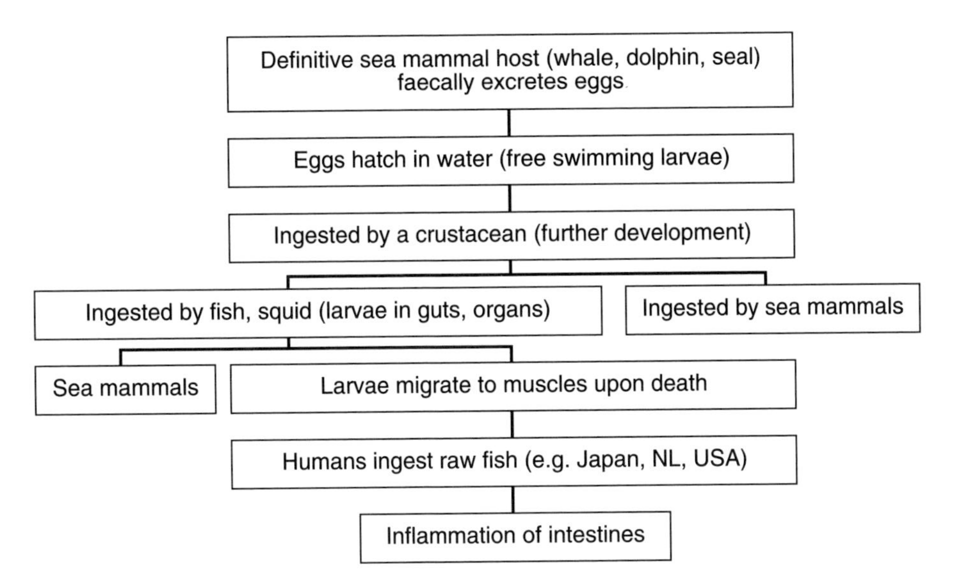

Fig. 9.8. Life cycle of *Anisakis simplex*.

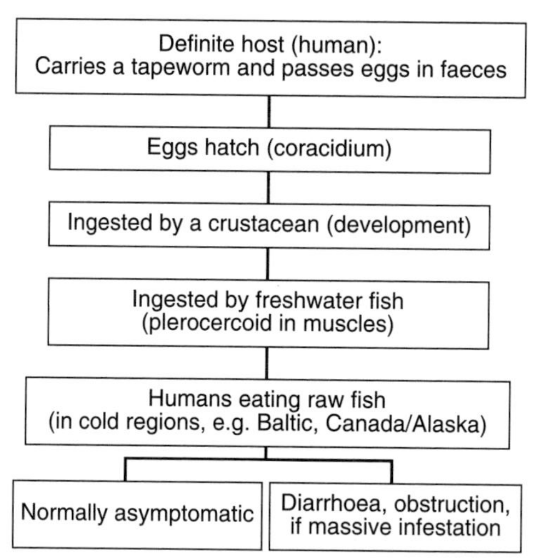

Fig. 9.9. Life cycle of *Diphyllobothrium latum.*

Algal toxins from shellfish

Algal toxins can cause paralytic shellfish poisoning (PSP) and other intoxications in humans (Fig. 9.10). Shellfish are filter-feeders, and consequently they concentrate algal toxins within their liver. Shellfish are normally eaten whole, so the livers, together with toxins, are subsequently consumed. The problem of algal blooming is increasing world-wide, due to factors including increased run-off from farms and carriage of phosphate-based fertilizers into coastal waters, thus enabling algal growth. Therefore, waters must be monitored regularly for pollution and for the presence and type of algae, since climactic conditions, farming and environmental practices affect the quality of coastal waters. Bans on shellfish harvesting must be enforced in affected areas. Cooking does not destroy algal toxins, which are heat-stable.

Summary of preventative measures to control fish-borne diseases

- Monitor and control the hygienic status (pollution, bacterial pathogens, toxic algae) of coastal waters.
- Prevent/reduce microbial growth and activity in/on fish after catching and during processing (heat-stable histamine) by good hygienic practice, refrigeration and freezing.
- Prevent post-cooking cross-contamination.
- Implement HACCP-based hygiene system in fish/seafood production chain to control *L. monocytogenes* and *Cl. Botulinum*.
- Avoid eating unfrozen and uncooked fish, which can contain pathogens or parasites.

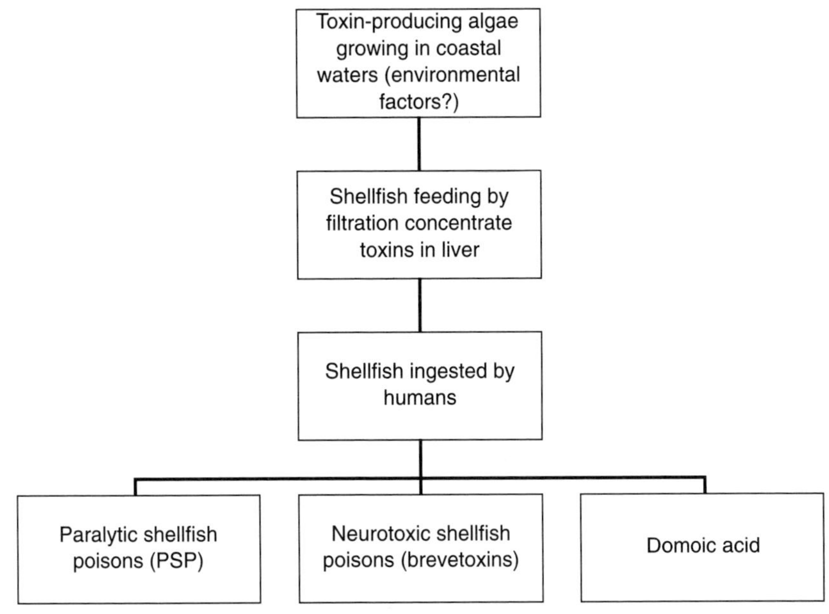

Fig. 9.10. Toxic algal poisoning via shellfish.

Further Reading

Huss, H.H. (1997) Control of indigenous pathogenic bacteria in seafood. *Food Control* 8, 91–98.

ICMSF (1980) *Microbial Ecology of Foods: Vol. II: Food Commodities*. Academic Press, New York.

Lund, B., Baird-Parker, J. and Gould, G. (2000) *The Microbiological Safety and Quality of Food*. Aspen Publishers, London.

9.4 Hygiene of Honey

The main components of honey are simple sugars (Table 9.15). Since the water activity is very low, and the product is relatively acidic, growth of microorganisms in honey is inhibited.

Initial Microflora of Honey

Microbial levels in honey are very low – usually up to 10^2 CFU/g, but exceptionally counts can be up to 10^4 CFU/g. Potential sources of microflora in honey include flower nectar (sterile) and pollen (non-sterile), but the primary source of microorganisms in honey is the gastrointestinal tract of the bee. Secondary contamination occurs via the processing environment and originates from humans, equipment, dust and insects.

The predominant bacteria in honey are *Bacillus* spp., some of which can be detected in bee larvae, and can cause 'foul brood' disease. *Cl. botulinum* spores may be present in honey, although they cannot germinate. Moulds and yeasts are relatively acid-resistant, so they can be present in higher numbers than can bacteria. Moulds (*Aspergillus*, *Penicillium*) can be harboured in bee intestines and in hives. The predominant yeasts are *Saccharomyces*. Osmophilic yeasts, such as *Zygosaccharomyces* in honey, originate from flowers, soil and equipment. These organisms can grow in honey, and numbers may reach 10^6 CFU/g.

Honey Processing

Basic steps in honey processing are the following:

1. Frames are stored at 32–35°C for 1 day.
2. Combs are uncapped either manually or mechanically.
3. Honey is extracted using centrifugation.

Table 9.15. Average composition and pH of honey.

Attribute	Percentage (w/w)
Sugars	80
Fructose	37
Glucose	30
Sucrose, maltose	13
Organic acids, minerals, proteins, enzymes	Substantial amounts
Water	17
Water activity	0.5–0.6
pH	3.9

4. Honey is recovered into sump tanks, which are heated to 46°C to overcome cooling and improve settling.
5. Warm honey is strained through cloths or screens.
6. Liquefied in hot air at 60–70°C.
7. Product is bulk-stored in a dry environment; air humidity of 60% is suitable for honey containing 17–18% moisture.
8. Packing.

Public Health Hazards in Honey and Their Control

Chemical agents can occur in honey, including antibiotics and antiparasitics. Honey production is less regulated with respect to these agents than are many other agricultural industries. Agricultural use of pesticides and industrial pollutants – such as heavy metals – can result in contamination of honey in hives with these agents.

Cl. botulinum is the main public health concern in honey. If honey containing spores is fed to infants, the spores can germinate in the intestine and produce toxin. The resulting toxicoinfection, infant botulism, can be a serious condition requiring hospitalization. Therefore, honey should not be fed to infants less than 12 months of age. Also, some pathogenic types of Enterobacteriaceae may occur in honey, but these are at low levels and do not normally present a public health risk.

The primary safety factor in honey is the hygroscopic environment with very low water activity: ≤ 0.65. Heating honey to <100°C reduces the already low microbial content. However, the extent of heating is limited by the formation of hydroxymethylfurfuraldehyde (HMF), which causes undesirable colour changes in the product. Sterilization of honey at >100°C significantly reduces or eliminates microbial populations, but is only used if honey is diluted.

Further Reading

Crane, E. (1979) *Honey, a Comprehensive Survey*. Heinemann, London.
Lund, B., Baird-Parker, J. and Gould, G. (2000) *The Microbiological Safety and Quality of Food*. Aspen Publishers, London.

10 Food Hygiene and Safety at the Retail–Consumer Phase

10.1 Food Hygiene at Retail–Consumer Level

Carol-Ann Wilkin (née Reid)

After processing, foods may have numerous stages to go through before reaching the consumer, with the possibility of the food becoming contaminated at any of these stages, e.g. packaging, storage, transport, retail display, and cooking within restaurants and cafes.

Food producers, retailers and caterers have a responsibility to supply safe food of good quality to the consumer. However, it is also the responsibility of the consumers themselves to ensure that foods continue to be handled, prepared and cooked in a safe manner. This chapter summarizes the responsibilities of the retailer – and ultimately the consumer – in ensuring food quality and safety. The retail industry covers a wide range of different types of outlets dealing with different types of foods, including butchers, grocers, greengrocers and bakers, supermarkets and catering establishments.

Food Safety at the Retail Level

Food legislation

In the UK, all those involved in the production of foods – including retail and catering establishments – are governed by The Food Safety Act, 1990. Other pieces of food regulations also exist, related to food-handling establishments excluding abattoirs (Food Safety, General Food Hygiene, Regulations, 1995). In addition, other guidelines are also available, such as various Codes of Practice, the use of Good Manufacturing Practice (GMP) and the use of Hazard Analysis and Critical Control Point (HACCP). However, all the individual food regulations are to be superseded on 1 January 2006, by the new EU Hygiene Regulations (H1–3). These cover regulations for the hygiene of all foods (H1), additional rules for foods of animal origin (H2) and official controls including the tasks of the Official Veterinary Surgeon (H3).

The retailer – shops and supermarkets

These are responsible for providing a wide range of products directly to the consumer, from a wide range of sources. In order to ensure the highest degree of safety and quality, only food items from reputable suppliers should be bought. The food must be properly labelled and packaged, with all packaging intact (particularly tin cans). The temperature of the food upon arrival should be checked to ensure it has not passed an acceptable level, i.e. chilled food $<10°C$, frozen food $<-12°C$. If foods have surpassed these temperatures, they should not be accepted onto the premises. Upon arrival at the retail outlet, all foods should be stored at the correct temperature and handled appropriately throughout.

Product shelf life

During storage, food products will start to lose their quality, as they all have an inherent life-span (meats and dairy being shorter than dry goods), known as the shelf life. The shelf life of a food product can be affected by changes in the environment in which it is stored, the packaging in which it is wrapped, and by internal changes in the food product itself. Environmental factors that can alter the life of food products include: light, oxygen, temperature, moisture levels, pests and chemicals stored near to food products that may cause flavour exchanges. In terms of packaging, there could be certain interactions between the product and the packaging material, with chemicals form the packaging leaching into the food product. The food product itself will undergo various changes over time, such as physical, chemical and biochemical, that can alter food quality. Possibly the most important factor that affects the shelf life of a product is the growth of any microbes present, which can result in spoilage of the food, but also more importantly, a reduction in the safety of the food by the growth of pathogenic bacteria.

In order to ensure that the food that reaches the customer is safe and of good quality, in terms of microorganisms, each new product is tested and given a maximum shelf life by the retailer. Batches of samples are tested for bacterial numbers at various stages of storage under controlled environmental conditions. When the food starts to become unacceptable in terms of quality, this is termed the maximum shelf life of the product. If any modifications are made to a food product, the maximum shelf life must be recalculated. Predictive modelling is one tool that can be used to predict maximum shelf life by the retailer.

Date-marking of foods

Once the maximum shelf life of a product is known, this has to be displayed on the product in order to alert the consumer – and indeed the retailer – as to when the product should be consumed in order to retain maximum quality and safety. This is known as date-marking, and there are several which can be displayed on a product.

The 'sell-by' date is for the retailer's reference only, and enables the vendor to carry out proper stock control. This gives information on the display life of the product.

The 'best-before' date must be displayed on a product for retail sale. This is the date up to which the product should retain its particular properties when stored under the correct conditions, and is required by UK legislation.

The 'use-by' date has been determined by the manufacturer of the product and is the last recommended day on which the food should be consumed in order to be of good quality. This date must be used for foods which are highly perishable and likely to pose a risk to human health, e.g. for meats and dairy products. Foods must not be sold once the use-by date has elapsed.

Display of foods for retail

Chilled and frozen foods

When wrapped foods for retail sale are stored under chilled or frozen conditions, they must be solely foods and food products that were delivered to the retail outlet under these conditions. These types of food will be displayed for sale in lit cabinets which should be properly temperature controlled to ensure they do not rise above an unacceptable temperature, i.e. chilled units should operate at $<7°C$ and frozen units at $<-18°C$, due to customers opening the doors to remove food items. Cabinets should also be placed away from direct sunlight, high-intensity lights and heating units within the retail outlet. The display cabinet should not be overstocked with products and should be stocked only with items at the correct temperature, i.e. frozen or chilled temperatures. The air inlets should not be blocked, and foods that have the shortest shelf life should be placed at the front, i.e. first in, first out.

Raw and cooked meats

In some retail outlets, such as butcher shops or butcher counters within supermarkets, raw and cooked meats can be displayed and sold together. The biggest risk factor from these types of foods is the cross-contamination of microorganisms between the raw and cooked products. In order to minimize this, a number of good hygienic practices should be observed. The same utensils, knifes and cutting boards should not be used for both raw and cooked products – colour-coded chopping boards can be used to handle raw and cooked products separately. The meat should be displayed in properly chilled cabinets that should be temperature-checked regularly throughout the day. There should be a physical separation between raw and cooked products during display. Staff handling the products should be properly trained in basic food safety and hygiene, and should observe proper hygienic practices throughout. However, the most important practice is to thoroughly wash one's hands with soap and water after handling raw foods, or after handling money from the customer. Staff can spread microorganisms onto foods due to poor personal hygiene, especially when showing signs of illness. Therefore, staff should not handle foods if they have sickness or diarrhoea or have had those symptoms in the previous 48 h. Food handlers should be free of symptoms for at least 48 h before their return to work.

Delicatessen foods

Delicatessen counters sell a wide range of unpackaged, ready-to-eat foods which have a short shelf life – usually 1 working day, such as cooked meats, pies, cheeses and salads. These will be displayed in a chilled cabinet in the same way as the raw and cooked meats above, and hence the same precautions as above should be taken. Again cross-contamination is the biggest risk factor with these foods, and so to reduce this risk separate tongs should be used for each food type, disposable gloves should be worn by the staff and a separate piece of paper should be used on the scales when weighing out each item of food. When replacing food products that have been sold, all of that particular food should be used and then completely replaced – not just topped up. Staff working on this counter should be trained in food hygiene and safety, and should follow the same guidelines as written in the 'raw and cooked meats' section.

Catering establishments

This type of retail outlet is responsible for selling food that has been prepared and cooked on the premises. Some of the points outlined above in the previous retail sections are also relevant here. Only foods of good quality and from reputable sources should be purchased, stored at the correct temperatures and handled correctly throughout. Steps should be put in place to avoid the risk of cross-contamination of raw and cooked products, both during storage and preparation. Staff should carry out all procedures hygienically as described above and be properly trained in food hygiene and safety.

However, additional precautions are required as the food is to be prepared and served immediately to the consumer – any improper practices could result in large-scale food poisoning. Hand towels and tea towels are known to harbour microorganisms which can be transferred to the food, and so those should be used appropriately in the kitchen and changed regularly.

Another area of concern in catering establishments is the chilling and re-heating of foods prepared in advance in large batches. Cooked foods should be chilled immediately, with the core temperature reaching <10°C within 2.5 h. In order to achieve this quickly, it may be beneficial to split the food into smaller portions. When foods need to be reheated prior to serving, they must reach an internal temperature of 70°C, be served within 30 min and only be reheated once.

Food Safety at the Consumer Level

Once the food item has been purchased from the retail outlet, it is then the responsibility of the consumer to transport, store and prepare the item in an appropriate manner in order to avoid the risk of food poisoning. The home is the only food preparation area where food is not governed by legislation, and consumers handle raw foods that harbour microorganisms without any formal training or education of the dangers. The home is the source for 50–80% of food-borne outbreaks within Europe, and most of the outbreaks of salmonellosis in the UK are attributed to the home. The foods most associated with outbreaks of food-borne disease in the home, according to data from the UK Health Protection Agency, are indicated in Fig. 10.1.

Food-borne outbreaks in the home

The main causes of food-borne outbreaks in the home have been identified as inadequate storage, inadequate cooking and cross-contamination.

Inadequate storage

Food bought by the consumer can be subjected to temperature abuse due to incorrect storage. As discussed earlier, a rise in temperature allows

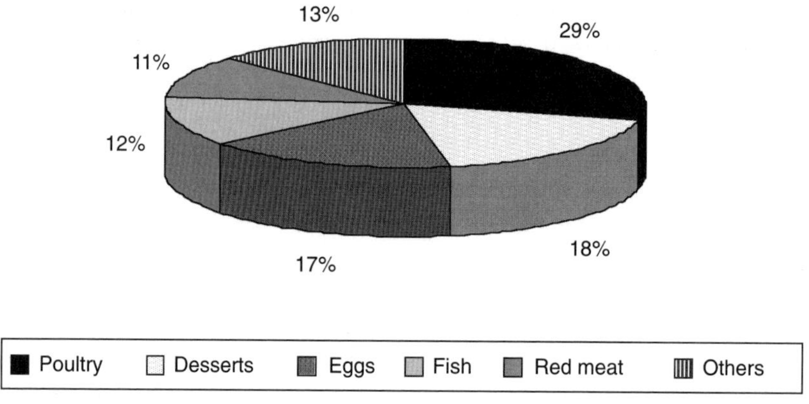

Fig. 10.1. Food-borne outbreaks from foods consumed at home 1992–1999 (the UK HPA data).

growth of microorganisms, which can result in implications for food safety. In order to minimize this, it is recommended that the consumer pick up chilled or frozen foods last when shopping, and should transport these foods home using a cool bag. A survey of 252 households in the south-west of England showed that only 12.7% of people transport chilled or frozen foods home using a cool bag (Evans *et al.*, 1991). In the same study, the effects of not storing food in a cool box were demonstrated: the temperature reached within an hour by the foods not stored in a cool box (raw chicken, cooked chicken, prawns) reached values (24–37°C) – more than sufficient to support the growth of microorganisms.

Once the chilled food has been transported home it should be placed in the refrigerator as soon as possible, to reduce the likelihood of temperature increase and the time at which the food spends at an increased temperature. In the same survey conducted by Evans *et al.*, the operational temperature of 252 household refrigerators was measured. The range was between 0.9°C and 11.4°C, with an average temperature of 6°C – only 1.6% of the refrigerators operated below 5°C. Nearly all the participants in the study were unaware that the correct operational temperature of a refrigerator is <8°C. The temperature variation within the refrigerators was also measured. The warmest place in 69.9% of refrigerators was the top, and the coolest place was the middle shelf of 45.1% of the refrigerators in the study. Therefore, food will be subjected to varying temperatures depending on which part of the refrigerator it is stored in.

Inadequate cooking

This can be due to several factors, such as misreading cooking times and temperatures, food not reaching the core temperature of 70°C, etc., but is increasingly becoming a problem due to the increased use of microwaves. Microwave ovens cook food rapidly, but also unevenly, leaving 'cold spots' in the food where bacteria may be able to survive. Food should ideally be stirred half way through cooking to dissipate the heat throughout the product. Another important factor is the standing time of the product, which should be observed, as this is required to complete cooking.

Microwave ovens may also be used to defrost foods prior to cooking. If this is the case, the food should be defrosted thoroughly and should then be cooked immediately.

Cross-contamination

In addition to those factors previously discussed in the retail and catering sections, other factors that contribute to cross-contamination within the consumer environment are dishcloths, sponges and tea/hand towels. The same sponge/cloth can be used to wipe several different surfaces, utensils and the refrigerator, within the kitchen as well as to wash dishes. Dishcloths and sponges are then left wet in a warm environment that is ideal for the growth of bacteria. Studies have shown that the bacteria present on dishcloths can increase from 10^2 to 10^6 (100–1,000,000) CFU after only 3 days of normal use. Dishcloths do not seem to be changed very regularly and so any bacteria present will increase to large numbers, but can also be spread round the kitchen environment time and time again. A recent study found that 60% of people change them at least once a month, 14% of consumers change their dishcloths every 1–3 months, and 5% of consumers change their dishcloths every 6–12 months. Bacteria such as *E. coli*, *Salmonella* spp. and *Listeria monocytogenes* have all been isolated from dishcloths in previous studies. These organisms will usually be picked up initially from raw food and can then be spread around the kitchen environment. Pathogenic bacteria have been often isolated from kitchen refrigerators. Data from the National Food Centre (Ireland) showed the presence of *S. aureus* in 40% of domestic refrigerators, *Salmonella* spp. 7%, *L. monocytogenes* 6%, *E. coli* 6% and *Y. enterocolitica* 2%.

Pets in the kitchen

Another area of potential cross-contamination in the kitchen is from domestic pets. These animals, particularly cats and dogs, can carry *Campylobacter* spp., *Salmonella* spp., *E. coli* O157, *Helicobacter pylori*, *Toxicara*, etc., which can be passed to man (see Chapter 10.5). Pets can spread these organisms by jumping on to food preparation areas, eating from containers used for human food, using utensils used to prepare human food and defaecating within the kitchen area. Hands should be thoroughly washed after handling animals and prior to preparing food, and litter trays should not be kept in the kitchen.

Further Reading

Bolton, D.J. and Maunsell, B. (2004) *Guidelines for Food Safety Control in European Restaurants.* Teagasc – The National Food Centre, Dublin.

Evans, G.I., Stanton, J.L., Russell, S.L. and James, S.J. (1991) *Consumer Handling of Chilled Foods: A Survey of Time and Temperature Conditions.* MAFF, London.

10.2 Microbiological Criteria for Foods

RIITTA MAIJALA

Introduction

The level of microbiological safety of a food portion at the time of consumption is a consequence of several factors. These include occurrence of microbes at the different steps of production, mixing and dividing of lots, contamination, growth and inactivation of microbes, as well as temperatures and time during processing and storage. In addition to the contamination frequency and level, the serving size, method of serving, frequency of consumption, dose–response and the susceptibility of the consumer all affect the microbiological risk caused by food at the time of consumption. Due to this complexity, the safety of a food at the time of consumption is based on multiple events and decisions made throughout the whole production chain.

The safety of foodstuffs should be ensured by preventive approach such as product design, implementation of good hygiene practice (GHP) and application of the principles of hazard analysis and critical control point (HACCP) throughout production, processing, handling, distribution, storage, sale, preparation and use. This type of control throughout the whole production chain can assure that the level of protection is met in many circumstances where end-production testing alone realistically cannot.

One of the management options available for usage, in order to improve food safety or to verify the safety status of a food lot, is microbiological criteria. However, it should be kept in mind that the microbiological safety of many foods can be assessed by a variety of methods besides microbiological testing (e.g. process or product characteristics). Microbiological criteria cannot be applied without microbiological testing, although testing itself can be used for many different purposes which may or may not be connected to microbiological criteria. The main targets for microbiological testing in food production are:

- acceptance of a lot of raw materials, food ingredients or end products;
- establishment of shelf life of certain foods;
- monitoring of the production lines;
- monitoring of the hygienic status of the processing environment;
- verification of GHP and HACCP;
- baseline studies for the occurrence of specific microbes at a specific step(s) of production;
- surveillance at a specific step of production; and
- outbreak investigations.

The purpose of testing is to determine the type of sample (raw materials, ingredients, processing line, environment, end product, etc.), target of sampling (indicators or pathogens) and the method used (rapidity, accuracy, repeatability, reproducibility, etc.). It is impossible to test all the raw materials, environment and end products in food production, and many factors in the history of the target intended for testing – laboratory capacity as well as practical aspects and costs – influence whether actual testing will be done or not. Since the traditional microbiological procedures applied on a sample of products cannot verify the absence of pathogens in a food lot, the use and interpretation of microbiological criteria are currently under discussion. In addition, the impact of ALOP (Appropriate Level of Protection) and FSO (Food Safety Objective) on microbiological criteria must be resolved in the near future.

Microbiological Criteria

According to the definition of the Codex Alimentarius Commission (1997), a microbiological criterion defines the acceptability of a product or a food lot, based either on the absence or presence, or number of microorganisms, including parasites, and/or on the quantity of their toxins/metabolites, per unit(s), volume, area or lot. It can be focused on pathogens, indicator or index organisms, microbial metabolism or specific genetic sequences, and it can be either qualitative or quantitative. Some of the basic terms in the field of microbiological criteria are presented in Table 10.1.

Microbiological criteria can be either mandatory or advisory, and they usually fall into three categories: namely standards, guidelines and specifications:

1. Standards (also termed mandatory criteria) are based on legal requirements and may result in reprocessing, rejection or destruction of a lot.
2. Guidelines can be applied during production and processing or on the end products, and they are intended for verification of safe and hygienic production or shelf life, and usually result in corrective actions.
3. Specifications are criteria used for contractual purposes by food businesses.

ICMSF (2002) has described these different types of criteria as follows:

1. Microbiological standards are used to determine the acceptability of a food with regard to a regulation or policy. These standards are established by regulatory authorities and they define the microbiological content that foods must meet to be in compliance with a regulation or policy. Foods not meeting the standard are in violation of the regulation or policy and are subject to removal form the market.

Table 10.1. Some terms defined in the field of microbiological criteria.

Term	Definition	Reference
Microbiological criterion	1. The acceptability of a product or a food lot, based on the absence, presence or number of microorganisms, including parasites, and/or quantity of their toxins/metabolites per unit(s), volume, area or lot.	Codex Alimentarius Commission, 1997
	2. The acceptability of a process, product or a food lot, based on the absence or presence, number of microorganisms, and/or quantity of their toxins/metabolites per unit(s), volume or area.	EC, 1999
	3. A yardstick on which a judgement or decision can be made: a microbiological criterion will stipulate that a type of microorganism, group of microorganisms or toxin produced by a microorganism must either not be present at all, be present in only a limited number of samples, or be present at less than a specified number or amount in a given quantity of a food or food ingredient.	NRC, 1985
	4. Is not a regulatory standard but a benchmark for evaluating test results.	FSIS, 1996
Acceptance criterion	Statement of conditions that differentiate acceptable from unacceptable food operations/lots. They can involve a variety of parameters (sensory, physical, chemical, biological); usually fall into three categories: standards, guidelines and specifications.	ICMSF, 2002
Microbiological standard	A mandatory criterion that is part of a law or ordinance. Used to determine the acceptability of food with regard to a regulation or policy.	ICMSF, 2002
Microbiological guideline	1. An advisory criterion issued by a control authority, industry association or food producer to indicate what might be expected when best practices are applied.	ICMSF, 2002
	2. A criterion that is often used by the food industry or a regulatory agency to monitor a manufacturing process. Guidelines function as alert mechanisms to signal whether microbiological conditions prevailing at critical control points or in the finished product are within the normal range.	NRC, 1985
Microbiological specification	1. Part of a purchasing agreement between a buyer and supplier of a food; such criteria may be mandatory or advisory according to use.	ICMSF, 2002
	2. A microbiological criterion that is used as a purchase requirement, whereby conformance with it becomes a condition of purchase between a buyer and vendor of a food or ingredient; such criteria may be either mandatory or advisory.	NRC 1985

Continued

Table 10.1. *Continued.*

Term	Definition	Reference
Performance criterion	1. The required outcome of one or more control measures at a step or combination of steps that contribute to ensuring the safety of a food.	ICMSF, 2002
	2. The effect in the frequency and/or concentration of a hazard in a food that must be achieved by the application of one or more control measures to provide or contribute to a PO[a] or an FSO[b].	Codex Committee on Food Hygiene, 2004
Performance standard	Prescribe the objectives or levels of performance (such as pathogen reduction standards for raw products) establishments must achieve.	FSIS, 1996
Process criterion	1. Control parameters of a control measure that if properly applied has been establishing as meeting, either alone or in combination with, other control measures, a performance criterion.	Codex Committee on Food Hygiene, 2004
	2. Control parameters (e.g. time, temperature, pH) at a step or combination of steps that can be applied to achieve a performance criterion.	ICMSF, 2002
	3. Consists of parameters that ensure that the level of a hazard does not increase to unacceptable levels before preparation or consumption. Can also be used to assess the acceptability of a food.	ICMSF, 2002
Product criterion	A physical or chemical attribute of a product that if properly applied as a control measure has been established as meeting, either alone or in combination with other control measures, a performance criterion.	Codex Committee on Food Hygiene, 2004
Default criterion	Conservative value established to ensure the safety of a process or a food.	ICMSF, 2002

2. Microbiological guidelines are usually established by either regulatory authorities, industrial trade associations or companies, to indicate the expected microbial content of a food when best practices are applied. Food companies use microbiological guidelines as a basis to design their control systems. These guidelines are advisory in nature and may not necessarily lead to rejection of a food.
3. Microbiological specifications are used by buyers of a food or ingredient to reduce the likelihood of purchasing a product that may be of unacceptable safety or quality. Microbiological specifications can define the microbiological limits for an ingredient so that, when it is used, the final product will meet all the requirements for safety and quality. Buyers throughout the food systems establish microbiological specifications for materials they purchase. In most cases, specifications are advisory and the materials are sampled periodically. When microbiologically sensitive ingredients are purchased, each incoming lot may be sampled and tested.

For a criterion, it must be defined exactly what type of hazard (e.g. *Staphylococcus aureus* or coagulase-positive staphylococci) and food category, production or processing steps are involved; the sampling plan, the analytical method accepted and the acceptable frequency of positive samples – as well as the consequences from positive test results are all essential components also.

There are two widely accepted types of sampling plans: the two-class plan (e.g. n = 5, 10, 15, 20 or more and c usually = 0) and the three-class plan (e.g. n = 5, c = 2, m = 10^3, M = 10^4) (ICMSF, 2002). In this notation n is the number of sample units (chosen separately and independently) examined from a lot and c is the maximum allowable number of defective sample units (two-class plan) or marginally acceptable sample units (three-class plan). In two-class plans m separates good quality form defective quality, and in three-class plans good quality from marginally acceptable quality. Consequently, M is used in three-class plans to separate marginally acceptable quality from defective quality.

The two-class plan is used mainly for pathogens and/or where a presence/absence test is to be performed, whereas a three-class plan is frequently used to examine for hygiene indicators where enumeration of microbes in a unit/volume or mass is possible. An example of a three-class plan would be coagulase-positive *Staphylococci* in milk powder with five samples to be taken (n), two samples (c) allowed to fall between 10 cfu/g (m) and 100 cfu/g (M). If these limits are not met when testing a food lot, it can be reprocessed, rejected or destroyed and/or further investigations made to determine appropriate actions to be taken. The results can also result in checking the efficiency of heat treatment and prevention of recontamination. What actions are to be taken with this kind of microbial criterion depends on its status (standard, guideline or specification) and the actions defined in the criterion.

Since many microbiological criteria are currently under revision, a list of them is not presented in this chapter. However, several reports and books have listed microbiological criteria for different foodstuffs (e.g. EC, 1998, ICMSF, 2002, FNB, 2003) and, for example, the European Commission is planning to have established a new set of microbiological criteria in 2006. The new code of Codex (2004) on microbiological risk management will most probably have a great influence on the development of criteria in future.

Interpretation of test results

In practice, the interpretation of microbiological results after testing is often made just by comparison with the microbiological criteria. However, it is important to keep in mind that confidence in a test result depends on many factors, e.g. lots selected for sampling, number of samples/units tested, homogeneity of the microbe distribution in the lot, randomization of sampling, time/temperature history of the samples at the time of analysis in the laboratory, true prevalence of microbe in the lot, sensitivity and specificity of the testing method and method validation and laboratory accreditation. Ensuring product safety by end product testing has a number of inherent weaknesses, not least the statistical problems associated with selecting samples for analysis. In fact, no sampling plan can assure the absence of a pathogen from a lot.

These factors are often neglected in decision-making, and it may be forgotten that, e.g. one sample analysed with a method with poor sensitivity can lead to a false sense of product security.

Setting microbiological criteria

When current and planned microbiological criteria are studied, it can be seen that there are several factors which influence the setting of a criterion:

1. New trends and prerequisites for food control;
2. Different aims for microbiological testing;
3. Reality factors; and
4. The actual content of a criterion (Fig. 10.2).

A final microbiological criterion is always a compromise of all these factors, e.g. it may be set without a clear connection to FSO or without formal risk assessment procedure.

Microbiological criteria should be based on scientific knowledge and take into account the practical, economical, etc. aspects. Therefore, the first decision to be made before setting a criterion is its aim. If it will be applied to international trade as a mandatory criterion, the need for solid and transparent scientific background information is much higher compared to the setting of a specification between two companies.

The traditional use of microbiological criteria to assess the safety of a specific lot or consignment is increasingly changing its focus to verifying

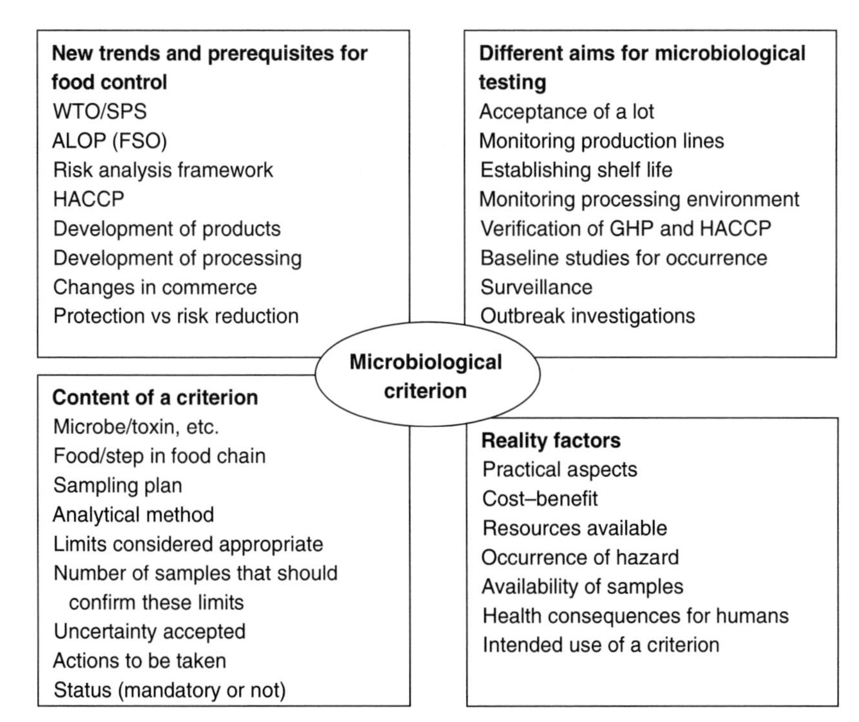

Fig. 10.2. Factors affecting the setting of a microbiological criterion.

the effectiveness of all or part of a food safety control system. In this context, microbiological criteria should be used only when they will have an impact on public health. In principle, they should, therefore, be one of the means to achieve the Appropriate Level of Protection (ALOP), which is, by definition, the level of protection deemed appropriate by the (WTO) member country establishing a sanitary or phytosanitary measure to protect human, animal or plant life or health within its territory (WTO, 1995).

Since ALOP is a broad public health goal, it cannot directly be related to microbiological criteria. However, if the relationship between ALOP and the different sources of infection are known, a Food Safety Objective (FSO) can be defined. FSO is the maximum frequency and/or concentration of a microbiological hazard in a food at the time of consumption that provides the ALOP. In this way, FSO articulates the overall performance expected of a food chain in order to reach a stated or implied public health goal.

Interpreting the concepts of ALOP and FSO is not so easy, and many different views still exist. However, current work ongoing in the Codex Alimentarius Commission on microbiological risk management will hopefully solve some of these problems. At the draft version of November 2004, the Codex Committee on Food Hygiene (CCFH) described how ALOP and FSO could be connected to risk management and introduced the concepts of Performance Objective (PO) and Performance Criteria (PC).

PO would articulate the maximum frequency and/or concentration of a hazard in a food at a specific step in the food chain before the time of consumption that provides or contributes to an FSO or ALOP, as applicable. PC would be the effect on the frequency and/or concentration of a hazard in a food that must be achieved by the application of one or more control measures to provide or contribute to a PO or an FSO. The primary role of microbiological criteria would then be to provide objective means of verifying – at a specified level of confidence – that a PO or PC (or FSO) is met. PCs could then be translated to process and product criteria. This proposal can also be seen as presented in Fig. 10.3.

Challenges in setting microbiological criteria

There are several challenges in setting criteria, the least one being the change in attitude from end product testing to validation/verification use of criteria. In addition to the actual content of a criterion, there are some specific questions which should always be solved when a microbiological criterion will be set:

1. If a criterion is set, will it have an impact on public health?

Optimally, the relationships between ALOP and FSO – as well as between FSO and microbiological criteria – should be known before a microbiological criterion is set. This can only be done by bringing scientific knowledge to bear on this question and should be based on risk assessment.

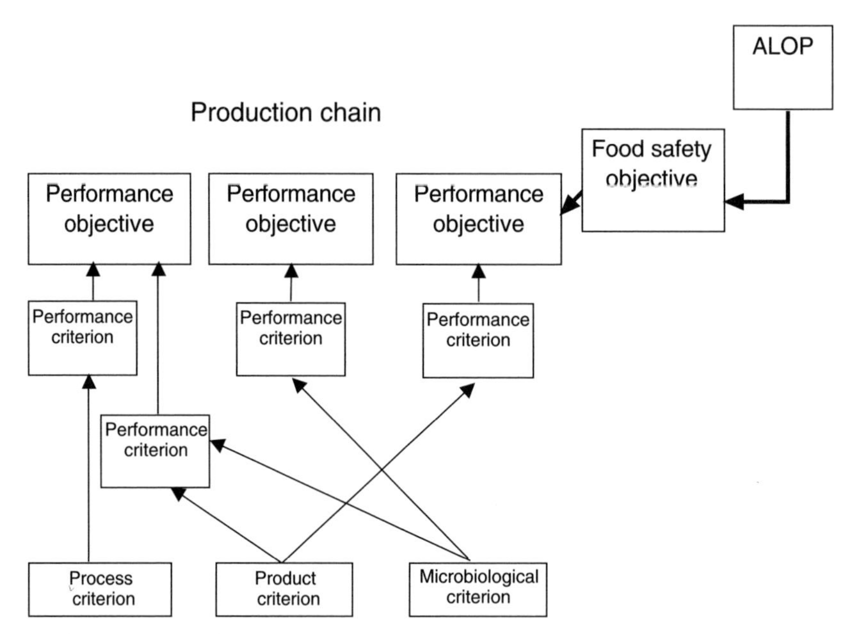

Fig. 10.3. An example of how the Codex proposal (2004) could be interpreted as connecting ALOP to microbiological criteria.

2. Is a criterion intended for risk reduction or protection in a risky situation (e.g. outbreak)?

In practice, end product testing hardly ever significantly reduces the risk caused by a microbiological hazard in a food lot. Therefore, the most useful use of a criterion from the public health point of view is to validate the GHP and HACCP. The role of epidemiological investigations of outbreaks becomes more important when there are fewer standards for end products. This is especially difficult if a criterion is quantitative (e.g. 1000 cfu/g), and the authorities must set a limit on that special case to withdraw the lot from the market. It is much easier if a standard exists for that particular kind of foodstuff. However, food-borne outbreaks are often caused by failures and using such an end product standard regularly would not decrease the public health risk.

3. Who should establish a criterion: authorities or industry?

The trend is to decrease the criteria set by authorities. Mandatory standards should be focused on those situations only where there is enough reasoning to believe that setting of a standard clearly decreases the public health risk.

4. What happens if a country runs a national control programme and an international standard gives lower protection?

According to the SPS agreement (WTO, 1995) if a country wants to have higher level of protection, it should be based on risk assessment.

Further Reading

Codex Alimentarius Commission (1997) *Principles for the Establishment and Application of Microbiological Criteria for Foods*, CAC/GL 21-1997.

Codex Alimentarius Committee on Food Hygiene (2004) *Proposed Draft and Guidelines for the Conduct of Microbiological Risk Management (MRM)*. Available at http://www.codexalimentarius.net/web/index_en.jsp

EC Regulation 178/2002 (2002) Official Journal of the European Communities L031, 1–24.

European Commission (1998) *Microbiological Criteria. Collation of Scientific and Methodological Information with a View to the Assessment of Microbiological Risk for Certain Foodstuffs*. Report EUR 17638 EN.

European Commission (1999) *The Evaluation of Microbiological Criteria for Food Products of Animal Origin for Human Consumption*. Available at http//europa.eu.int/comm./food/fs/scv/out26_en.pdf.

European Food Safety Authority (2004) *Opinion Adopted by the BIOHAZ Panel Related to the Microbiological Risks in Infant Formulae and Follow-on Formulae. Adopted 9th September 2004*. Available at http://www.efsa.eu.int/science/biohaz/giohaz_opinions/691_en.html

Food Nutrition Board (2003) *Scientific Criteria to Ensure Safe Food*. Committee on the Review of the Use of Scientific Criteria and Performance standards for Safe Food. Food Nutrition Board, Institute of Medicine and Board on Agriculture and Natural Resources. The National Academic Press, Washington DC. Available at http://books.nap.edu/openbook/030908928X/html/R1.html#pagetop

FSIS (Food Safety and Inspection Services) (1996) Pathogen reduction: hazard analysis and critical control point (HACCP) systems. Final Rule. *Food Register* 61, 38805–38855.

Harwig, J., Sharpe, A.N. and Dodds, K. (1998) *Guidance Concerning Microbiological Criteria,*

Microbiological Testing and Associated Methods for the Food Industry and Regulatory Agencies in Canada. Available at http://www.hc-sc-gc-ca/food-aliment/mh-dm/mhe-dme/compendium/volume_1/e_guidance01.html

Health Protection Agency (HPA) (1999) Available at www.hpa.org.uk

ICMSF (1986) International Commission on Microbiological Specifications for Foods. Micro-organisms in Foods 2. *Sampling for Microbiological Analysis. Principles and Specific Applications*, 2nd edn. Blackwell Science, Oxford, UK.

ICMSF (2002) International Commission on Microbiological Specifications for Foods. Micro-organisms in Foods 7: *Microbiological Testing in Food Safety Management*. Kluwer Academic/Plenum Publishers, New York.

ILSI (2004) *Food Safety Objectives – Role in Microbiological Food Safety Management*. Summary report of a workshop held in April 2003 at Marseille, France. International Life Sciences Institute, 36 pp.

Lindgren, S., Linqvist, R. and Norberg, P. (2003) *Microbiological Criteria for Food*. A summary of two Nordic Workshops in Sigtuna and Uppsala, Sweden. Livsmedelsverket report 22/2003. National Food Administration, Sweden.

NRC (National Research Council) (1985) An Evaluation of the Role of Microbiological Criteria for Foods and Food Ingredients. National Academy Press, Washington, DC. Available at http://www.nap.edu/openbook/0309034973/html/R1.html#pagetop

World Trade Organization (WTO) (1995) *The WTO Agreement on the Application of Sanitary and Phytosanitary Measures (SPS Agreement)*. Available at http://www.wto.org/english/tratop_e/sps_e/spsagr_e.htm

10.3 Food-borne Outbreak Investigation

SARAH O'BRIEN

Outbreak investigation is a core skill for public health practitioners. They occur locally, regionally or even nationally. Outbreaks are unwelcome, inconvenient and potentially stressful. They are also excellent opportunities to hone field epidemiology skills, learn more about the epidemiology and natural history of infectious diseases and to take action to prevent further illness. Outbreak investigation is truly public health in action.

Defining an Outbreak

There are several definitions of an outbreak:

- two or more related (i.e. epidemiologically linked) cases of a similar disease – this situation is commonly identified following a discrete event like a celebratory dinner;
- an increase in the observed incidence of cases over expected within a given time period – in this instance an outbreak might be detected through a rise in routine laboratory reports. Although the onset is less dramatic, the implications are more serious than in the first example since the source is unknown and the extent of further cases not yet quantified; and
- a single case of a serious disease – for example a single case of food-borne botulism represents a public health emergency, initiating a very intensive investigation.

Objectives of Outbreak Investigation

The main aims of epidemic/outbreak investigation are to:

- identify the causative agent;
- define the route of transmission;
- establish the risk factors;
- develop and implement control and prevention strategies; and
- advise on preventing similar events in the future.

An outbreak investigation is usually led by a Consultant in Health Protection (formerly known as a Consultant in Communicable Disease Control, or CCDC).

Technical Steps in Outbreak Investigation

Verify that an outbreak exists

Local knowledge, coupled with scrutiny of routine surveillance data, is usually enough to verify the existence of an outbreak. However, there are several reasons for pseudo-outbreaks and these include:

- Changes in reporting practice – have people suddenly started to report infections that they had not done previously?
- Introduction of new microbiological methods – are diseases that were previously undetectable now being reported because of improvements in diagnostics?
- Increasing awareness of an infection in the community leading to increased reports – might people be seeking advice from their doctor because they have already heard about a problem?
- A laboratory contamination incident – it happens! It is as well for this to be checked out before everyone gets embarrassed, but ask nicely!

Substantiating the diagnosis

This means arranging for appropriate samples to be collected and tested. The advice of an expert in microbiology is invaluable in deciding what to collect and what the target pathogens are. In a food-borne disease outbreak faecal samples are always collected but, in certain circumstances, there may be value in looking for serum or salivary antibodies. It is also courteous to warn laboratory staff of an imminent influx of specimens. This permits them to organize their work and prioritize outbreak samples. Outbreak-related samples need to be flagged in some way so that laboratory staff can pick them out from amongst their routine workload. However, laboratory diagnosis takes time and waiting for results must not cause delays. In the meantime, the investigation can proceed once a case definition has been created.

Generating a case definition

The case definition comprises clinical criteria, which should be simple and objective, with limitations on time, place and person. Sometimes various levels of case definition will be needed:

- Suspected cases = people with signs and symptoms and an incubation period clinically compatible with the suspected infection, but in whom the diagnosis is negative, awaited or incomplete.
- Presumptive cases = people with signs and symptoms compatible with the suspected infection but in whom diagnostic information is incomplete.

- Confirmed cases = people with signs and symptoms compatible with the suspected infection and in whom a diagnosis has been confirmed. This may be by either isolation of the pathogen from an appropriate clinical sample or by demonstration of a fourfold rise in antibody titre serologically.

The case definition usually includes temporal, geographical and personal criteria. For example, in an outbreak of multi-resistant *Salmonella typhimurium* definitive phage types 104 the initial case definition was as follows: any person resident in England or Wales from whom *S. typhimurium* DT104 resistant to ampicillin, chloramphenicol, streptomycin, sulphonamides, spectinomycin and tetracycline (*S. typhimurium* DT104 R-type ACSSuSpT) was isolated since 1 August.

Case finding

Where an outbreak follows a circumscribed event (e.g. a wedding breakfast or conference dinner) it is relatively straightforward to obtain the guest list and contact everyone who might have been exposed, and then to find out if they have symptoms. Where the extent of the outbreak is a less well-defined trawl there are several options, including:

- Asking local General Practitioners to report everyone with compatible symptoms. This is easier where syndromes are rare, but for diarrhoeal disease, which is common, differentiating those people that might be part of an outbreak from the background disease incidence is difficult.
- Asking microbiologists to look out for samples containing certain organisms, and to prioritize these for strain identification and further characterization at a reference laboratory.
- Asking relevant clinicians to inform about cases, e.g. reporting of cases of haemolytic uraemic syndrome by paediatricians.

Whatever method of case-finding is adopted, it is important that the case definition is applied without bias. Data from cases are usually documented in a questionnaire:

- Personal demographic data such as name, address, date of birth, sex and occupation.
- Clinical details, including date of onset of illness, predominant symptoms, duration of illness, time off work, details of any admission to hospital and outcome of illness.
- Depending upon the exact nature of the outbreak there may also be questions on travel history, exposure history (food, water, recreational, environmental, places visited, shopping habits, contact with other ill people or contact with animals).

Outlining the epidemic curve

Having organized the data from cases the next step involves plotting the number of cases over time on a graph to create an epidemic curve. Conventionally, cases are depicted as square boxes. The shape of the epidemic curve provides evidence of the nature of the outbreak. A point-source epidemic curve, where exposure has been limited in time, usually shows a sharp rise to a peak and a fairly rapid tailing off (Fig. 10.4). In a propagated, or continuing source, epidemic curve the shape of the curve is flatter and cases persist over a much longer period of time (Fig. 10.5). In an outbreak transmitted from person to person epidemic waves can be seen (Fig. 10.6). The epidemic curve should be updated on a daily basis. Note that the index case in an outbreak is the first case that comes to medical attention. This may or may not be the first person who has become ill in the outbreak, i.e. the primary case may pre-date the index case. It is important to choose an appropriate time interval for the *x*-axis (i.e. hours or days depending upon the organism/intoxication) and to make sure that there is at least one incubation period at either end of the outbreak curve to avoid missing any cases.

Plotting cases on a map may also help to pinpoint a source. This is particularly helpful where an environmental source is being considered. In outbreaks of Vero cytotoxin-producing *Escherichia coli* O157, mapping cases has proved valuable. Remember also that the cases might have been exposed to an organism a long way from where they live.

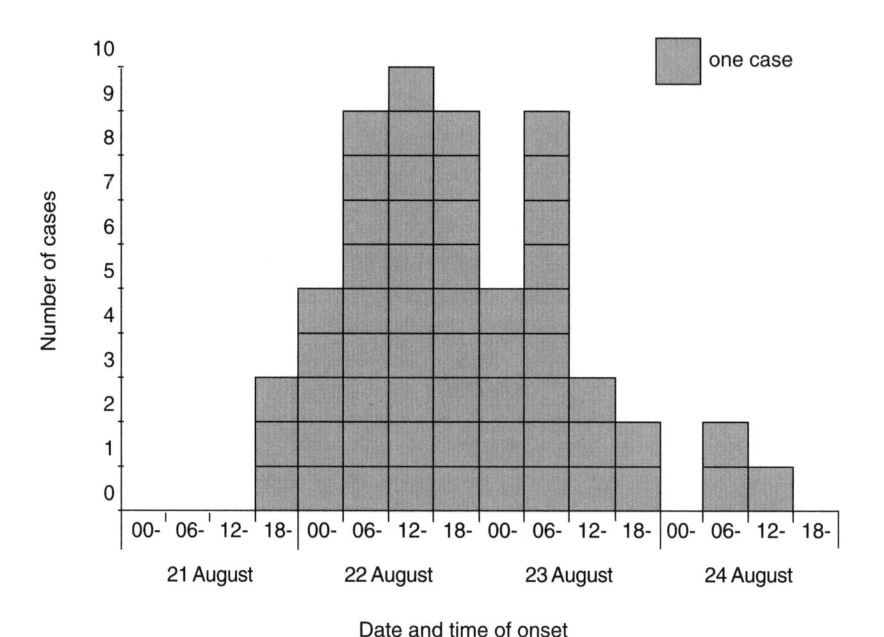

Fig. 10.4. Point source epidemic curve.

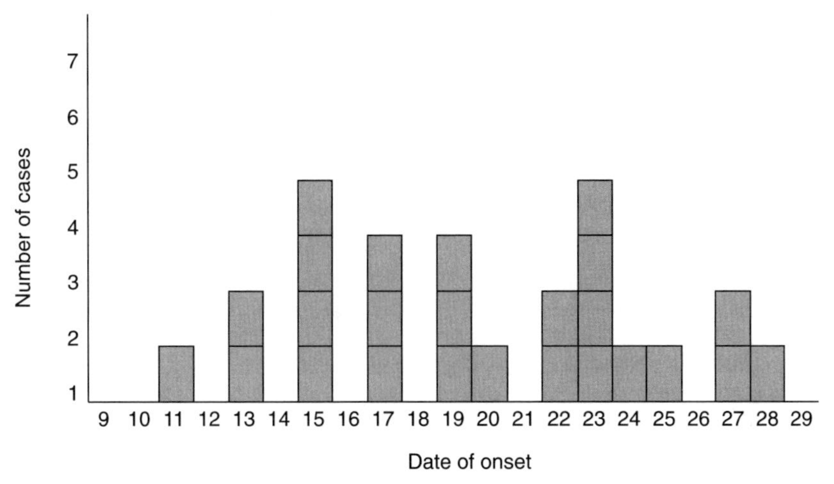

Fig. 10.5. Continuing source epidemic curve.

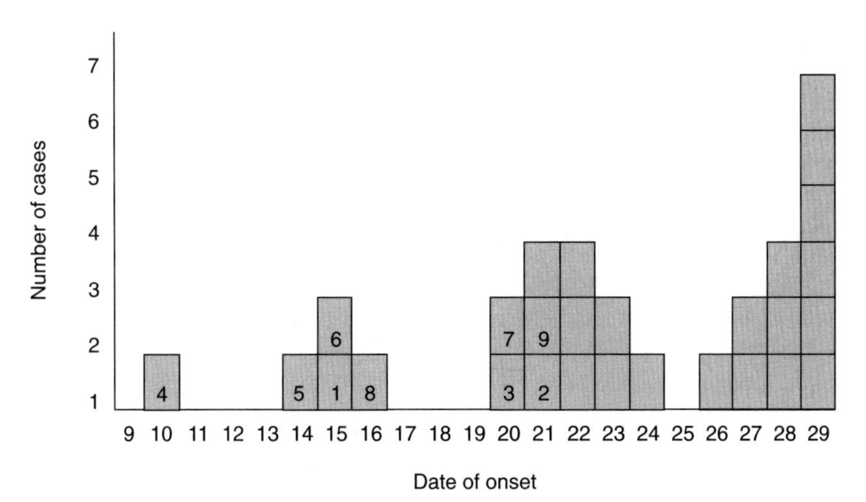

Fig. 10.6. Person-to-person epidemic curve.

Working out who is at risk

In certain circumstances this is obvious, e.g. a food poisoning outbreak at a wedding breakfast where those at risk are the guests. Often, certainly in large and/or national outbreaks, the extent of the population is much less easily defined. In this instance it may be necessary to include the whole population as potentially at risk. This is especially true where a nationally distributed food is suspected. However, it might still be possible to limit the extent of the enquiry. For example, where a type of baby food is suspected the population at risk may be children under 1 year of age, as opposed to the entire population.

Developing and testing hypotheses for exposure

Collate information about symptoms, circumstances and diagnosis to form a hypothesis about the cause of an outbreak. The hypothesis/(es) may be tested using analytical epidemiology, but do not use cases that were interviewed to form the hypothesis. Decide on the appropriate study design. If the event is so well delineated that all those at risk, both ill and well, can be identified, then a cohort study is appropriate. If all those at risk cannot be delineated, e.g. where a general excess of disease is apparent in the community but its origin is not, a case-control study is appropriate.

- Data capture: from the cohort, cases and controls, and usually employs standardly structured questionnaire. Often questionnaires are paper-based but, if possible, developing questionnaires on the worldwide web avoids the need for separate data entry, but make sure that data are secure. E-mailing questionnaires also achieves rapid responses.
- Control selection (case-control study): Controls must have had the opportunity of exposure to the hypothesized source and, in a community outbreak, the controls should be selected from that community. Consider the need for matching (e.g. within 10% for age), but overmatching should be avoided. Matching on too many variables leaves nothing to test for because, by definition, cases and controls are identical with respect to matched variables. Controls can be nominated by cases or recruited at random (e.g. random digit dialling).
- Data analysis: In a cohort study, where denominators are known, it is possible to compare the attack rates in those who consumed a given food with the attack rate in those who did not, to generate relative risks (Table 10.2). In a case-control study the odds of becoming ill are compared (Table 10.3). In each instance 95% confidence intervals should be calculated and an appropriate statistical test used (seek expert advice from a statistician if necessary). If more than one exposure is significantly associated with illness, then strategies for dealing with confounding will need to be explored, e.g. stratified analysis or logistic regression modelling.

Considering what additional evidence is needed

Corroborating evidence from a variety of sources can be garnered. For example in a food poisoning outbreak, Environmental Health Officers will collect important details such as food preparation and storage practices and carry out an inspection of the implicated premises. In an outbreak of VTEC O157 or salmonellosis where farm premises are implicated, a detailed veterinary investigation is indicated. Similarly, an inspection by a Health and Safety Executive officer may be needed.

Combining information from the epidemiological, environmental and microbiological investigations allows the investigating team to develop a picture of what went wrong and why, and helps them formulate both

Table 10.2. Analysis of data generated in a retrospective cohort study.

Variable	Ate?	Ill	Not ill	Attack rate (%)	Relative risk
Food vehicle	Yes No	a c	b d	a/(a+b) c/(c+d)	a/(a+b) c/(c+d)
Quiche Lorraine	Yes No	26 4	25 12	51 25	2.04
Ham salad	Yes No	27 3	24 13	53 19	2.79
Strawberry cheesecake	Yes No	15 15	36 1	29 93	0.31
Lemon gateau	Yes No	23 7	28 9	45 43	1.04
Orange juice	Yes No	22 8	29 8	43 50	0.86

Table 10.3. Analysis of data generated in a retrospective case-control study.

Variable	Ate?	Ill	Not ill	Odds of illness	Relative risk
Food vehicle	Yes No	a c	b d	a/c (for ill people) b/d (for well people)	a/c b/d Alternatively ad bc
Quiche Lorraine	Yes No	26 4	25 12		3.12
Ham salad	Yes No	27 3	24 13		4.88
Strawberry cheesecake	Yes No	15 15	36 1		0.03
Lemon gateau	Yes No	23 7	28 9		1.33
Orange juice	Yes No	22 8	29 8		0.76

immediate control measures and measures to prevent a recurrence in the longer term. This is, after all, one of the main aims of investigating outbreaks in the first place.

Implementing control measures

These can be initiated at any stage of the investigation, as soon as there is sufficient evidence to act upon, and specialist advice can be sought if necessary. Common sense needs to be used here. As soon as it becomes obvious what needs to be done – action should be taken. For example it would be completely unprofessional to wait for sufficient cases to occur to perform an analytical study if control measures can be implemented. A good example of this occurred in the Central Scotland outbreak of VTEC O157, where control measures were implemented very speedily, on the basis of good descriptive epidemiology, and an analytical study was never carried out.

Write an outbreak control team report

It is important both to keep contemporaneous notes as the investigation progresses and to write up the findings in an outbreak control team report once the team has concluded its study. As well as serving as a record of process of investigation and its findings, lessons learned should be highlighted so that others may learn from what happened.

Further Reading

Giesecke, J. (2002) *Modern Infectious Diseases Epidemiology* (2nd edn). Arnold Publishing, London.

Gregg, M.B. (1996) *Field Epidemiology*. Oxford University Press, Oxford, UK.

International Association of Food Protection. *Procedures to Investigate Foodborne Illness*. (5th edn). Available at: http://www.foodprotection.org/ (accessed 23 March 2005).

Palmer, S.R. (1995) Outbreak investigation: the need for 'quick and clean' epidemiology. *International Journal of Epidemiology* 24 Suppl. 1, S34–S38.

10.4 Surveillance of Food-borne Diseases

SARAH O'BRIEN

Introduction

The global burden of food-borne disease in humans is large, and many of the causative pathogens are zoonoses. In the United States alone there are an estimated 76 million cases of food-borne illness annually (Mead *et al.*, 1999). In England and Wales in 2000 there were an estimated 1.3 million cases of food-borne disease (Adak *et al.*, 2002). These figures have been compiled, at least in part, using a variety of routine sources of food-borne diseases surveillance data. The main objectives of food-borne disease surveillance are to establish the degree to which food acts as a route of transmission for specific pathogens, and to identify high-risk foods, practices and populations (Borgdorff and Motarjemi, 1997). The following sections outline some of the major systems for the surveillance of food-borne disease in humans in the United Kingdom and some of the dangers when interpreting surveillance data (see also O'Brien *et al.*, 2004).

What is Surveillance?

A commonly used definition of surveillance is:

> the ongoing systematic collection, analysis and interpretation of health data essential to the planning, implementation, and evaluation of public health practice, closely integrated with the timely dissemination of these data to those who need to know so that an action can result.
>
> (Thacker *et al.*, 1983)

This is often abridged to 'information for action'. The objectives of surveillance are to:

- predict epidemics;
- detect outbreaks;
- identify groups in the population at risk of developing certain diseases;
- evaluate the effectiveness of interventions;
- set priorities for allocating resources; and
- generate hypotheses that can be tested through the use of analytical epidemiology.

These objectives are achieved through monitoring disease trends, although, as the definition implies, surveillance activities importantly involve a feedback loop.

How is Surveillance Undertaken?

Population-based information on food-borne disease is collated from various sources (Wall *et al.*, 1996). Although in this chapter we will concentrate on surveillance in the UK, similar schemes exist in most European countries.

Surveillance of food-borne disease involves a range of people – clinicians, laboratory staff, public health department officials, environmental health officers (sanitarians), veterinarians and their colleagues. In the United Kingdom data on human disease are ultimately collated nationally at:

- The Communicable Disease Surveillance Centre (CDSC) of the Health Protection Agency's Centre for Infections in England and Wales; or
- Health Protection Scotland (in Scotland); or
- CDSC (Northern Ireland) in Northern Ireland.

The feedback loop is achieved routinely by means of regional and national surveillance bulletins. The national bulletins for these bodies are, respectively, CDR Weekly (http://www.hpa.org.uk/cdr/index.html), the HPS Weekly Report (http://www.show.scot.nhs.uk/scieh/) and the Communicable Disease Monthly Report Northern Ireland edition (http://www.cdscni.org.uk/). Food-borne disease surveillance data are also published in the annual United Kingdom Zoonoses Report (http://www.defra.gov.uk/animalh/diseases/zoonoses/reports.htm) and in peer-reviewed scientific papers.

What are the UK Sources of Data on Food-borne Disease?

Fig. 10.7 summarizes the main sources of food-borne disease surveillance data in the UK.

Food poisoning notification

This is the only statutory means of collating data on food poisoning. Food poisoning was first made notifiable in England and Wales in 1949, but the most recent legislation governing notification in England and Wales are the Public Health (Infectious Diseases) Regulations 1988 (McCormick, 1993). Every registered medical practitioner is legally obliged to notify the Proper Officer (usually a Consultant in Communicable Disease Control) of a Local Authority of any case of food poisoning, on clinical suspicion alone. A confirmed diagnosis is not required in order to notify a case of food poisoning. Since food poisoning can be difficult to distinguish from other causes of gastroenteritis clinically, the Advisory Committee on the Microbiological Safety of Food recommended a standard definition of food poisoning in 1992. This was 'any condition of an infectious or toxic nature, caused by, or thought to be caused by contaminated food or water' (Calman, 1992).

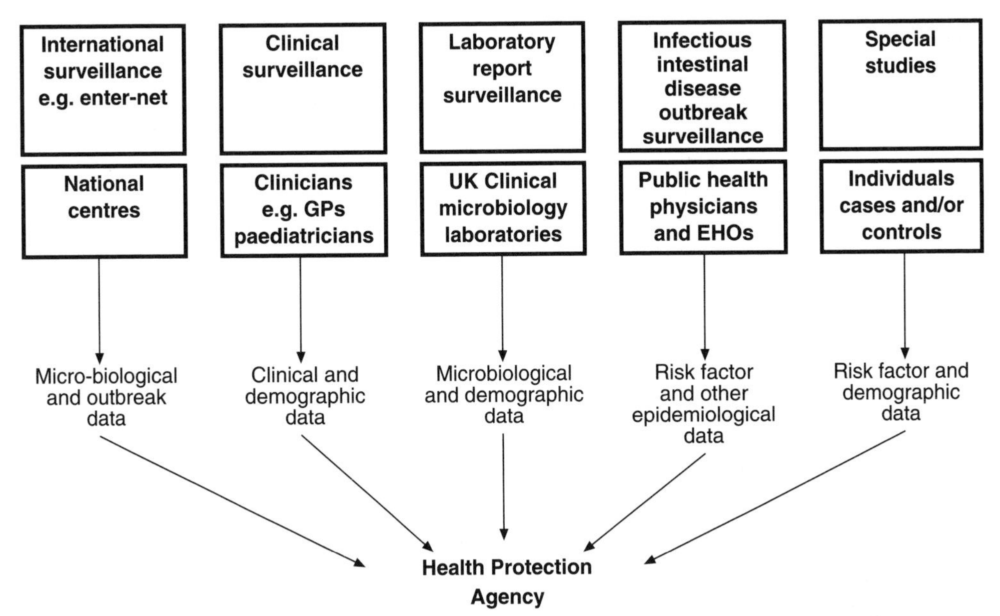

Fig. 10.7. Sources of data on food-borne disease in the UK (source: Health Protection Agency).

Laboratory report surveillance

This is generally regarded as the most useful system for monitoring long-term trends in food-borne disease, identifying outbreaks and assessing the impact of interventions. Data from clinical diagnostic laboratories are enhanced with information from national microbiology reference laboratories and collated at the three national centres. As can be seen from Fig. 10.8, *Campylobacter* and *Salmonella* in England and Wales clearly exceed other gastrointestinal pathogens reported through the laboratory system.

Surveillance of general outbreaks of infectious intestinal disease

In England and Wales, systematic surveillance of completed outbreak investigations has been undertaken since 1992 (O'Brien *et al.*, 2004). The objectives of outbreak surveillance are to:

- describe the impact of outbreaks of infectious intestinal disease (IID);
- identify transmission routes;
- identify trends in pathogens causing outbreaks;
- identify trends in food vehicles implicated in outbreaks;
- detect new pathogens or food vehicles; and
- identify the impact of outbreaks in different settings (O'Brien *et al.*, 2004).

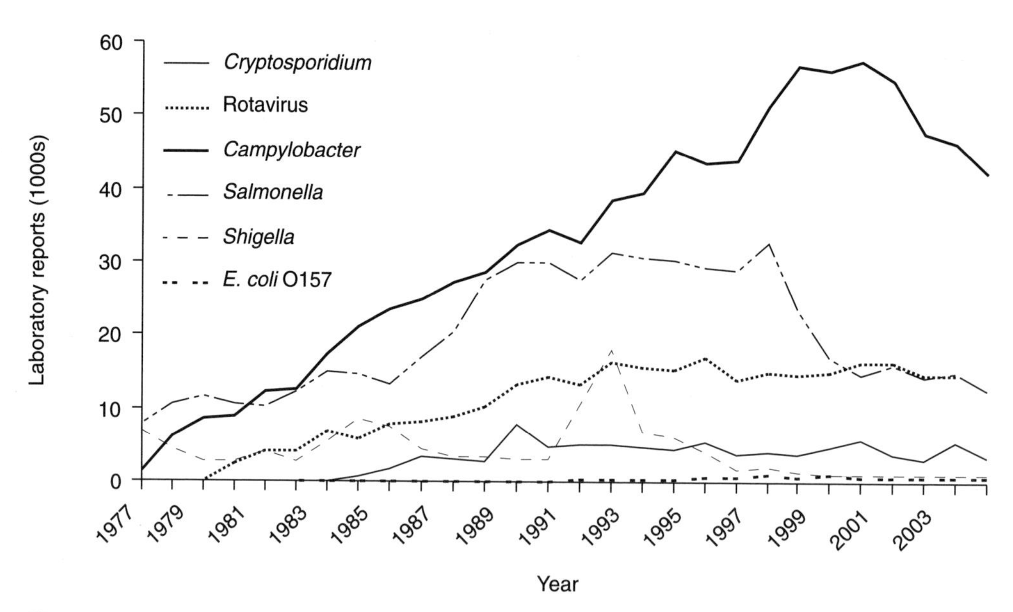

Fig. 10.8. Laboratory reporting of selected GI pathogens in England and Wales, 1977–2004 (source: Health Protection Agency).

The results of epidemiological, environmental and microbiological investigations are brought together in this system (O'Brien *et al.*, 2004). The outbreak dataset includes the setting, mode of transmission, causative organism and any suspected food vehicle, including the type of evidence upon which suspicion is based (i.e. epidemiological, microbiological and/or environmental – including food inspections). Fashions in catering can be detected, e.g. a penchant for cooking chicken livers 'pink' (a risk for *Campylobacter* infection), as well as changes in distribution of pathogens causing food-borne disease outbreaks.

Clinical surveillance

Certain food-borne infections can lead to very serious consequences. Undertaking surveillance involving clinicians responsible for the management of individual patients means that the clinical impact of infection can be more fully appreciated in both the short and longer term.

International surveillance

The national surveillance centres in the UK all feed into an international surveillance network for salmonellosis and VTEC called 'Enter-net', which has been funded by the European Commission to respond rapidly to international outbreaks involving these organisms (Fisher, 1999).

What are the Pitfalls in Interpreting Surveillance Data?

There are many reasons why what is reported at national level does not accurately reflect disease burden in the population. It is essential to understand why this occurs so that surveillance data are not misused.

A notification of food poisoning does not necessarily imply that infection was the cause

The definition of food poisoning, described above, is very broad. In particular, it does not guide the notifying clinician towards a suspected aetiology. Chemical intoxication may also lead to symptoms of gastroenteritis, so that not all that is notified is necessarily due to food-borne infection. Having said that, it is interesting to note that trends in food poisoning notifications tend to mirror clinical microbiology results (Atkinson and Maguire, 1998), particularly those of *Salmonella* and *Campylobacter*. This implies that clinicians are awaiting a diagnosis before completing a notification form.

Laboratory reporting underestimates the true population burden of food-borne disease

For a case of laboratory-confirmed infection to appear in national statistics several steps need to be fulfilled:

- the case must consult their General Practitioner (GP). (If an infected individual does not present to their GP they cannot be counted in national statistics);
- the GP must conclude that the case's gastroenteritis might be due to food poisoning. (At this point the case should be notified. In fact, only a very small proportion of cases are notified in this way);
- the GP must request a faecal sample from the patient. (Note that in order to manage individual cases of food poisoning the GP does not necessarily need to know the definitive diagnosis since the clinical management is likely to be the same, no matter what the infecting organisms. S/he might not, therefore, request a specimen);
- the patient must provide the sample to the GP;
- the sample must be sent through to a clinical laboratory under the correct conditions, i.e. so that any pathogen, if present, does not die off in transit;
- the microbiologist must examine the specimen for the pathogen using appropriate microbiological techniques;
- the microbiologist must report any positive results back to the GP and also to their Consultant in Communicable Disease Control (CCDC). (This may be done electronically or via a paper report);

- the microbiologist must send an isolate to a national reference laboratory, if appropriate;
- the information on the positive specimen results from the microbiologist must be reported to the regional surveillance unit and thence to national surveillance databases; and
- information from the national reference laboratory, if appropriate, must be linked with the clinical isolate.

Thus, it can be seen that there are many stages where valuable information can be lost. By far the greatest loss of data occurs before patients present to their GP. Many food-borne illnesses are relatively short-lived and those who consult their GP tend to perceive their symptoms as being more severe and are more likely to have returned recently from a trip overseas (Tam *et al.*, 2003).

Variations in clinical practice (i.e. the likelihood of requesting a specimen from an ill patient) and differences in laboratory practice will also influence how much disease is reported. Not all laboratories use the same battery of tests (Evans *et al.*, 2000), so that 'nothing abnormal detected' is not necessarily the same as 'nothing abnormal detectable'. Added to this, it should be remembered that a negative laboratory result might have several explanations:

- the patient had symptoms of gastroenteritis but was not suffering from an infection; or
- the patient had an infection but the sample was obtained too late to yield a pathogen; or
- the patient had an infection with an organism for which the laboratory did not examine the specimen; or
- the patient had an infection but the laboratory used a method which would not necessarily have detected the organism; or
- the patient had an infection with an emerging pathogen for which a routine diagnostic test has not yet been developed.

The infectious intestinal diseases (IID) study in England allowed surveillance specialists to work out the relationship between what is officially recorded and the true disease burden in the community. For every case of IID reported to national surveillance they worked out that 136 cases will have occurred in the community. For *Campylobacter* infection the ratio of disease in the community to national surveillance reports is around 8 to 1, and for *Salmonella* it is approximately 3 to 1 (Wheeler *et al.*, 1999).

The fact that surveillance systems underestimate the true population burden of food-borne infection does not necessarily matter if the main aim is to describe trends in the longer term. Provided that there have not been major changes in the methods of data collection over time, then trend interpretation is possible and a correction for under-ascertainment can be made. Thus, for long term-trend description consistency of reporting is more important than accurately description of the disease burden.

There is variation in the follow-up of sporadic cases of food-borne disease

Once a patient has a laboratory-confirmed infection, the extent to which further public health investigations are undertaken varies (Rooney *et al.*, 2000). Investigation of *Salmonella* spp. and VTEC O157 appears to have a higher priority amongst local authority environmental health officers investigating sporadic cases than investigation of either *Campylobacter* infection or viral gastroenteritis.

There is variation in the follow-up of outbreaks

As mentioned above, systematic surveillance of general outbreaks of infectious intestinal disease in England and Wales is designed to provide unbiased information on causative organisms, sources or vehicles of infection and modes of transmission. A spin-off from this systematic data collection is that investigation techniques and patterns of evidence can also be monitored (O'Brien *et al.*, 2004).

Weaving together strands of evidence from microbiological, environmental, epidemiological and (sometimes) veterinary investigations helps to unravel the cause of a food-borne disease outbreak. However, the extent to which all four of these strands are employed varies according to the type of outbreak (O'Brien *et al.*, 2002). Veterinary investigations may form a crucial part of investigating outbreaks of salmonellosis, cryptosporidiosis or VTEC O157 infection.

Conclusions

Surveillance is key to understanding the epidemiology of food-borne disease. Equally important is to appreciate the biases that occur in surveillance data so that the information generated is not over-interpreted.

Acknowledgements

The author would like to thank the consultants in communicable disease control, public health physicians, microbiologists, environmental health officers, infection control nurses and all the staff at the Health Protection Agency and National Health Service laboratories, without whose work the various surveillance schemes would not function, and to Mrs S. Le Baigue, Miss C. Hopcroft and Miss C. Penman, who maintain the databases at CDSC.

References

Adak, G.K., Long, S.M., O'Brien, S.J. (2002) Trends in indigenous food-borne disease (IFD) and deaths, England and Wales – 1992–2000. *Gut* 51, 832–841.

Atkinson, P. and Maguire, H. (1998) Is food poisoning a clinical or a laboratory diagnosis? A survey of local authority practices in the south Thames region. *Communicable Disease and Public Health* 1, 161–164.

Borgdorff, M.W. and Motarjemi, Y. (1997) Surveillance of Foodborne Diseases: what are the options? *World Health Statistics Quarterly* 50, 12–23.

Calman, K.C. (1992) Definition of food poisoning. Letter from the Chief Medical Officer, Department of Health (PL/CMO(92)4), London.

Evans, C.J., Cowden, J.M., Breen, D. and Thomson-Carter, F. (2000) Investigation and management of sporadic gastrointestinal infections with potentially Vero cytotoxin producing *Escherichia coli* in Scotland. *Communicable Disease and Public Health* 3, 201–7.

Fisher, I.S.T. (1999) The Enter-net international surveillance network – how it works. *Euro Surveill* 4, 52–55.

McCormick, A. (1993) The notification of infectious diseases in England and Wales. *Communicable Disease Report, CDR Review* 3, R19–R25.

Mead, P.S., Slutsker, L. and Dietz, V. *et al.* (1999) Food-related illness and death in the United States. *Emerging Infectious Diseases* 5, 607–625.

O'Brien, S.J., Elson, R., Adak, G.K., Gillespie, I.A. and Cowden, J.M. (2002). Surveillance of foodborne outbreaks of infectious intestinal disease in England and Wales 1992–1999: contributing to evidence-based food policy? *Public Health* 116, 75–80.

O'Brien, S.J., Gillespie, I.A. and Adak, G.K. (2004) Foodborne disease surveillance for policy-making. *Food Safety and Veterinary Public Health* 3, 33–52.

Rooney, R., O'Brien, S.J., Mitchell, R., Stanwell-Smith, R. and Cook, P.E. (2000) Survey of local authority approaches to investigating sporadic cases of suspected food poisoning. *Communicable Disease and Public Health* 3, 101–105.

Tam, C.C., Rodrigues, L.C. and O'Brien, S.J. (2003) The study of infectious intestinal disease in England: what risk factors for presentation to general practice tell us about potential for selection bias in case-control studies of reported cases of diarrhoea. *International Journal of Epidemiology* 32, 99–105.

Wall, P.G., de Louvois, J., Gilbert, R.J. and Rowe, B. (1996) Food poisoning: notifications, laboratory reports, and outbreaks – where do the statistics come from and what do they mean? *Communicable Disease Report, CDR Review* 6, R93–R100.

Wheeler, J.G., Sethi, D., Cowden, J.M. *et al.* (1999) Study of infectious intestinal disease in England: rates in the community, presenting to general practice, and reported to national surveillance. The Infectious Intestinal Disease Study Executive. *British Medical Journal* 318, 1046–1050.

10.5 Companion Animals and Public Health

ALISON SMALL

Man's relationship with animals as providers of food, beasts of burden and assistants in agriculture, transport and hunting has developed over a large number of centuries. Recently, the role of animals as companions, as pets or as leisure animals has become increasingly important. In any situation where humans and animals interact, there are public health considerations, as the health and behaviour of the animal can impact upon that of humans.

Behavioural Considerations

Keeping animals as pets can have many beneficial effects on public health. It has been shown that the mere act of stroking an animal can reduce stress and aid convalescence. Caring for another living being can be rewarding, boost self-esteem and distract attention from minor problems and stresses within the life of the carer. Many pets are important companions to those who live alone, or whose families have moved away. In such cases, the bond between owner and pet can be so great that the loss of the pet is as devastating as the loss of a family member.

When sharing one's life with another person, human beings use many behavioural forms of communication, otherwise known as 'body language', as well as speech, to communicate. With animals, although many pet owners aver that their pets do 'talk' to them, communication must be via body language, and when that language is misunderstood or ignored, the human may be injured as the animal continues its behavioural 'conversation' as it perceives to be appropriate. From the animal's point of view, its reactions are a justified defence against attack by the human, which is invading its personal space, or even a natural stage in a game, the example being the dog which nips at the owner's hand whilst 'wrestling'. In this case, the dog is joining in the game as though the human is a littermate, and the canine rules allow gentle nips. A dog's definition of gentle, however, may be different from the human's. Many bites, kicks and scratches received by animal handlers could be avoided through understanding the animal's behavioural signals.

Bites

Around 50% of people will receive a dog or cat bite at some point in their lifetime, and of these 1% will require hospitalization either due to the severity of the injury or, more commonly, to wound infection. Almost half of dog bites seen by doctors are perpetrated by the family's own dog, and children below the age of 12 years are most likely to be bitten. Men are three times more likely to be bitten by a dog than women, but women are three times more likely to be bitten by a cat. The animal mouth is far from sterile, and teeth carry a variety of organisms, which contribute to infection of bite wounds. Local cellulitis and abscess formation is common, and bacteraemia can occur with potentially serious sequelae. Commonly implicated organisms include:

- *Pasteurella multocida* – implicated as a major pathogen in 20–50% of dog bites and over 50% of cat bites. This organism is a common commensal of the oral cavity of the dog (60%) and cat (90%). The syndrome is normally self limiting, with local inflammation being seen about 48 h after the initial bite, but abscesses and systemic spread must be treated with antibiotic preparations;
- *Staphylococcus intermedius*;
- *Streptococcus* spp.;
- *Erysipelas rhusiopatiae* – has been isolated from cat bites; can cause systemic illness and endocardiosis;
- *Serratia marcescens* – associated with bites from reptiles such as iguanas;
- *Halomonas vensuta* – associated with bites from saltwater fish;
- *Streptobacillus moniliformis*; and
- *Spirillium minus* – associated with 'rat bite fever', a syndrome of fever, muscle and joint pain, lymphadenitis and a purplish rash, which develops days to weeks after the initial bite wound has healed. The organism is excreted in the urine and saliva of rats, so illness could also be contracted from contaminated milk, food or water. If untreated, this disease results in a mortality of 10%, and can show long-term sequelae such as endocarditis, or relapses.

Animal bites may also be the route of transmission of other zoonotic pathogens, e.g. rabies.

Cat scratch disease (CSD)

This illness is seen most commonly in children; up to 80% of cases occur in young people under the age of 21 years. It manifests first as a series of papules or pustules around a cat scratch after 3–14 days' incubation. Between 1 and 7 weeks later a regional lymphadenopathy develops affecting nodes proximal to the cat scratch, and conjunctivitis with peri-auricular lymphadenitis may be seen. The illness is usually self-limiting over a period of 4 months, but it may progress to fever, rash, muscle pains, weight loss and splenomegaly. Severe disease with systemic complications may occur in the immunocompromised individual, or in small children. Often the illness becomes recurrent over a period of 2 years.

The organism associated with CSD is *Bartonella henselae*, which produces a prolonged (22 months) bacteraemia in cats. Kittens pose a greater risk of carrying the organism than older cats, and although the infection can be diagnosed serologically in cats, its response to antimicrobial therapy is very variable. Direct cat–cat transmission of the organism has not been demonstrated, suggesting that the infection may be vector-borne, and the organism has been isolated from fleas. It is not known whether fleas can transmit the illness to humans, but 25% of CSD patients do not report having been bitten or scratched by a cat, although they have had some kind of contact with cats.

Zoonotic Diseases

All animals pose the risk of becoming infected with a zoonosis, a disease that can be transmitted naturally between animals and man. Some of these are very rare, but the more common conditions are mentioned here.

Psittacosis

Psittacosis, otherwise known as ornithosis, chlamydiosis or parrot fever, is a febrile bacterial disease caused by the organism *Chlamydia psittaci*. The disease is acquired by contact with infected birds, through inhalation of contaminated dust. It is most commonly associated with psittacine birds (parrots, parakeets and cockatiels), and is excreted in the faeces and nasal discharges of affected birds. In birds, the condition may be asymptomatic, but fever, diarrhoea, conjunctivitis and nasal discharge are common. In humans, a flu-like illness with fever, headache, joint and muscle pains begins some 4–15 days after infection, and persists for a few days. Occasional cases develop atypical bronchopneumonia, endocarditis and hepatitis that may last for several weeks. Fatalities are rare, but sheep can carry an abortifacient strain of the organism which, if contracted by pregnant women, can be life threatening, and results in late abortion, neonatal death and disseminated intravascular coagulation in the mother. Psittacosis in birds responds well to tetracycline or erythromycin therapy, and imported birds should be treated for prolonged periods to eliminate carriage of the organism. Pregnant women should avoid contact with sheep during the lambing period.

Tularaemia

This disease, also known as Francis' Disease, Deer-fly Fever, Rabbit Fever or O'Hara's Disease, is primarily associated with bites from small wild mammals such as rabbits, hares and rodents. The causal organism, *Francisella tularensis*, has also been isolated from wild birds, and around 2% of human cases are associated with bites or scratches from infected cats.

Transmission may be through an animal or insect bite, or via contaminated food or water. Affected cats show fever, malaise, anorexia and purulent lymphadenitis. They may develop ulcers in the mouth, hepatitis and enterocolitis. The disease varies from mild to fatal.

In humans, there is an incubation period of 1–10 days, after which there is a sudden onset of fever, headache and prostration, which may persist for several weeks. Where the organism has gained access to the body via a bite, an indolent ulcer may form, with local lymphadenitis and abscess formation. Further symptoms may include pneumonia, pharyngitis, conjunctivitis, corneal ulceration, abdominal pain with vomiting and diarrhoea, and a chronic purulent lymphadenitis. The response to antibacterial therapy is variable, recovery is prolonged and fatalities are around 2%, resulting from systemic involvement. Post-mortem examination reveals necrotic foci in the liver, spleen and lymph nodes.

Ringworm

Ringworm, otherwise known as Dermatophytosis, Dermatomycosis, Tinea, Trichophytosis or Microsporosis, is a fungal skin disease acquired by direct or indirect contact with infectious humans or animals. The organisms involve include *Trichophyton* spp. (associated with horses) and *Microsporum* spp. (associated with dogs and cats). The incubation period is 4–14 days in humans, but 1–4 weeks in animals. The classical manifestation of the disease is a ring-shaped, crusty lesion that slowly enlarges, and these are commonly seen on housed cattle and affected humans. In animals, particularly in horses, all that may be seen is a small, grey, crusty scab. It is a chronic, benign condition that responds well to topical anti-fungal therapy, but secondary bacterial infection can lead to scarring. The disease is more commonly acquired from animals than directly from another human being, and the role of fomites (inanimate objects) in the transmission of this condition is very important, as the fungal spores remain viable for long periods on carrier animals, their grooming equipment, harness and environment.

Bordetella bronchiseptica

This organism is one of the many organisms implicated in the canine respiratory syndrome Kennel Cough, and has also been associated with respiratory disease in cats and rabbits. Its true pathogenicity and role in human disease is not known, but it has been isolated from respiratory tract infections, from sinusitis to pneumonia, particularly in immunocompromised hosts. In immunocompetent individuals a 'whooping cough'-like syndrome has been reported, although true 'whooping cough' is normally associated with the related organism *Bordetella pertussis*.

Influenza

Influenza virus is a worldwide problem, with reservoirs of infection found in humans, birds, horses and pigs. The individual viruses appear to be species specific, but there are sporadic cases of human disease resultant from avian or pig strains. Influenza virus has the ability to undergo antigen shift whilst circulating in an animal population, and may suddenly develop the ability to cause pandemic illness in the human population. Transmission of the virus is by inhalation of droplets produced by coughing or sneezing, and convalescent carriers remain a reservoir of infection between epidemics. During epidemics, there is a high fatality rate amongst elderly and debilitated patients.

Endoparasites

A number of parasites of animals can affect humans, humans often being the accidental intermediate hosts of these parasites. Transmission is by the faecal–oral route, and the eggs have been found on animal coats. For more detail see Chapter 2.2.

- *Toxocara canis/cati*;
- *Multiceps multiceps*;
- *Multiceps serialis*;
- *Echinococcus granulosus*; and
- *Diphyllobothrium latum*.

Carriage of Human Disease Agents

Toxoplasma gondii

This protozoan parasite is a common inhabitant of most animals, birds and man. It occurs worldwide, and the condition is normally asymptomatic. Systemic illness can occur, which manifests as fever, headache, cough and lymphadenopathy, and rare sequelae include myocarditis, encephalitis and pneumonitis. Latent infection can reactivate in immunocompromised individuals, with serious consequences. *Toxoplasma gondii* is a common intestinal coccidian of cats. Infection of sheep can cause systemic disease and abortion. The greatest risk for humans is to the unborn child. Infection during pregnancy causes abortion, and can have long-term effects on the fertility of the woman. When infection occurs during the second trimester of pregnancy, congenital Central Nervous System disorders arise. Transmission is via the faecal–oral route from cat faeces, or indirectly via contamination of foods.

Cowpox

Cowpox, a benign viral skin disease originally associated with cattle, can be carried by cats and small rodents. The condition is self-limiting and manifests as vesicles and pustules on the skin. Rarely there is fever and lymphadenitis, and secondary infection could lead to scarring.

Helicobacter pylori

This organism has been associated with gastrointestinal illness in humans, manifesting as severe abdominal cramps, flatulence, diarrhoea and gastric ulceration. Isolation of the organisms is more common in older patients, and a link to intestinal neoplasia has been demonstrated. *H. pylori* has been isolated from faeces, salivary secretions and dental plaque of naturally infected cats, and also from houseflies. The epidemiology and transmission of this organism is not yet fully understood, but feline isolates are genetically similar to human isolates. It may be the case that humans are the primary reservoir of this organism, infecting the cats secondarily. In the cat, the condition may be asymptomatic, but it has been associated with lymphofollicular gastritis. Dogs also carry *Helicobacter* spp., but these tend not to be *H. pylori*.

Food-borne disease agents

Animals can be the asymptomatic carriers of many organisms commonly associated with food poisoning or water contamination. The organisms are excreted in the faeces of the animal and may be found on the coat. Transmission is by direct faecal–oral transfer, or indirectly via foods prepared using contaminated hands or utensils. Some examples of such organisms are listed below.

- *Campylobacter* spp.;
- *Salmonella* spp.;
- *Giardia lamblia*; and
- *Cryptosporidia parvum*.

For more information on these pathogens, see Chapters 1.2 and 2.2.

IV Stable-to-Table Concept

11 Principles of Longitudinal and Integrated Food Safety Assurance

11.1 LISA Concept and its Main Elements

General Framework of Modern Food Safety Assurance Systems

Historically, the main approaches to assuring that food is safe to eat included: (i) food inspection; and/or (ii) end product laboratory testing.

Food inspection – for example veterinary meat inspection – has contributed immensely to human health over the past 150 years through organoleptically detecting classical zoonotic diseases in slaughtered animals and eliminating them from the food supply. However, with the passage of time, the nature of meat safety problems has changed. Classical zoonotic diseases became eradicated or very infrequent. Unfortunately, microbial pathogens now causing the majority of food-borne diseases (e.g. *Salmonella*, *Campylobacter*, *E. coli* O157) can be shed by animals showing no clinical symptoms and these diseases are undetectable by conventional meat inspection. They may be detected by another approach, end product (carcass) laboratory testing, but this has been shown to be largely ineffective, the reasons for this including: not every food item can be tested for all pathogens; available testing methods are often insufficiently sensitive; the results obtained are too late to be of use; and such testing does not indicate the root of any problem. In one way or another, these two traditional food safety approaches are reactive, i.e. they deal with problems only after they have appeared.

The basis of our modern food safety assurance system is a novel approach designed to address potential food safety problems before they actually appear (proactively; preventatively), and at points of the food chain where they are expected to appear. Health hazards (harmful agents) enter the food chain at different, sometimes multiple, points; they have to be dealt with at each of those points. However, because events at one point affect the adjacent points of the chain (*longitudinal* effect), activities at any individual point cannot be effective if applied in isolation. Instead, hazards have to be controlled at relevant, multiple points in a coordinated (*integrated*) way. Where they cannot be totally eliminated, public health risks can be reduced; it is possible to achieve a 'summation effect' of risk reductions in such a longitudinal and integrated system that results in an ultimate risk reduction (i.e. at the moment of food consumption) that would be unachievable using other methods. Understandably, because participants in the food chain are numerous, diverse in profile and activities, the development and application of this 'farm-to-fork' system must be both multidisciplinary and science-based.

The commercial basis of the LISA concept lies in the fact that the final product of all individual producers in the food chain (feed producer, farmer, abattoir, processor, and retailer) is the same – food. Unless the produced food is safe, no participant can be economically viable. Therefore, the commercial frame of the LISA concept can be illustrated by using existing examples of longitudinal integration of production operations from farm to supermarket, e.g. the poultry meat chain and the milk/dairy chain; they are often driven by large retailer chains.

Operational Aspects of LISA Concept

The main operational aspect of, and tools for, application of LISA concept are summarized in Fig. 11.1.

To start dealing with public health hazards, it is first necessary to know whether, and where, they exist in the food chain. This information can normally be obtained through monitoring and surveillance programmes that target hazards with both local pre-history and potential newly introduced hazards. In the EU, Directive 2003/99/EC describes conditions and methods of monitoring and surveillance for: (i) zoonoses and zoonotic agents; (ii) antimicrobial resistent agents; (iii) investigation of food-borne outbreaks; and (iv) exchange of information on zoonoses and these agents.

Further, using risk assessment methodology, public health risks from hazards need to be quantified, which enables their ranking. Then, the largest proportion of available scientific and financial resources can be rationally directed towards development and implementation of control systems for hazards posing the highest risks.

Presently, the best available control systems are based on Good Hygiene Practice (GHP) and Hazard Analysis and Critical Control Points (HACCP) principles. These principles can be used globally, i.e. when considering the whole food chain, with identification of global control measures available along it (Fig. 11.1). Furthermore, specific controls applied at individual points are based on development and implementation of GHP and HACCP programmes specifically tailored for each individual producer. Food safety management is, along with food quality management, part of the Total Quality Management system (TQM; Fig. 11.2). The effectiveness of food safety systems, at both food chain- and individual point-level, need to be continuously evaluated after their implementation. This can be achieved, for example, through monitoring and surveillance of hazards targeted by the systems, so as to verify that public health risk reductions for targeted hazards have been achieved, as well as to note any emerging new hazard not yet targeted by existing systems.

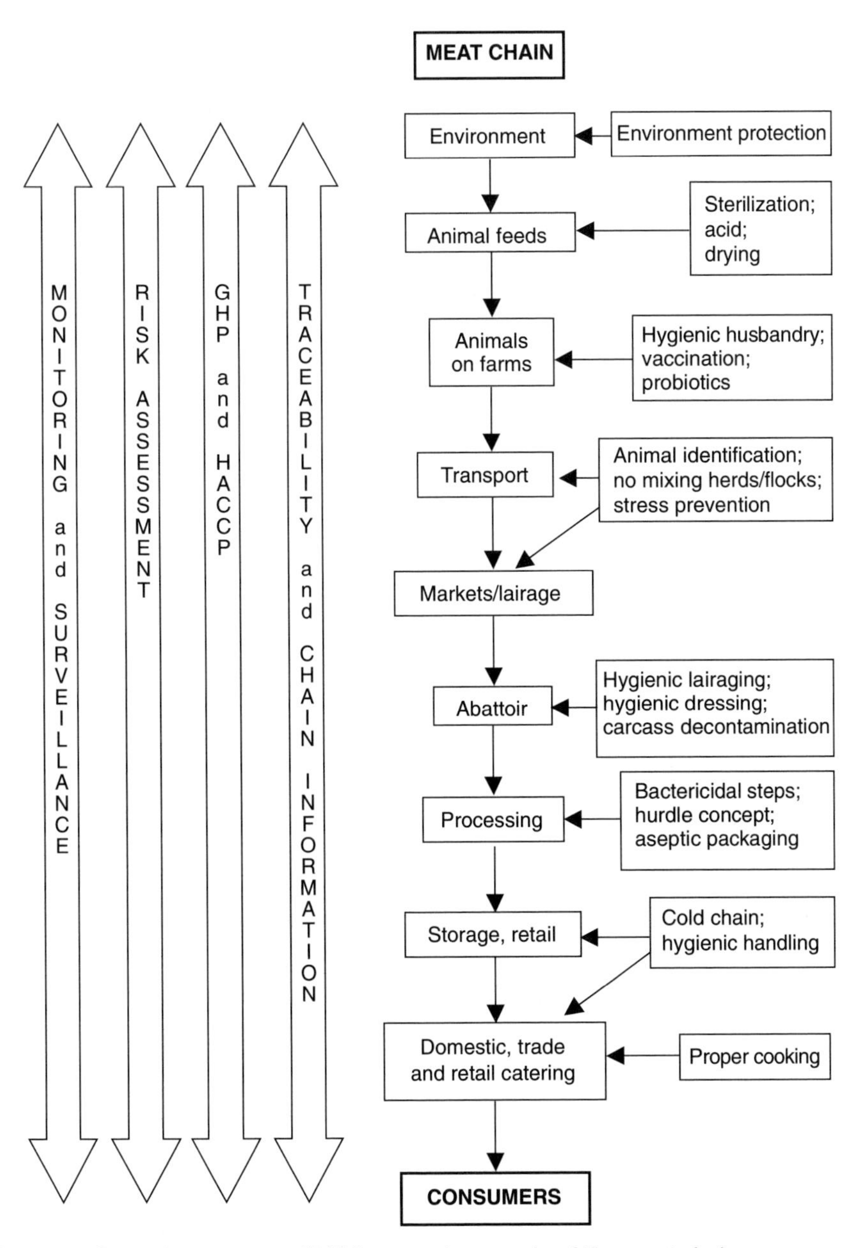

Fig. 11.1. Operative aspects of LISA concept: example of the meat chain.

At each point of the food chain, information on the pre-history of the products (or components) entering that point (i.e. Food Chain Information (FCI)) needs to be available, so that these products can be grouped according to the level of risks from particular hazards which they pose, and then handled accordingly. For food safety systems to be effective, both at the global (i.e. food chain) and individual point (i.e. producer) level,

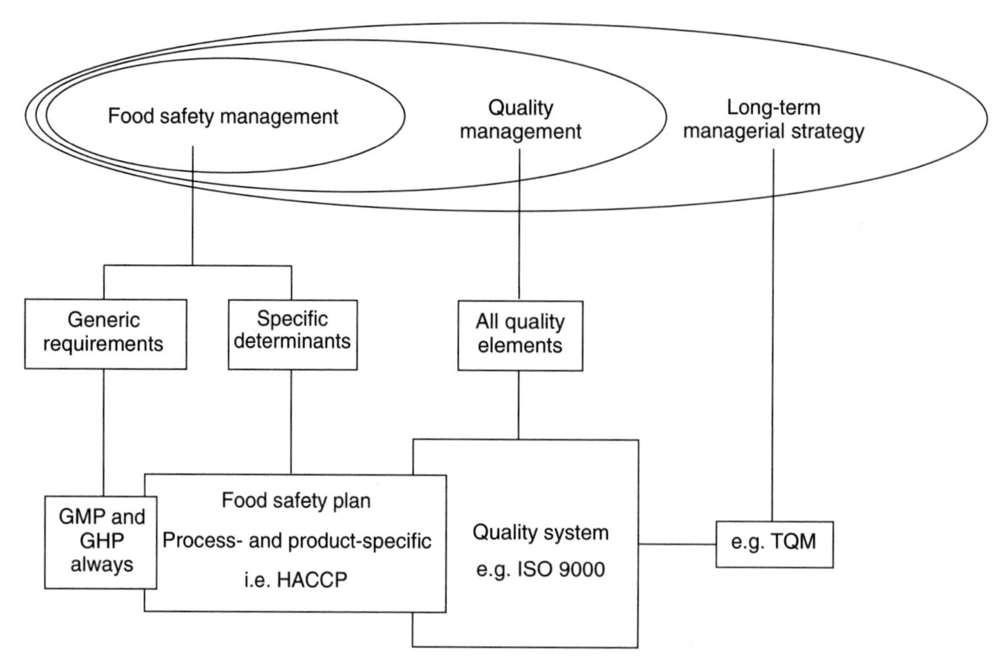

Fig. 11.2. Relationship between food safety management and food quality management systems.

product traceability along the whole food chain is a necessary prerequisite. For effective traceability, a product identification system is necessary, enabling correlation of all product components that enter and leave any point of the food chain, as well as between-points (both 'forward' and 'backward') product correlation. One of the key elements of the LISA concept is timely and two-directional (forward and feedback) flow of information on all relevant aspects of the product to be finally consumed, between all relevant participants in the food chain.

11.2 Risk Assessment of *Campylobacter* in Poultry

BIRGIT NØRRUNG

Introduction

Campylobacter is the leading cause of zoonotic enteric human infections in most developed countries (Anon., 2001). The human cases are usually caused by *C. jejuni*, and to a lesser extent by *C. coli*. The high prevalence rates in chicken meat at retail (Anon., 2001), and the fact that case-control studies conducted worldwide repeatedly have identified handling raw poultry and eating poultry products as important risk factors for sporadic campylobacteriosis, seem to support the fact that chickens play an important role in the transfer of *Campylobacter* to humans.

Quantitative risk assessment can be used as a tool to provide risk managers with information on the influence of different mitigation strategies on the number of human cases associated with thermophilic *Campylobacter* species in chickens. In this chapter we try, in broad lines, to illustrate the elements and applicability of a formal quantitative risk assessment of human campylobacteriosis caused by chickens.

Risk Assessment Framework

A formal risk assessment includes the steps: (i) hazard identification, which aims to identify the risk of campylobacteriosis associated with thermophilic *Campylobacter* in chickens; (ii) hazard characterization, which focuses on evaluating the nature of adverse health effects associated with food-borne *Campylobacter* spp. and the dose–response relationships; (iii) exposure assessment, in which the likelihood and magnitude of exposures to *Campylobacter* as a result of consumption of a chicken meal are estimated; and (iv) risk characterization, which estimates the risk of campylobacteriosis in a given population for a given set of input data.

A risk model, based on a farm-to-fork approach, was developed to estimate the exposure to *Campylobacter* from chickens and the number of human cases associated with this exposure (see Fig. 11.3; Rosenquist *et al.*, 2003).

This model details the changes in prevalence and number of *Campylobacter* on chickens throughout the production line from slaughter to consumption. Module 1 models the transfer and spread of *Campylobacter* through a chicken slaughterhouse. Module 2 describes the transfer and spread of *Campylobacter* during food handling in private kitchens and the different consumption patterns. Output distributions from Module 1 were used as input to Module 2, and output distributions from Module 2 were then integrated with the dose-response relationship to estimate the number of human cases associated with thermophilic *Campylobacter* species in chickens.

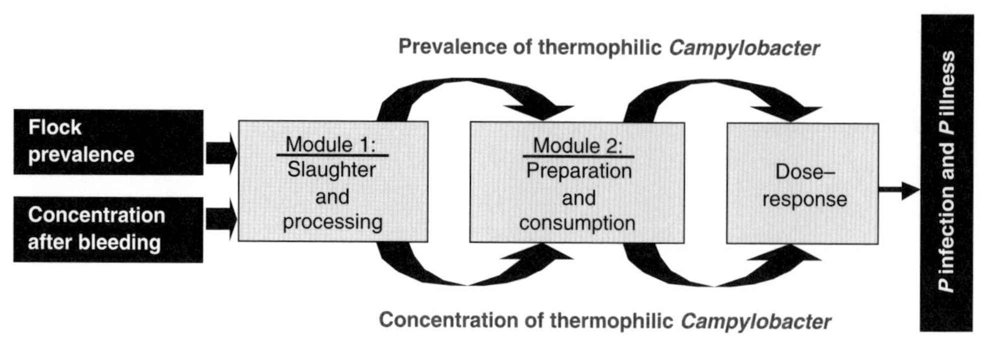

Fig. 11.3. Framework of the risk model. Concentration and number of *Campylobacter* in chickens or in chicken meals.

An overview of the different steps from farm to fork in Danish broiler production can be seen from Fig. 11.4. In the quantitative risk assessment of *Campylobacter* presented here, only the non-shaded areas are taken into account.

Hazard identification and hazard characterization

As described in the introduction, eating poultry products has been identified as an important risk factor for campylobacteriosis in humans. Thus, having identified the hazard, the next step is to characterize this hazard. Hazard characterization focuses on evaluating the nature of adverse health effects associated with food-borne *Campylobacter* spp. and on describing the dose–response relationships.

Enteropathogenic *Campylobacter* may cause an acute enterocolitis, the main symptoms being malaise, fever, severe abdominal pain and watery to bloody diarrhoea. The incubation period varies from 1 to 11 days, typically 1–3 days. In most cases the diarrhoea is self-limiting and may persist for up to a week (Allos and Blaser, 1995). *Campylobacter* infections may be followed by rare, but severe, non-gastrointestinal sequelae: (i) reactive arthritis, a sterile post-infectious process affecting multiple joints, which is often associated with the tissue phenotype HLA-B27; (ii) the Guillain-Barré syndrome, a demyelinating disorder of the peripheral nervous system resulting in weakness – usually symmetrical – of the limbs, weakness of the respiratory muscles and loss of reflexes, that may become chronic or even mortal; and (iii) the Miller Fisher Syndrome, a variant of the Guillain-Barré syndrome characterized by opthalmoplegia, ataxia and areflexia. Development of antimicrobial resistance, such as the emergence of fluoroquinolone-resistant *C. jejuni* in humans, may compromise treatment of patients in severe cases where drug treatment is required. In severe cases the drug of choice is usually erythromycin, though fluoroquinolones such as ciprofloxacin and norfloxacin are also used.

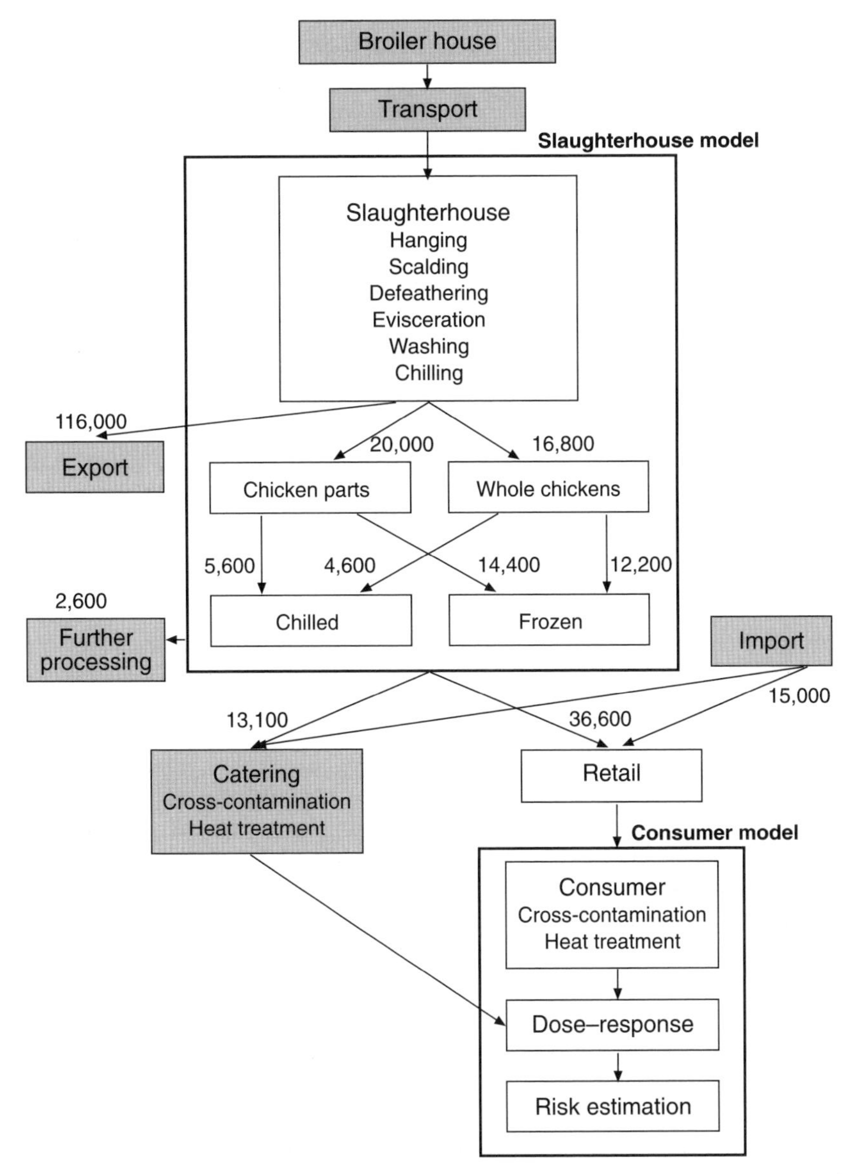

Fig. 11.4. Overview of the steps describing the flow of Danish broilers/chickens from farm to fork. Shaded areas are not included in the QRA model. The numbers are the amount of whole chickens in tons in 1998.

Only a few studies describing the human response to a known dose of *Campylobacter* exist. In one experiment a dose of 500 organisms ingested with milk caused illness in one volunteer. In another experiment involving 111 healthy young adults from Baltimore, Ohio, doses ranging from 800 to 20,000,000 organisms caused diarrhoeal illness (Black *et al.*, 1988). Rates of infection increased with dose, but development of illness did not show a clear dose relation. In an outbreak at a restaurant, the number of *C. jejuni* in the causative chicken meal was estimated to range from 53 to 750/g. These few investigations indicate that the infective dose of *C. jejuni* may be relatively low. The data generated by Black *et al.* (1988) have formed the basis of a dose–response model, which translates the number of organisms an individual is exposed to into an estimate of the individual's probability of acquiring infection and illness. This estimate is dependent on: (i) the numbers of organisms ingested; (ii) the probability of each individual organism of surviving and infecting the host once it is ingested; and (iii) the probability that the host will become ill once infected. The estimate is also influenced by the virulence of the ingested strain, the vehicle with which it is ingested (Black *et al.*, 1988) and the susceptibility of the individual, e.g. immune status, age and stomach contents.

Exposure assessment

Data on flock prevalence and number of *Campylobacter* on skin surface throughout the processes of scalding, defeathering, evisceration, washing and chilling are available. In addition, data on the prevalence of *Campylobacter*-contaminated broilers and on the number of *Campylobacter* on either chilled or frozen whole carcasses are available.

Two successive mathematical models (Module 1 and Module 2 in Fig. 11.3) were developed to estimate the likelihood and magnitude of exposures to *Campylobacter* as a result of consumption of a chicken meal. These detailed the prevalence and the number of *Campylobacter* on chickens throughout the production line, from slaughter to consumption, and the consumption patterns of the consumers. No growth models were included in the exposure assessment, as thermophilic *Campylobacter* species do not multiply below 32°C (ICMSF, 1996).

After processing, carcasses for sale are stored as either chilled or frozen products. While chilled storage (at 4°C) does not seem to affect the number of *Campylobacter* considerably, the number of *Campylobacter* will be reduced due to freezing at −20°C (approximately 0.5–2.5 log units) (Yogasundram and Shane, 1986). No further changes in the number of *Campylobacter* during transport and storage were considered in the model. The ratio of chilled compared to frozen chicken products sold in retail stores was included.

The transfer of *Campylobacter* from a *Campylobacter*-contaminated chicken to the consumer may occur via several contamination routes. Humans may become infected by direct contact, i.e. by licking hands that have been in contact with a chicken or, indirectly, by consuming an undercooked chicken meal or a food item, e.g. salad or prepared chicken, which has been cross-contaminated during handling or preparation of a raw chicken. Since *Campylobacter* is rather sensitive to heat, the transfer of *Campylobacter* to humans due to undercooking is assumed to be a rather insignificant event. To simplify the process, only the transfer caused by cross-contamination via unwashed cutting boards was included in the module, as this pathway was assumed to be the most important route of transfer. Hence, Module 2 in the risk model quantifies the transfer of *Campylobacter* from a contaminated raw chicken to preparation surfaces, and subsequently from these surfaces to ready-to-eat food (salad and prepared chicken). It was assumed that washing the cutting boards, immediately after handling of the raw chicken, would eliminate the risk of cross-contamination. In contrast, if the cutting boards were not washed, there would be a risk of transferring *Campylobacter*.

Risk characterization

In the risk characterization part, the estimated exposure is integrated with the dose–response model to provide a risk estimate. In most cases the risk estimate itself is not very interesting. Also, there will often be major uncertainties concerning the estimate. However, the ability to run simulations and to observe how the risk estimate changes when different mitigation strategies are applied is a very useful exercise in establishing efficient risk management strategies.

Four different mitigation strategies to reduce the incidence of campylobacteriosis associated with the consumption of chicken meals have been compared, by running Monte Carlo simulations on the quantitative risk model developed to detail the probability of exposure to *Campylobacter* and the likelihood of campylobacteriosis associated with this exposure.

The simulations indicated that the incidence of campylobacteriosis associated with consumption of chicken meals could be reduced 30 times by introducing a 2-log reduction of the number of *Campylobacter* on the chicken carcasses. To obtain a similar reduction of the incidence of campylobacteriosis, the flock prevalence should be reduced approximately 30 times (e.g. from 60% to 2%) or the kitchen hygiene improved approximately 30 times (e.g. from 21% not washing the cutting board to 0.7%).

Risk management options

Several countries have implemented, or are at the point of implementing, strategies to reduce the number of *Campylobacter*-contaminated broiler flocks. Until now establishment of 'strict hygienic barriers' or 'biosecurity zones' at each poultry house seemed to be the only preventive option shown to work in practice (Reiersen *et al.*, 2001).

The numbers of *Campylobacter* on chickens may be reduced by introducing different techniques during processing. It is well known that, for example, freezing meat leads to a drop in the concentration of approximately 2 log units (Yogasundram and Shane, 1986). If broiler flocks are examined for *Campylobacter* prior to delivery to the slaughterhouse, and if a flock is tested positive, then such meat could be sold as a frozen product while *Campylobacter*-negative flocks could be sold as fresh chicken. This intervention would, according to the risk assessment, be very efficient in lowering the number of human cases of campylobacteriosis.

Other techniques that might have a positive effect on removal or inactivation of *Campylobacter* are: (i) increasing the scalding temperature; (ii) improving evisceration techniques (to avoid faecal contamination of the meat); (iii) using more water throughout the entire slaughter line; (iv) using forced air-chilling; and (v) introducing disinfectants.

Education of consumers to obtain a reduction of cross-contamination during food handling was included in the model by changing the number of people who did not wash their cutting board during food handling. From the simulations it was obvious that an improvement of the hygiene level in private kitchens (i.e. by washing the cutting board) could reduce the incidence of campylobacteriosis. There was a linear one-to-one relationship between the occurrence of not washing the cutting board and the number of human cases. This means that efforts, directed at improving the frequency of washing the cutting board, for example by a factor of two, would result in a reduction of the incidence of campylobacteriosis by a factor of two.

References

Allos, B.M. and Blaser, M.J. (1995) *Campylobacter jejuni* and the expanding spectrum of related infections. *Clinical Infectious Diseases* 20, 1092–1101.

Anon. (2001) *Trends and Sources of Zoonotic Agents in Animals, Feeding Stuff, Food and Man in the European Union and Norway in 1999*. Part 1. Document No. SANCO/1069/2001 of the European Commission, Community Reference Laboratory on the Epidemiology of Zoonoses, BgVV, Berlin, Germany.

Black, R.E., Levine, M.M., Clements, M.L., Hughes, T.P. and Blaser, M. (1988) Experimental *Campylobacter jejuni* infection in humans. *Journal of Infectious Diseases* 157, 472–479.

ICMSF (1996) *Micro-organisms in Foods 5. Characteristics of Microbial Pathogens*. Blackie Academic and Professional, London, pp. 45–65.

Reiersen, J., Briem, H., Hardardottir, H., Gunnarsson, E., Georgsson, F. and Kristinsson, K.G. (2001) Human campylobacteriosis epidemic in Iceland 1998–2000 and effect of interventions aimed at poultry and humans. *International Journal of Medical Microbiology* 291 (Suppl. 31), 153.

Rosenquist, H., Sommer, H., Nielsen, N.L., Nørrung, B. and Christensen, B. (2003) Risk assessment of human illness related to *Campylobacter jejuni* in Chicken. *International Journal of Food Microbiology* 83, 87–103.

Yogasundram, K. and Shane, S.M. (1986) The viability of *Campylobacter jejuni* on refrigerated chicken drumsticks. *Veterinary Research Communications* 10, 479–486.

11.3 Risk Assessment of *Salmonella* in Pigs

Søren Aabo

Introduction

A marked increase in human cases caused by *Salmonella typhimurium* DT104 resistant to ampicillin, chloramphenicol (florfenicol), streptomycin (spectinomycin), sulphonamide and tetracycline (R-type ACSSuT) (MRDT104) was recognized from the early 1990s in England (Threlfall *et al.*, 1997). Since, it has spread in animal production in many countries and has become a significant food-borne pathogen internationally (Threlfall *et al.*, 1996; Wall *et al.*, 1997; Tauxe, 1999). In 1996 MRDT104 was isolated for the first time in Denmark from an infected Danish pig herd. The Danish Bacon and Meat Council (DBMC) reacted by deciding to stamp out MRDT104-infected pig herds. The Danish Veterinary and Food Administration (DVFA) followed with a 'DT104 order' in 1997, which made the detection of MRDT104 in food animals notifiable and introduced, for the first time, zero tolerance for a pathogen in primary production and in food–including raw meat.

A significant increase in the number of MRDT104-infected herds in Denmark in 1999 and 2000 forced DBMC to stop the destruction strategy for economic reasons. Following this, surveillance was intensified and a Zoonosis Restriction Order was implemented. An important part of the order was the restriction on trade with live animals coming from MRDT104-infected herds. Also, all carcasses from MRDT104-infected slaughter herds should be showered with 80°C hot water for 15 s (called hot water treatment: HWT), which allowed the fresh meat to be distributed for retail. Otherwise, all the meat should be heat processed or condemned. In Fig. 11.5, a schematic presentation is given of the allocation of pigs with *Salmonella* and MRDT104-infected herds for slaughter in Denmark up to 2003.

In 2002, DBMC applied for a change in the MRDT104 management strategy in primary pig production. The most critical change was a lifting of the trade restrictions for MRDT104-infected herds. This would have been most likely to lead to an increased spread of MRDT104 through piglets produced by MRDT104-infected sow herds. In Denmark, more than 10,000,000 live pigs, mostly piglets, are traded each year. Trade, as such, is a risk factor for spread of pathogens between herds. More than 23,000,000 Danish pigs are slaughtered each year.

The occurrence of MRDT104 is still rather restricted in Denmark. Since the introduction of MRDT104 in Denmark in 1996, very few poultry flocks and cattle herds have been positive for MRDT104. In contrast, more than 100 pig herds have been recognized as MRDT104 infected. In a 1-year period from mid-2001 to mid-2002, 35 pig herds were detected positive for MRDT104, and for the same period The Danish Zoonosis

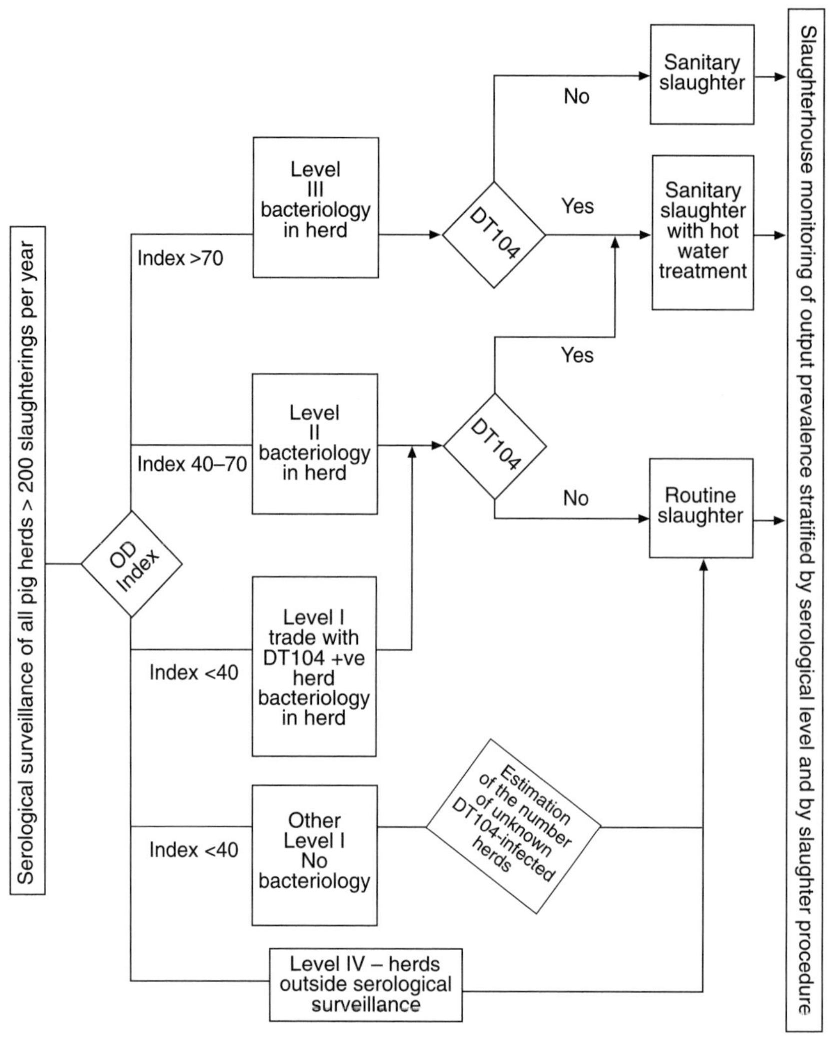

Fig. 11.5. Schematic representation of the allocation of slaughter pigs for slaughter based on the serological *Salmonella* surveillance system, which includes bacteriological investigation of Level II and III herds and herds with trade contact with MRDT104-infected herds.

Centre estimated that Danish pork was responsible for approximately 200 human cases of salmonellosis, with MRDT104 from pork being estimated to be responsible for only two human registered cases.

In 2002, Danish risk managers decided to initiate a quantitative risk assessment of MRDT104 in pigs in Denmark and of the effect of lifting trade sanctions on MRDT104-infected herds, and particularly important, MRDT104-infected piglet-producing sow herds. Even though the number of human MRDT104 cases related to pork has been low, the authorities needed documentation of the increase in consumer risk (also in light of the zero tolerance policy) on which to base any lifting of trade sanctions.

This chapter provides a short description of a formal quantitative risk assessment of *Salmonella typhimurium* DT104 in Danish pork on the human health impact of a lifting of trade restrictions for pigs from *S. typhimurium* DT104-infected herds. The chapter will focus on the impact on food safety of MRDT104 specifically, and not deal with food safety aspects of *Salmonella* in pork in general.

Overview of the Risk Assessment

The four main components of this are described in Chapters 1.5 and 11.2.

Normally, quantitative risk assessment modelling is based on quantitative data from the food production chain in order to be able to model the number of pathogenic bacteria ingested by the consumer per meal. By linking the number of bacteria to dose-response models, the probability of developing disease per single serving and for all servings in a population for a given time period can be estimated. This approach has been used in the risk assessment of *Campylobacter* in chickens (see Chapter 11.2).

However, in order to estimate the likely change in the number of human cases of *Salmonella typhimurium* DT104 from pork due to changes in the trade of live pigs, only very few quantitative data were available. Therefore, it was necessary to develop an alternative risk model, based on qualitative data from the farm-to-fork chain. From all parts of the pork-producing chain an overwhelming amount of qualitative data have been generated on *Salmonella*, which was used as a basis for the risk assessment. This approach was also made possible due to the development of a prevalence-based human risk model (Hald *et al.*, 2001, 2003).

The risk assessment comprised three main elements: (i) a hazard characterization of MRDT104; (ii) an exposure modelling of the effect of lifting trade restrictions; and (iii) a risk characterization based on the exposure estimate. For an account of the full risk assessment see Sommer *et al.* (2003).

Hazard characterization

Antibiotic resistance in *Salmonella typhimurium* may cause increased morbidity and mortality in humans through different mechanisms:

1. Increased transmission and occurrence among persons on antibiotic therapy.
2. Increased risk of outbreaks in hospitals and other places where antibiotics are used.
3. Spreading of resistance genes to other bacteria.
4. Risk of reduced effect of early empirical treatment (before results from culturing and testing possible resistance are available.
5. Limitations in the treatment options after results of resistance testing become available.

In relation to points 1 and 2, it has been shown that persons on antibiotic treatment are 3.7 times more likely to become infected with resistant *Salmonella* compared to persons who were not on treatment before exposure (Barza and Travers, 2002). A more recent study by Glynn *et al.* (2003) confirmed that treatment with antibiotics prior to exposure increased the risk of *Salmonella typhimurium* MRDT104. From the meta-analysis (Barza and Travers, 2002) and the study by Glynn *et al.* (2003), it can be derived that the morbidity may increase two to three times if a resistant *Salmonella* type is introduced to a setting where some 40% of the patients are being treated with antibiotics, compared to exposure to the same organism among persons who are not being treated with antibiotics. The risks of invasive infection and hospitalization have recently been determined in the United States. Seven per cent of *S. typhimurium* R-type ACSSuT was isolated from blood, compared to 3% of fully sensitive strains (Mølbak *et al.*, 2002). Based on these results we estimated that 7.1 Danish cases per 100 of MRDT104 would develop bacteraemia, of which three would be attributed to the *Salmonella* infection in general and 4.1 to the carriage of antibiotic resistance.

A study by Varma *et al.* (2002) estimated the risk of hospitalization among US patients who were infected with resistant *Salmonella* strains compared to the risk for patients infected with pan-susceptible strains. Provided that the *S. typhimurium* R-typeACSSuT*a* strains increase the risk of hospitalization similarly to other resistant *Salmonella* strains, and that the US data are comparable to Danish data, it can be estimated that 28 Danish MRDT104 cases per 100 were likely to be hospitalized: 21 because of the *Salmonella* infection in general and seven as an effect of antibiotic resistance. A recent register-based study has also documented an excess mortality associated with antimicribial drug-resistant *Salmonella typhimurium* 1–2 years after infection (Helms *et al.*, 2002, 2003).

Exposure assessment

A prevalence–response risk model, developed at the Danish Zoonosis Centre, combines *Salmonella* prevalence data with human consumption data for the modelling of the relative and absolute impact of different food sources on human salmonellosis in Denmark – also termed the Zoonosis Source Account (Anon., 2002). By this model, the Danish Zoonosis Centre has estimated that among the 40–50 registered sporadic human cases of MRDT104 in Denmark, approximately only two cases were attributable to Danish pork in 2001 (unpublished data). This model allowed us to employ prevalence estimates of MRDT104-contaminated carcasses on the slaughter line as the basis for a human risk modelling, taking into account the *Salmonella* serology level of the herd and whether HWT was used or not. Thus, we were able to provide quantitative estimates of the number of human cases (risk characterization) based on estimates on MRDT104-positive carcasses leaving Danish slaughterhouses without modelling the number of *Salmonella* bacteria and subsequent dose–response modelling.

Estimation of the total number of MRDT104-contaminated carcasses from known and from unknown MRDT104-infected herds used general *Salmonella* data to substitute for insufficient MRDT104 data.

The main parameters for estimating the total number of MRDT104 contaminated carcasses were:

1. The prevalence of *Salmonella*-contaminated carcasses after slaughtering for herds belonging to each of the serological Levels I, II and III.
2. The prevalence of *Salmonella*-contaminated carcasses after HWT slaughtering for herds belonging to each serological level.
3. The average number of herds belonging to each serological level.
4. The average number of pigs delivered to slaughter per month for herds belonging to each serological level.
5. The prevalence of *Salmonella*-positive herds per month for herds belonging to each serological level.
6. The proportion of MRDT104-infected herds (including an estimate of those MRDT104-infected herds which are unrecognized) among all *Salmonella*-infected herds.

In Denmark, all pig herds which produce more than 200 pigs a year are monitored serologically for *Salmonella*. The system allocates the slaughter pig herds into three serological levels. Levels I, II and III are herds with low or no *Salmonella* problems, intermediate *Salmonella* problems and severe *Salmonella* problems, respectively. A level IV was included in this study to include herds outside the serological surveillance.

The estimation of the number of MRDT104-infected herds was stratified into three categories: (i) herds producing pigs for slaughter (some of them also have sows); (ii) piglet-producing sow herds; and (iii) breeder and multiplier herds. The spread of MRDT104 related to trade between these herd categories was modelled and used to estimate the number of recognized and unrecognized MRDT104-infected slaughter pig herds under the present trade sanctions and after a lift of trade sanctions. By summing up herds from the four different serological levels for the 1-year period 2001–2002, 35 herds were recognized as MRDT104-positive and the number of unrecognized herds was estimated to be 61, giving a total of 96 slaughter pig herds positive for MRDT104 if trade restrictions were maintained. If trade restrictions were lifted the number of recognized herds was estimated to increase to 111, and the number of unrecognized herds to increase to 268, giving a total number of MRDT104-positive slaughter pig herds of 379 (Korsgaard *et al.*, 2002). These numbers are mean numbers and the number of herds may vary considerably. Thus, a significant higher number of infected herds can be expected if more herds in the breeding system become infected than assumed in this model.

The prevalence of MRDT104-positive carcasses was established for herds for each serological level considering that recognized MRDT104 herds are HTW treated and unrecognized MRDT104 herds are being routinely slaughtered without HWT (Mølbak *et al.*, 2002) (see Figs 11.6 and 11.7). This approach made it possible to avoid the very complex modelling through the slaughterline process.

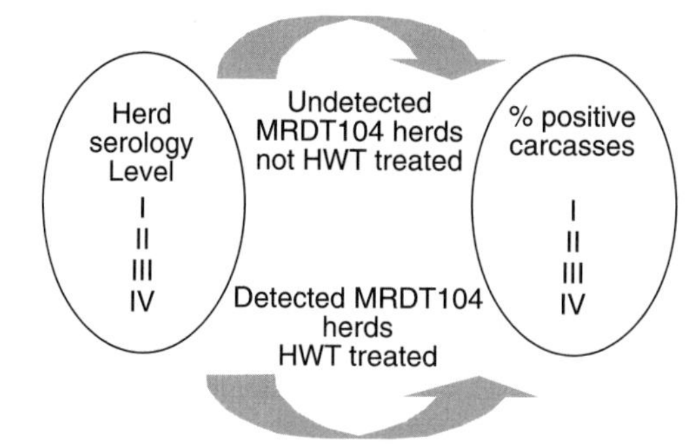

Fig. 11.6. The herd serology level is linked to an average prevalence of *Salmonella*-positive carcasses from detected and undetected MRDT104-infected herds. Level IV denotes herds outside the serological surveillance.

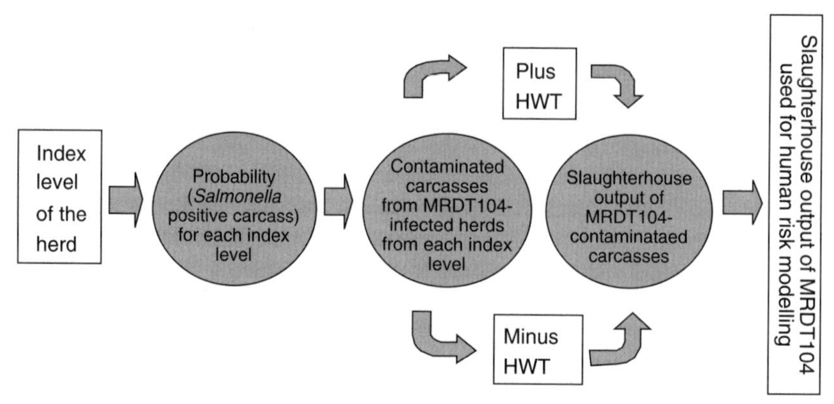

Fig. 11.7. Schematic representation of risk modelling based on output prevalence and number of MRDT104-contaminated carcasses from Danish slaughterhouses. HWT denotes Hot water treatment, which comprises showering of carcasses with hot water at 80°C for 15 sec.

The prevalences of *Salmonella*-contaminated carcasses after slaughtering without using HTW were 1.76, 3.84, 5.07 and 6.40 for herds belonging to each of the serological Levels I, II, III and IV, respectively. For herds subjected to HWT the prevalence of *Salmonella*-positive carcasses was reduced approximately 50-fold.

Now, having estimated the outcome of *Salmonella* from each serological level, this was combined with the mean delivery sizes for herds for each serological level per month in order to estimate the mean output of *Salmonella*-positive carcasses per delivery. This was adjusted for the relative proportion of MRDT104 in order to estimate the mean output of MRDT104-positive carcasses per delivery from MRDT104 slaughter pig herds.

The mean delivery size per month per herd for each serological level was deduced from registered production data. A mean delivery size of 237, 319 and 133 animals was found for herds of Levels I, II and III, respectively. These herd sizes were also regarded as mean herd sizes for the MRDT104-infected herds.

The total number of infected carcasses from MRDT104-infected herds was estimated to be 3354 per year under maintained trade restriction. If trade restrictions were lifted, the number was estimated to increase to 10,759 MRDT104-positive carcasses per year. It appeared that the major fraction (approximately 95%) of MRDT104-positive carcasses originated from undetected MRDT104 herds regardless of lifting trade or not. The number of carcasses being HWT treated was estimated to increase from 72,109 to 303,013 per year if trade sanctions were lifted.

A total of 21,553,315 pigs were slaughtered in Denmark in 2001. We could then calculate the prevalences of MRDT104-contaminated carcasses to be 0.016% (3,354/21,553,315) if trade sanctions were maintained, and 0.050% (10,759/21,553,315) if trade sanctions were lifted. The prevalences were used as inputs in the risk characterization model (Hald *et al.*, 2001, 2003).

Risk characterization

This provides an estimation of the number of human registered cases. Since 1988, the Danish Zoonosis Centre has applied a method for estimation of the number of human cases attributable to each of the major animal food sources (Hald *et al.*; 2002). The basic principle of the method is to compare *Salmonella* (sero- and phage) types isolated from animals and foods with *Salmonella* types isolated from humans. In brief, types of *Salmonella* which are exclusively (or almost exclusively) found in a particular food animal reservoir or food type ('unique types') are used as 'anchor points' for distribution of types occurring in several reservoirs/sources. It is assumed that all human infections caused by the unique types are associated with the indicated food type or derived from the indicated food animal reservoir (e.g. pork, beef, chicken or eggs). *Salmonella* types which occur in several reservoirs are distributed relative to the prevalence of unique types in a given reservoir/food type. Thus, detailed knowledge of the distribution of *Salmonella* types in all relevant food animals and food types, generated through intensive and continuous monitoring, is an essential prerequisite for the analysis.

The model calculates the number of registered domestic sporadic cases caused by different *Salmonella* sero- and phage types as a function of the prevalence of those *Salmonella* types in the animal food sources and the amount of food source consumed. The number of domestic and sporadic cases is obtained by subtracting the estimated number of travel- and outbreak-associated cases from the total number of reported cases, i.e. the observed data.

For the purpose of estimating the number of human cases that would occur due to changes in trade strategy, the prevalence estimates of MRDT104-positive carcasses, which were estimated in the present exposure model, were used as input.

For the present trade strategy, an independent estimate of 1.9 human MRDT104 cases relating to Danish pork for the period 1 August 2002 to

31 July 2003 has been generated using the model by Hald *et al.* (2003). When anchoring the number of human cases to 1.9, we estimated the mean number of human cases after a lift of trade restrictions to increase to 5.9 cases per year (3.2 times).

Discussion and Conclusions

The present risk assessment estimates the human health impact of proposed changes in MRDT104 trade strategy in Denmark, using qualitative data from the Danish *Salmonella* surveillance and control programme. The key prerequisite for this approach was the available prevalence-based risk characterization model (Hald *et al.*, 2001, 2002) and numerous available *Salmonella* data generated in the primary production and at slaughterhouses. The risk assessment estimated that lifting of trade sanctions would lead to a threefold increase in the number of human registered MRDT104 cases. The absolute number of MRDT104 cases related to Danish pork was estimated to be as low as two cases in 2001. Thus, the absolute average increase in human cases related to a change in MRDT104 strategy would increase from two cases to approximately six cases, on average. If a higher number of the breeder and supplier herds are infected with MRDT104 than assumed in this model, the number of human cases may increase to significantly higher numbers.

According to the risk assessment, it was, in particular, the number of unrecognized MRDT104-infected herds which was responsible for the human exposure, as these herds provided 90–95% of all MRDT104-positive carcasses. If the risk managers require that consumer exposure is not allowed due to the zero tolerance policy in Denmark, then any lifting of trade sanctions must be followed by a significantly improved system for identifying MRDT104-infected herds. This would ensure that an increased and sufficient number of MRDT104-contaminated carcasses will be subjected to HWT.

The output from the model estimates the number of sporadic human cases, and it does not take into consideration the probability of food-borne outbreaks. No outbreak models are available, and incorporation into the risk assessment awaits the establishment of such models.

References

Anon. (2002) Annual Report on Zoonosis in Denmark 2002. The Danish Ministry of Food, Agriculture and Fisheries, Copenhagen.

Barza, M. and Travers, K. (2002) Excess infections due to antimicrobial resistance: the 'Attributable Fraction'. *Clinical Infectious Diseases* 34: Suppl 3, S126–130.

Glynn, M.K., Reddy, V., Hutwagner, L., Rabatsky-Ehr, T., Shiferaw, B., Vugia, D.J., *et al.* (2004). Emerging infectious program: FoodNet Working Group. Prior antimicrobial agent use increases the risk of sporadic infections with multidrug-resistant *Salmonella enterica* serotype Typhimurium: a FoodNet case-control study, 1996–1997. *Clinical Infectious Diseases* 38: Suppl. 3, S227–S236.

Hald, T., Vose, D. and Wegener, H.C. (2001) Quantifying the contribution of animal-food sources to human salmonellosis in Denmark in 1999. In: *Proceedings of the 4th International Symposium on the Epidemiology and Control of Salmonella and Other Food Borne Pathogens in Pork*, pp. 349–351.

Hald, T., Vose, D., Wegener, H.C. and Koupeev, T. (2004) A Bayesian approach to quantify the contribution of animal-food sources to human salmonellosis. *Risk Analysis* 24, 55–69.

Helms, M., Vastrup, P., Gerner-Smidt, P. and Mølbak, K. (2002) Excess mortality associated with antimicribial drug-resistant *Salmonella typhimurium. Emerging Infectious Diseases* 8, 590–495.

Helms, M., Vastrup, P., Gerner-Smidt, P. and Mølbak, K. (2003) Short and long term mortality associated with food-borne bacterial gastrointestinal infections; a registry-based study. *British Medical Journal* 326, 57–61.

Korsgaard, H. *et al.* (2002) Assessment of the effect of proposed changes to the management of multi-resistant *Salmonella* Typhimurium DT104 in primary food animal production in Denmark. Report, DVI, Denmark.

Mølbak, K., Varma, J., Rossiter, S., Lay, J., Joyce, K., Stamey, K. *et al.* (2002) Antimicrobial resistance in *Salmonella* serotype Typhimurium, R-type ACSSuT, is associated with bacteremia; NARMS, 1996–2000. *Proceedings of the International Conference of Emerging Infectious Diseases*, 24–27 March, Atlanta, Georgia (http://www.cdc.gov/iceid/).

Sommer, H.M., Aabo, S., Christensen, B.B., Saadbye, P., Nielsen, N.L. and Nørrung, B. (2003) Risk assessment of the impact on human health related to multiresistant *Salmonella typhimurium* DT104 from slaughter pigs – with an assessment of the impact of possible risk management changes. Report. IFSE, Denmark (also at www.foldevaredirektoratet.dk.foldeare.mikrobiologiske_forureninger/Salmonella).

Tauxe, R.V. (1999) *Salmonella enteritidis* and *Salmonella typhimurium* DT104: Successful subtypes in the modern world. In: Scheld, W.M. *et al.* (eds) *Emerging Infections 3*. ASM Press, Washington, DC.

Threlfall, J.E., Frost, J.A., Ward, L. and Rowe, B. (1996) Increasing spectrum of resistance in multiresistant *Salmonella typhimurium. Lancet* 347, 1053–1054.

Threlfall, E.J., Ward, L.R., Skinner, J.A. and Rowe, B. (1997) Increase in multiple antibiotic resistance in nontyphoidal salmonellas from humans in England and Wales: a comparison of data for 1994 and 1996. *Microbial Drug Resistance* 3(3), 263–266.

Varma, J.K., Mølbak, K., Rossiter, S., Hawkins, M.A., Jones, T.F., Mauvais, S.H. *et al.* (2002) Antimicrobial resistance in *Salmonella* is associated with increased hospitalization; NARMS 1996–2000. *Proceedings of the International Conference of Emerging Infectious Diseases*, 24–27 March, Atlanta, Georgia (http://www.cdc.gov/iceid/).

Wall, P.G., Ross, D., van Someren, P., Ward, L., Threlfall, J.E. and Rowe, B. (1997) Features of the epidemiology of multidrug resistant *Salmonella typhimurium* DT104 in England and Wales. In: Colin, P. *et al.* (eds) *Proceedings, Salmonella and Salmonellosis '97*. Zoopole, Ploufragan, France, pp. 565–567.

Index